Lecture Notes in Biomathematics

Managing Editor: S. Levin

42

George W. Swan

Optimization of Human Cancer Radiotherapy

Springer-Verlag
Berlin Heidelberg New York 1981

Author

George W. Swan
14125 62nd Drive W,
Edmonds, WA 98020, USA

AMS Subject Classifications (1981): 92-02

ISBN 3-540-10865-3 Springer-Verlag Berlin Heidelberg New York
ISBN 0-387-10865-3 Springer-Verlag New York Heidelberg Berlin

Printing and binding: Beltz Offsetdruck, Hemsbach/Bergstr.
2141/3140-543210

To: My mother, Margaret
My wife, Edith
My daughters, Melanie
Katrina

whose diverse minds with such creative abilities are an unending source of pleasure to me.

PREFACE

The mathematical models in this book are concerned with a variety of approaches to the manner in which the clinical radiologic treatment of human neoplasms can be improved. These improvements comprise ways of delivering radiation to the malignancies so as to create considerable damage to tumor cells while sparing neighboring normal tissues. There is no unique way of dealing with these improvements. Accordingly, in this book a number of different presentations are given. Each presentation has as its goal some aspect of the improvement, or optimization, of radiotherapy.

This book is a collection of current ideas concerned with the optimization of human cancer radiotherapy. It is hoped that readers will build on this collection and develop superior approaches for the understanding of the ways to improve therapy.

The author owes a special debt of thanks to Kathy Prindle who breezed through the typing of this book with considerable dexterity.

TABLE OF CONTENTS

Chapter 1
GENERAL INTRODUCTION

1.1 Introduction

The author, by training and design, is an applied mathematician in the British sense. That is, he is interested in the formulation, development and solution of mathematical models which in some sense, are approximations to the biological problems of interest. Accordingly then it is the opinion of the author that the main content of this book is not concerned with theories but rather with mathematical models of the response of biological material to X-irradiation.

A brief synopsis of the history of cancer and its treatment by radiotherapy is presented in Section 1.2. In these modern times it seems that many of us tend to forget the impact on society of the discovery and application of X-rays. The interested reader can use the numerous references given in that section to construct an in-depth understanding of the progress that has been made during the last eighty-five years.

The author's book, Swan (1977), provides a useful illustration of the variety and complexity of many current mathematical models in cancer research, and is recommended as background reading in connection with Section 1.3. In this section there is a description of mathematical models which attempt to approximate the gross characteristics of tumor growth, that is, give some measure of tumor burden as measured, say, by tumor volume, or the number of tumor cells.

During radiation treatment of a tumor it is important to know the spatial distribution of the radiation dose. This situation is examined in Section 1.4.

It seems to be worthwhile to generate some of the well-known results in what are commonly referred to as the "hit" and "target" "theories". These classical results are usually produced by statistical approaches and give mathematical expressions for the surviving fraction of the population to a dose of X-irradiation.

The formal mathematical development of these models is presented in Chapter 2.

Historically, the basis for these models is as follows. Some particular molecule or biological structure such as a cell or part of it is regarded as being the _target_ of the incidence dosage of X-rays. These rays collide with electrons in or near the target and ionization is produced. A _hit_ refers to the production of some effective event in the target. One of the earliest viewpoints, Dessauer (1922), held that the form of the dose-effect curve is due to the fact that absorption of the radiation is not a continuous but a discrete process and follows Poisson statistics. In the same year Blau and Altenburger (1922) presented a formal mathematical description of this idea. However it was Crowther (1927) who gave a mathematical development of what is now properly called the _single-target multi-hit_ survival model; see Chapter 2, Section 2.6. He derived the theoretical result contained in (2.5). His work, Crowther (1924, 1926, 1927 and 1938), offered the possibility of calculalating a volume from the dose-effect curve. This volume, see Section 2.3, is the target within which, for a given probability, the required number of absorption events occur. Zimmer (1961, pp. 13-15) has given a good description of a number of specific applications which have followed from Crowther's work. Other pertinent reviews are contained in Crowther (1938), Lea (1955), and Elkind and Whitmore (1967).

Since the main survival expressions in Chapter 2 have been known for a number of years there is the strong temptation to believe in them. Also, their derivation is straightforward and does not require "more complicated" mathematics such as differential equations. Many papers have been written discussing many aspects of the probabilistic approach to the derivation of survival curves. The net conclusion is that the hit and target models are unsatisfactory for a number of reasons. Some of these include the following: Dose-effect curves are not adequately represented at low doses; the "volume" used in these models, in a majority of experimental situations, does not have any relationship whatever to the actual physical space occupied by any of the atoms or molecules taking part in the reaction. Also, dynamic processes are occurring within the irradiated cell and these strongly influence the production of a lethal species (leading ultimately to cell death) as well as the cell's capacity to undertake restitution and repair.

However it is useful to develop some of the approaches to the optimization of human cancer radiotherapy in which some of the survival expressions of the hit and target "theory" are used for illustrative purposes.

In dramatic contrast to the strictly probabilistic models of Chapter 2 is the introduction in Chapter 3 of a molecular model which allows for the determination of survival expressions based on single and double strand breaks in the DNA molecule. Although the development of a theory at the molecular level may correspond closely with nature, there will be splitting of the cell population into varying levels of damage, which appears to require some kind of statistical approach. There is a growing body of evidence in support of the survival expression (3.1).

The hit and target models have enjoyed a long reign. During this period, however, there has been developing a growing awareness of the need to take the transient behavior of radiation mechanisms and events into consideration in order to reach more appropriate levels of understanding of the phenomena involved. One result of this activity is the usage of a time variable, instead of the absorbed energy dose, as the fundamental variable in the overall descriptions, which lead to survival expressions.

The investigation of the time scale of events as they occur in the living cell presents a major challenge and only very limited progress in this area has been made so far. An early paper which employs time as an independent variable is by Reboul (1939), who deals with cellular recovery. Then Sievert (1941) introduced the concept of a "latent period" depending on radiosensitivity and the presence and speed of reconstitution of important reserves in the cell. His work involved the use of a differential-delay equation for the behavior of the concentration with time of some substance within the cell. Dittrich (1957) also used time in a recovery model. Then in the mid 1960's a number of papers appeared which used time: Hug and Kellerer (1966), Sacher and Trucco (1966), and Dienes (1966); the work of this latter author is examined in detail in Chapter 4.

Delattre (1974) has also noted the importance of separating the time from other variables used to analyze the irradiated system. In elementary courses in systems analysis one locates elements of a system (often referred to as states with each state represented by a little circle) together with the transformations which take one state into another. Each circle is connected by one or more straight lines, each line with a directed arrow. The resulting picture is termed a transformation graph. Delattre's paper is written in terms of the descriptions and jargon of present day systems analysis. Section IV of Delattre's paper considers possible transformation graphs for the single-target, multihit survival expression (2.5) as well as some graphs for radiation effects and subsequent biological recovery. To date systems analyses of the above type do not appear to be as useful as the kinetic schemes of Chapter 4.

It is interesting that in the recent monograph by Mayneord and Clarke (1975) the theoretical developments do not proceed directly with usage of the absorbed dose D as a fundamental variable.

Chapter 4 presents some of the material of the kinetic approach of Dienes (1966); with subsequent extensions to fractionation schemes in (1971). The kinetic approach is based on time as the fundamental variable and provides a useful framework from which one can derive survival expressions. The work of Kappos and Pohlit (1973), and the extension of the kinetic approach to deal with age-specific compartments in the cell cycle, see, e.g. Scott (1977), are also examined in Chapter 4.

It seems worthwhile to identify other papers which have appeared in recent years and which serve to augment the kinetic approach. Some of these include the following: Curtis et al. (1973) present a mathematical model of tumor growth and regression based on experimental results of cellular kinetics and radiation survival of cells of a rhabdomyosarcoma in a rat. Brown et al. (1974) deal with radiation strategy; see Section 5.5 for more details on their work. Payne and Garrett (1975) consider both irreversible and reversible lesions can be formed by the radiation products from an energy-loss event. The development is in terms of the kinetic approach. Brannen (1975) considers an extension of the hit and target models of Chapter 2 to include temperature and dose rate effects. His approach is similar to that of Dienes (1966) with the principle differences being the use of inverse proportionality in the dose-rate effects and the inclusion of temperature-insensitive rate constants. Epp et al. (1976) examine recent advances in the experimental and theoretical approaches involving single and double pulses of high intensity ionizing radiation delivered to cultured bacterial and mammalian cells. Garrett and Payne

(1978) consider the modeling of several cell survival experiments with regard to the repair effects on survival of various cell types. Their equations represent an extension of the Dienes (1966) approach.

There is an increase in the number of investigations concerning the use of hyperthermia as a possible therapeutic modality for the treatment of a number of human tumors. It has been suggested that temperatures in the range of 42 to 45° C are lethal to cancer cells, can be combined with X-irradiation in such a way as to improve the therapeutic outcome, and can stop the recovery of cells from sub-lethal and potentially lethal radiation damage, while enhancing the levels of lethal damage. A major advance in the interpretations of recent experimental work on hyperthermia is by Bronk (1976). His theoretical approach, see Section 4.9, is based on the kinetic schemes produced by Dienes (1966). Accordingly Bronk's work provides more support for use of a kinetic-based approach.

Current radiation therapy is based on giving doses of radiation at the end of discrete intervals of time. This is the concept of a fractionation scheme. In between doses the normal cell population is assumed to recover at a faster rate than the tumor cells. The simplest mathematical approach to describe a fractionation scheme is to assume that, at the instant of time when the radiation dose is given, there is an <u>instantaneous</u> drop in the level of tumor cells. The behavior of the normal and tumor cell populations can be described mathematically. However during the regrowth phase it is necessary to utilize a mathematical model of tumor growth. A number of possible models for approximating tumor growth, e.g. exponential, logistic, Gompertz etc., are developed in Section 1.3. For purposes of illustration only exponential growth is used in Section 5.2. Recovery of the normal cell population is modeled by logistic growth in Section 5.3.

The type of fractionation scheme described at the beginning of Chapter 5 is the basis of the clinical applications by Cohen and coworkers. His work in characterizing a number of kinetic parameters in tumors is collected together in one place and examined. Furthermore Section 5.4 provides material on the content of Cohen's computer programs which give information on the determination of cell kinetic parameters.

The material in Section 5.5 is concerned with a model of radiation therapy involving radiation resistant and radiation sensitive cells. Some basic mathematical results for dose fractionation with general survival curves is given in Section 5.6.

Cohen's work in Chapter 5 involves the optimization of parameter values. That is, there is an on-going effort to obtain better estimates of cell kinetic data which can be used in models of fractionation schemes to predict the outcome of some course of radiation therapy.

A different kind of optimization occurs in Chapter 6. An empirical formula was given by Ellis (1969) from which a numerical value (the nominal standard dose or NSD) represents the normal connective tissue tolerance; see Lokajicek et al. (1979). The basic Ellis convention can be used in a mathematical model of a fractionation scheme which seeks to minimize the surviving fraction at the end of a course of therapy, and this is demonstrated in Section 6.2. The Ellis approach is still used by many people. However, Hethcote et al. (1976) examined and compared five different radiation fractionation models. They concluded that the Ellis empiricism was inadequate and judged that the exponential-quadratic survival expression (3.1) was one of the better models.

Other work which produces conclusions that are at variance with the Ellis approach appears in Fischer and Fischer (1977) and Herbert (1977). These two papers represent ways in which mathematical models are now being utilized in radiotherapy. They provoked an editorial by Keller (1977).

In this book there are a number of mathematical models which, in some sense, may approximate tumor growth. It does not matter what particular mathematical structure (e.g. differential equation, difference equation, etc.) is used. What is important, at least for this book, is that estimates can be made from a mathematical model of the number of tumor cells, or tumor volume. Also, in this book, a number of models which allow for mathematical expressions for survival functions have been developed.

With the combination of the model for tumor growth and a cell survival expression it is then possible to explore the consequences of using one type of fractionation scheme and compare it with another. Techniques of multi-variable calculus can be used to examine the minimization of the surviving fraction of tumor cells. This is shown in Sections 6.2 and 6.3.

Another different kind of mathematical optimization problem occurs when it is desired to reduce the tumor to less than one cell. The technique known as dynamic programming can be used. Problems of this type are analyzed in detail in Chapter 6. One of the models described in Section 6.4 involves a tumor model with hypoxic cells and a reoxygenation phase. This seems to be a reasonable problem to examine since hypoxic cells do not remain hypoxic throughout a course of treatment. Estimates are available from the literature, e.g. Denekamp et al. (1977), on the number of hypoxic cells in a certain type of human tumor. Much more work needs to be done, however, to include repair mechanisms and hypoxic effects in mathematical models; Orr et al. (1979).

These problems have some particular objective--it is desired to satisfy some criterion of performance. Also there is a discrete nature to the problem since dosages are given at the end of discrete intervals of time. In control theory terminology they are referred to as multistage optimal control problems. Chapter 7 develops a comprehensive background for this area and includes theoretical as well as numerical discussions of problems. That chapter should be adequate for an understanding of the difficulties that may be encountered when trying to use dynamic programming to solve the optimization problems in Sections 6.4 - 6.7.

Of course the selection of an appropriate performance criterion is a task in itself. One of the features in this book is that a number of different performance criteria are considered. When a mathematical model of a multistage process (such as a fractionation scheme), including a performance criterion, is known then application of the techniques of optimal control theory allows one to predict, on a rational basis, how a system will react to (a) external perturbations, and (b) internal structural changes. For example the models of Sections 6.4 - 6.7 are influenced by (a) the radiation dosages delivered, and (b) reoxygenation within the tumor as a result of disease.

However imperfect they may be mathematical models describing the response of cell populations must be constructed to make proper use of a variety of optimization procedures for giving insight into the consequences of using a certain treatment schedule.

As a desired clinical objective a number of clinicians suggest that one should try to maximize the ratio of benefit of treatment to cost of treatment. For example one might try to "optimize"

(i) $\dfrac{\text{percentage of tumor control}}{\text{percentage of necrosis}}$,

or (ii) $\dfrac{\text{probability of total cure, } P_c}{\text{probability of damage, } P_d}$.

A discussion of related treatment objectives is presented in the first part of Chapter 8.

In the whole area of cancer research it appears that Cohen (1960) gave the first published account of an optimization procedure for eradicating a given tumor. Cohen has since (1973a) updated his earlier work. It is interesting that, independently, Moore and Mendelsohn (1972) and Prewitt (1973) present similar ideas for treatment optimization. The features of this work are in Sections 8.1 - 8.3.

Age response functions are considered briefly in Section 8.4 Some recent attempts to compare all kinetic approaches are presented in Section 8.5

The more well-known approach to optimization in radiotherapy is the use of linear programming schemes to assist in finding the best arrangement of beams of radiation in order to produce a previously assigned dose distribution. It seems that mathematicians prefer to give the most cryptic and concise treatment of the most general type of linear programming problem without motivating the processes involved in seeking a solution. In Chapter 9 I have attempted to motivate the simplex method of solution and follow the approach of one of my teachers, Ben Noble, when I was an undergraduate.

Treatment planning has come a long way from its early days when much of the work was done by hand. There has been a considerable impact in radiology by the use of computers; Levene et al. (1978), Sternick (1978). The larger dimensional linear programming problems can be solved on a computer, although on occasions, because of the approximate nature of the problem, a solution may not always be found to satisfy the constraints. One objective, e.g. Bahr et al. (1968), is to minimize the integral dose over vulnerable regions. In addition one can introduce further constraints on the radiation dose. The problem becomes one for the determination of beam weightings, and, since each constraint is linear, it is natural to consider the application of linear programming. Other work in the decade of the seventies involving linear programming in radiotherapy is examined in Section 9.4.

Recently Kolata (1979) reported on a discovery by a Russian mathematician, L.G. Khachian, which is of great theoretical and probable practical importance--a new way to solve linear programming problems. Khachian's method has already been programmed on a pocket calculator to solve problems with six inequalities and six unknowns, and this is a considerable achievement. At this point in time one may be excused for suggesting that it will not be long before programmable pocket calculators in radiation oncology departments are being used with this new method to obtain rapid results for comparing different treatment plans.

Instead of linear constraints on dosage to the tumor and normal tissues it has been suggested, e.g. Redpath et al. (1975), that one should choose to minimize the variance of the doses to preselected points within the tumor. Limiting doses at certain points in the tumor provide linear constraints on the beam weights. The weights are found as the solution to a quadratic programming problem, which is a special case of a more general nonlinear programming problem. This work is presented in Section 9.5. What is of interest is that, once criteria on the desired dose distribution have been formulated, automatic optimization of the beam arrangement can generate treatment plans which are as good as or even better than those produced by a skilled human operator using "visual optimization" techniques such as working with a computer terminal with rapid calculation and display of dose distributions.

Also, in Section 9.5, is presented the work of McDonald and Rubin (1977) who developed a program for the optimization of dose via a quadratic programming problem. Some results are presented for the optimal dose distribution and beam configuration for a centrally-located brain tumor which is considered to be treated by Cobalt 60 γ-rays.

A further application involves the moving-strip technique.

It is worthwhile at this stage drawing attention to a number of points raised by Bjärngard (1977). He notes that the word "optimization" is being used with increasing frequency in the area of radiotherapy. In connection with external beam therapy he concluded that the automatic optimization of beam arrangement can be implemented clinically in various situations, such as finding the doses and beam angles in multiportal, isocentric techniques, where the dose distributions from different beam arrangements are similar. If one wishes to compare beam configurations such as wedged pairs and full rotations, that produce quite different dose distributions, it is necessary to assign relative risk factors or relative constraints to different types of complications. This is not straightforward, since the clinical objectives require to be defined in greater detail.

The last section of Chapter 9 deals with the work of Mistry and DeGinder (1978), who are concerned with estimating and diagramming cumulative biological effects resulting from various fractionation schemes used in external beam radiotherapy.

The X-ray photon energies that give the highest signal-to-noise ratios per unit of exposure or average dose in mammography are much larger than those used in current film/screen systems. Muntz et al. (1978) investigate the significance of photon energy control in mammography. They give some preliminary results on the use of electrostatic imaging systems, which can operate at optimum photon energy levels and so minimize either the dose or the exposure. Related work occurs in Muntz (1979).

This work by Muntz and coworkers illustrates an "optimization" application in diagnostic radiology. However our interests here lie in the direction of reconstructive tomography, which is the subject of Chapter 10. There are a number of excellent surveys of the theory and applications in reconstructive tomography--an area that has experienced explosive growth during the last ten years. My objective here is to describe some of the features involved in a reconstruction algorithm, based on using Fourier integral transforms and some of the properties of generalized functions. Early detection, extent of disease and tumor response are only three of the useful features that scanning techniques provide for patients. These new tomographic scanners can be used for treatment planning and an introduction to this area is in Section 10.4.

Section 10.5 is concerned with a number of possible ways in which dose reduction can be accomplished. The implementation of a number of these methods would certainly lead to a lower dosage to the patient than presently appears to be the case.

An overview of optimization techniques in human cancer radiotherapy is presented by the author, Swan (1981c).

1.2 History of Cancer and its Treatment by Radiotherapy

When I published my first book in cancer research, Swan (1977), I was surprised to find that there did not appear to be any definitive works dealing with the history of cancer in humans. Also, it comes as a surprise to many of my friends that cancer is not a modern disease that somehow came into being after the second world war. A number of scholars surmise that, before the onset of written history, many people died as a consequence of having cancer. Throughout written history there appear numerous accounts dealing with various cancers and treatments for them. During the last quarter of a century there has been a dramatic upsurge in investigations of all of the areas associated with cancer research.

An interesting brief history of cancer in humans is given by Bett (1957). More recently, Watson (1972) presents a history of the molecular biological developments in cancer research. A very readable account of occupational and environmental cancer in humans is in Chapter 4 of Harris (1976). The book by Rather (1978) traces and discusses many of the historical ideas concerning cancer.

The material in this book is concerned with X-rays and their usage in dealing with human cancer radiotherapy. X-rays were discovered by Röntgen (1895). Shortly thereafter came the work on radioactivity by Becquerel (1896) and on radium by the Curies (1898). By the early 1900's a number of people believed that these new rays could provide a cure for cancer.

The primitive state of knowledge of X-rays in the first quarter of this century was no deterrent to the practitioners who used them in cancer therapy. Radiation dose was not measured with any accuracy and there was no generally accepted unit of dose. It was thought that a single massive dose of irradiation was the way to treat tumors. As a consequence, physicians spent a considerable amount of time analyzing radiation injury.

The way in which X-rays are produced is as follows. Electrons come off a hot wire (the cathode) and, under the influence of an applied electrical potential difference, are accelerated towards a metal plate (the anode). The impact of an electron on the anode results in its kinetic energy being converted into an X-ray quantum, a photon. X-rays are one example of high-energy radiation. There is the possibility of damage to human tissue from the radiation insult of X-rays. This damage affects both normal and tumor tissue. Even though X-rays have been known since 1895 their mechanism of cell kill is still not known. When tissue gets irradiated the radiation produces an ionization effect, which in turn creates free radicals. It is thought that these free radicals mount a chemical attack on cellular deoxyribonucleic acid (DNA). Free radicals are highly reactive unstable compounds, containing an odd number of electrons, and have a brief existence in tissues.

The motivation for using radiation for the treatment of cancer is as follows. After a radiation insult the normal cell population is expected to recover at a much faster rate than the tumor cell population. It is interesting that the more undifferentiated the tumor, the more rapidly proliferating, and the more anaplastic (indicating a primitive or embryonic state) the better is the response to irradiation treatment. A number of tumors are radiation-resistant; slowly growing tumors are in this category.

Studies in Paris, in the early 1920's, by Regaud suggested that the testis with its high rate of cell turnover had some characteristics of the growth of a malignant tumor. He suggested that the radiation dosage be given in fractions and not as a single massive dose. That is, after the initial dose, a period of time passes (maybe a day, or several days) before the next dose is given. In between doses the normal cell population has a better chance of recovery. Although the tumor cells will also recover, a certain proportion of them will eventually die. Continuation of the fractionation scheme may result in cure of the patient. It did not take people too long to discover that Regaud's suggestion was sound. Current day radiotherapy procedures make use of fractionated therapy.

The unit of absorbed radiation dose is the rad and this was universally adopted in 1956. The rad is used in most of the scientific literature dealing with radiotherapy. However there is a recent recommendation that the unit, called the Gray, be adopted;

$$100 \text{ rads} = 1 \text{ Gray (Gy)}, \; 1 \text{ Gray} = 1 \text{ J kg}^{-1}.$$

The rad is used in this book and it is easy to convert into Grays, if needed.

To increase the depth of penetration of X-rays into tissue it was necessary to apply higher potential differences (and therefore higher voltages) in X-ray tubes. Coolidge (1913) introduced a vacuum X-ray tube which operated at energies approximating 200 kilovolts (kV). In a historical appraisal of radiotherapy, Buschke (1970) noted that the kilovoltage era was one of considerable achievement.

The pursuit of creating beams of even higher energies continued. Schultz (1975) chronicles the developments from the kilovoltage era to the megavoltage (MV) era. From nuclear fission reactions it is possible to obtain considerable quantities of radioactive cobalt, ^{60}Co. Eventually Cobalt 60 teletherapy equipment became available with beam energies equivalent to 3 MV X-rays.

In the mid fifties appeared reports on the clinical usefulness of the linear electron accelerator. These machines produced beams of megavoltage energies with the feature that peak ionization occurred at great depths beneath the skin surface. Since the dose limiting factor had been the radiation tolerance of the skin, use of these new devices effectively eliminated that restriction. The beams have considerable penetration and well defined lateral edges and so provide a powerful tool with which to deal with a number of tumor complications. Use of these beams has considerably improved the long-term survival and cure rates of a number of tumors. Accordingly it is not surprising that linear accelerators are part of the standard equipment in many radiation therapy treatment centers; see Karzmark and Pering (1973). See, also, Tapley (1976) and Lerch (1979).

This now brings us to the developments in radiobiology and radiation therapy during the last twenty-five years.

In radiobiology, quantitative studies of radiation dose-cell survival relationships were made. There is an initial shoulder portion to these exponential survival curves. Investigations, Elkind and Sutton (1960), indicated this initial shoulder was due to the recovery of mammalian cells from sublethal damage in the low-dose range. Kaplan (1968) reported on studies at the molecular level which demonstrated that the lethal effects of ionizing radiation in bacterial and mammalian cells are generally the result of breaks or other damage in the strands of DNA. See Kaplan (1979) for a recent historical review. A mathematical expression for the survival versus dose curve was constructed by Chadwick and Leenhouts (1973) from their molecular model of single and double strand DNA breaks.

Oxygen appears to be a key constituent in instantaneous reactions that convert the initially reversible forms of chemical alteration induced by ionization to irreversible secondary forms, and so fixes the radiation damage within a cell. Mammalian cells are known to have about a threefold reduction in their sensitivity when irradiated in an atmosphere of nitrogen rather than air or oxygen. Gray (1957) pointed out that, when tumors have exhausted their blood supply, and so robbed of the essential nutrient, oxygen, hypoxic foci exist and these will influence the successful outcome of radiation therapy. In fact many patients have been treated in hyperbaric chambers, but the procedure is very unwieldy and impractical. This has led to newer approaches involving the heavy particles and the use of cyclotrons. A consolidation of work in this area is reported in the 7th International Conference on Cyclotrons and Their Applications published by Birkhäuser Verlag (Basel), 1975. Proton and neutron therapy will undoubtedly take a more prominent role in the future; Catteral and Bewley (1979).

Meyn and Withers (1980) present many current papers in radiation biology.

A useful summary of the key concepts in radiotherapy over the last twenty-five years was given by Fletcher (1978). He noted that in 1949 the absolute concepts of radiotherapy were the following:

(1) all or none cancericidal dose linked with the histology of the disease;

(2) a homogeneous dose of irradiation to the target;

(3) the use of a single treatment modality, either irradiation or surgery;

(4) no use of elective postoperative irradiation, because of the concept that one had to wait for a recurrence so that one would have something tangible to irradiate;

(5) the need for a surgical procedure to be radical, called a "cancerwise" procedure.

The considerable changes from the 1949 concepts to the 1977 concepts of radiotherapy are:

(i) sensitivity is not linked to histology but to the volume of the cancer, and the concept of cancericidal dose must be revised due to the existence of a sigmoid response curve;

(ii) the dose does not necessarily have to be homogeneous in the target volume but should be gauged to varying volumes of cancer;

(iii) the fact that irradiation may not be the sole treatment in some tumors does not mean that it does not have a place in their management;

(iv) as a general rule, large tumors should not be treated with irradiation alone;

(v) since there is a dose-response curve for control rates and for complications, an optimum dose level, depending on the clinical situation, must be maintained;

(vi) one must think of the quality of life available to the patient.

In connection with (ii) above the treatment plans described in this book are each concerned with uniformity of dose distribution.

There are many different aspects of radiation biology and therapy and no attempt is made to include a synposis of them. Instead the author refers the reader to the following: Paterson (1963), Elkind and Whitmore (1967), Buschke and Parker (1972), Hall (1973), Nygaard et al. (1975), Gilbert and Kagan (1978), Christensen et al. (1978), Rubin (1978), Caldwell (1979), Hendee (1979), Moss et al. (1979) and Order et al. (1979). See also Walter and Miller (1959) and Walter (1977).

Recently Fowler (1979) presented a survey of future areas in radiation oncology. The article discusses the gains to be made in such areas as (a) physical dose distributions, (b) the development of new methods, (c) clinical trials, (d) fractionation, (e) ways to deal with hypoxic cells, (f) fractionated X-rays, neutrons and radiosensitizers, (g) hyperthermia, and (h) combinations of radiotherapy and chemotherapy.

Radiation therapy to the cancer patient is improving all the time and there are a number of areas which show promise for the future; see Fowler (1979). Some of these include the following:

(a) Combinations of radiotherapy and chemotherapy; Phillips and Fu (1976); Rubin and Carter (1976); Steel and Peckham (1979).

(b) The use of various drugs to radiosensitive hypoxic cells; Dische et al. (1978, 1979); Wasserman et al. (1979).

(c) The use of fast neutrons; Hall et al. (1979).

(d) Improved fractionation schemes; Withers (1975, 1977, 1978); Arcangeli et al. (1979).

(e) The utilization of techniques in reconstructive tomography, positron emission tomography, nuclear magnetic resonance to localize the tumor, make a study of it electronically, and follow the functioning of various body tissues.

1.3 Some Mathematical Models of Tumor Growth

Detailed presentations of many of the deterministic and some of the stochastic mathematical models currently in use as potential aids in the understanding of tumor growth appear in the author's book, Swan (1977). Mathematical models which involve simple deterministic differential equations take the general forms

$$\dot{L}(t) = Lf(L) \tag{1.1}$$

$$\text{and} \quad \dot{L}(t) = g(L(t),t), \tag{1.2}$$

where the notation $\dot{L}(t)$ means $dL(t)/dt$. The quantity $L(t) \equiv L$ is often interpreted as being the total number of tumor cells, or the level of tumor burden such as the volume of space occupied by the tumor. Whichever of these two mathematical models is chosen it is useful to bear in mind that they can only be (mathematically) valid so long as it is meaningful, in some sense, to talk about an instantaneous rate of change, which is probably true for large populations of cells, when L is thought of as being cell number. For "small" numbers of cells these ordinary differential equations may not adequately represent the tumor growth problem under investigation.

Simple exponential growth is given by $f(L) = \lambda(>0)$:

$$\dot{L}(t) = \lambda L,\ L(t) = L(t_o)e^{(t-t_o)\lambda}; \tag{1.3}$$

the solution being true when the specific growth rate λ is a constant. This growth situation continues so long as the population does not experience any apparent bound on its supply of essential nutrients, such as oxygen or necessary substrates.

As the cell population increases, but now with a limit to the available nutrient supply, then it experiences an inhibitory effect on its further growth. Mathematically, this is contained in the requirement that $df(L)/dL$ be negative. Some examples of this situation are now given.

Logistic growth is given by $f(L) = \lambda - \mu L$, where λ and μ are positive constants:

$$\dot{L}(t) = (\lambda - \mu L)L. \tag{1.4}$$

The right-hand side gives the growth rate as the product of potential rate of unbounded growth with that proportion of the greatest level (i.e. λ/μ) which is as yet unrealized. Graphs of the solutions of the logistic differential equation are shown in Fig. 5.2. An explicit mathematical formula for the solution is easily found by converting the nonlinear differential equation into a linear one by means of the transformation $u = 1/L$; see (5.10).

One extension of the case of logistic growth is provided by the equation

$$\dot{L}(t) = [\lambda(t) - \mu(t)L(t)]L(t). \tag{1.5}$$

The solution is readily obtained by use of the nonlinear transformation of the last paragraph and

$$L(t) = \frac{\rho(t)}{C + \int^t \mu(\xi)\rho(\xi)d\xi},\quad \rho(t) = \exp[\int^t \lambda(\xi)d\xi], \tag{1.6}$$

where C is an integration constant. A more complicated equation is

$$\dot{L}(t) = \{\lambda(t) - \mu(t)[L(t)]^{\alpha-1}\}L(t),\ \alpha > 1. \tag{1.7}$$

Introduce the nonlinear transformation $u(t) = g(t)/L(t)$, where

$$g(t) = \exp \int^t \lambda(\tau)d\tau.$$

Then

$$\frac{\dot{u}(t)}{u(t)} = \frac{\dot{g}(t)}{g(t)} - \lambda(t) + \mu(t)\left[\frac{g(t)}{u(t)}\right]^{\alpha - 1},$$

which simplifies to the variables-separable form

$$u^{\alpha-2}du = \mu(t)[\exp \int^t \lambda(\tau)d\tau]^{\alpha-1}\ dt.$$

Since $\alpha > 1$, integration of each side together with reorganization of expressions gives

$$L(t) = \frac{\exp \int^t \lambda(\tau)d\tau}{\{(\alpha - 1)[C_1 + \int^t \mu(t)(\exp \int^t \lambda(\tau)d\tau)^{\alpha-1}\ dt]\}^{1/(\alpha-1)}} \tag{1.8}$$

where C_1 is a constant of integration. A special case occurs when $\lambda(t) = \lambda$, and $\mu(t) = \mu$, where λ and μ are constants for then the last display simplifies to give

$$L(t) = \{\mu/\lambda + (\alpha -1)C_1 \exp[-(\alpha - 1)\lambda t]\}^{-1/(\alpha -1)}, \tag{1.9}$$

which is the general solution of

$$\dot{L}(t) = \{\lambda - \mu[L(t)]^{\alpha-1}\}L(t),\ \alpha > 1. \tag{1.10}$$

When $1 < \alpha < 2$ the solution (1.9) gives a sigmoid-shaped curve, which lies above the logistic curve and corresponds to rapid tumor growth; $\alpha > 2$ gives a curve which lies far to the right of the logistic curve and could possibly represent slowly growing tumors. See Swan (1977).

Gompertz growth is described by $f(L) = \lambda\ \ell n(\theta/L)$, where θ is the greatest size of the tumor and λ is a constant:

$$\dot{L}(t) = \lambda L\ \ell n(\theta/L). \tag{1.11}$$

This nonlinear equation is readily reduced to a linear one by means of the nonlinear transformation $Y = \ell n(\theta/L)$ and the solution can be written in the form

$$L(t) = \theta \exp\{-\exp[-\lambda(t - t_o)]\ell n(\theta/L_o)\}, \tag{1.12}$$

where $L_o \equiv L(t_o)$ is the tumor size at time $t = t_o$. The adoption of a Gompertz growth equation arose from the work of Laird (1964). She used the solution (1.12) to fit to tumor volume data for a number of experimental animals; the fit looked reasonable. Further impetus to use the Gompertz equation arose when Simpson-Herren and Lloyd (1970) published their results on the fit of the solution (1.12) to data from nine experimental tumors; the fit was "good".

Data on human multiple myeloma has been fitted to a Gompertz growth equation; e.g. Sullivan and Salmon (1972). Again, the fit of this mathematical model to clinical data, in this instance, is reasonable. So much so, that (1.11) and (1.12) are proposed by various investigators as being <u>the</u> mathematical model. At the present time, there is no apparent biological reasoning which leads to the Gompertz equation. Many investigators use (1.11) purely as a matter of convenience.

A variety of papers have appeared in the seventies dealing with experimental and clinical studies and the analysis of data in terms of a Gompertz equation. For a representative selection see Lloyd (1975), Swan (1975), Norton et al. (1976), Swan and Vincent (1977), Swan (1977), Brunton and Wheldon (1978), and Demicheli (1980).

With $f(L) = T^{-1} \ell n\, 2$ then a simple mathematical model of tumor growth is obtained:

$$L(t) = L(0)\, 2^{t/T}, \tag{1.13}$$

where T is the tumor doubling time. Note that $L(t + \tau) = 2^{\tau/T} L(t)$.

The selection of $f(L) = \lambda \exp(-\mu L)$, λ and μ constants, so that the tumor growth equation is

$$\dot{L}(t) = \lambda L \exp(-\mu L), \tag{1.14}$$

is introduced by Fischer (1971a). This equation does not have an explicit analytical solution, but of course can be easily integrated by numerical means.

One feature that each of the above mathematical models have in common is the assumption that the tumor is well oxygenated. The quantity $f(L)/\lambda$ can be interpreted as being the fraction of the total cells present which are well oxygenated. Also, λ^{-1} is a characteristic time constant for the growth of the tumor. Solid tumors are known to contain well oxygenated cells and hypoxic cells. Such a tumor is assumed to consist of a total of L cells of which $Lf(L)/\lambda$ are oxygenated and grow with rate constant λ, and $[1 - f(L)/\lambda]L$ which are poorly oxygenated (anoxic) and do not reproduce. The growth parameter λ describes the rate of increase of the well oxygenated cells overall but does not provide any detailed information about the fraction of cells within this group that are actually dividing.

Hypoxic cells tend to be resistant to ionizing radiations. A mathematical model which provides a theoretical analysis of some optimal treatment schedules when the tumor consists of well oxygenated and anoxic cells (a two level population model) is presented by Hethcote and Waltman (1973), and will be examined in greater detail in Section 6.5.

A four level population model for a tumor undergoing a scheme of irradiations is examined in Section 6.4.

There are a number of other simple mathematical models for unperturbed tumor growth and some of these include the use of difference equations or partial differential equations when age and/or maturity structure is needed. Useful stochastic models have also been developed to describe cellular response to ionizing radiations; see, e.g., Paskin et al. (1967), Bansal and Gupta (1978).

These mathematical models provide useful (albeit crude) approximations to a real viable tumor. For example a solid tumor consists of a macroscopically discernable volume consisting of heterogeneous material including dividing cells, non-dividing cells, dead cells not yet eliminated, solid stroma, blood and other cellular debris.

The mathematical models and corresponding equations so far introduced in this Section have been applied to total numbers of cells. However many scientists believe that it is important to go further and describe the events which take place within the cell cycle. This has led to many analyses of cell cycle kinetics. One of the best discussions of this area in connection with the growth kinetics of tumors is in the recent book by Steel (1977) which represents the culmination and synthesis of more than fifteen years of work.

Cellular kinetics refers to the transient events in the life history of a cell population which take place in relation to time, space, morphology and function. In the early 1950's dramatic progress was made in the understanding of the behavior of a normal cell as it goes through its various phases of development. These phases follow in sequence and are said to be located in the cell cycle. A key discovery was made by Howard and Pelc (1953) who showed the the deoxyribonucleic acid (DNA) is synthesized only in one limited stage of the cell cycle. Their work provided the structure for the interpretation of radio-isotope labeling experiments and also provided an underlying framework on which mathematical models of cellular kinetics could be built.

A commonly-used description of the cell cycle is due to Baserga (1965): For the normal cell there are assumed to be four distinct phases:

G_1: Here proteins and ribonucleic acid (RNA) are synthesized. This is also called the pre-DNA phase.

S : This is the DNA synthesis phase with duplication of DNA. Protein and RNA synthesis continues.

G_2: In this post-DNA phase there is no synthesis of DNA. However, protein and RNA synthesis continues.

M : Mitosis phase and leads to cell division.

The DNA synthesis produces the "daughter" chromosomes. There is a preparatory period (or gap) preceding S phase. After S phase is complete there is a further preparatory period before mitosis starts. These gap phases are also referred to as rest periods.

From within its local environment a cell may receive an adverse signal, indicating that there is a run-down in the supply of essential nutrients, or lack of serum with necessary growth factors. When this occurs, growth of the cell usually is arrested at a point soon after mitosis in early G_1.

For L_{1210} leukemia (an experimental tumor used in connection with laboratory animals such as rats) the total cycle time is of the order of 13 hours. For human acute lymphoblastic leukemia, when there is of the order of 10^{11} tumor cells, the total cycle time is 20 hours, with 12 hours being spent in S phase. For human melanoma the cell cycle time is approximately 100 hours.

Study has shown that the Howard-Pelc model refers only to the active portion of the cell cycle. Some slowly proliferating tissues apparently spend a long time (months and even years in other cases) prior to entering the G_1 phase. Lajtha (1963) and Quastler (1963) suggested that, for such tissue, there is an actual resting period G_o. From G_o the cells can be triggered to enter the mitotic cycle. Lajtha never suggested that the concept of the G_o state be applied to tumor cells. However the existence of cells in G_o for human tumor populations has been shown by Clarkson et al. (1967, 1969, 1970, 1977), Saunders and Mauer (1969) and Gabutti et al. (1969). Their conclusions appear to be true for leukemia. No experimental evidence seems to be available to support the hypothesis that cells can be in the G_o state for solid tumors. In fact Stoker (1976, p. 6) suggests that there does not appear to be any good evidence to indicate that out of cycle tumor cells are in fact resting, in the sense of normal cells.

Although a number of mathematical models of cellular kinetics have been utilized in cancer research, see Aroesty et al. (1973) and Swan (1977) for surveys, they have not enjoyed sustained success. Recently Tannock (1978) and Hill (1978) have presented critical reviews of cell kinetics studies and their relevance to cancer chemotherapy.

The cell cycle is divided into the four phases G_1, S, G_2, and M by Paskin et al. (1967), who assigned an average transit time $\overline{t}_i$ to each phase, with t_i the time spent by a cell in the ith phase. The four transit times were assumed to be independently distributed as Gaussians. They utilized a Monte Carlo technique to follow the life cycle of a cell and all of its progeny. Their stochastic model represented the cyclic characteristics of the cell proliferation process. This approach permitted quantitative and simultaneous treatment of the cell proliferative process together with external perturbation of the system and its recovery.

Tewfik et al. (1977) are interested in determining the minimal dose and the optimal time between fractionated exposures to produce the greatest amount of tumor control while minimizing damage to normal tissues.

A more recent study by Braunschweiger et al. (1979) deals with cell kinetics as a basis for effective radiotherapy. That article prompted an editorial from Steel (1979), who pointed out that there were four main lessons to be learned from the previous 20 years work on cell kinetics studies:

(1) Although the simpler experimental systems provide the best opportunities for research and lead to clear conclusions they are the least likely to provide conclusions of clinical importance.

(2) Mathematical models are at the extreme end of the spectrum of artificial-realistic models of cancer. While they can provide much intellectual stimulation one needs to critically assess their contribution in each case in applied cancer research.

(3) One should perhaps concentrate attention on those cells that survive with colony forming ability.

(4) In cancer therapy it is essential to consider, side by side, tumor response and normal tissue damage.

Earlier discussions in this section suggested the use of the mathematical model

$$\dot{L}(t) = Lf(L) \tag{1.15}$$

to represent tumor growth. To incorporate the effects of irradiation, chemotherapy, etc., on the tumor cell population a loss term can be introduced into the right-hand side of (1.15). However a representation for the loss term presents some difficulty.

If at time t a dose of radiation of size D rads is delivered to the tumor then one assumption is to consider that the action of the irradiation is proportional to the tumor population size at t and can be written as g(D)L. Equation (1.15) then takes the form

$$\dot{L}(t) = Lf(L) - g(D)L, \; L = L(0) \text{ at } t = 0. \tag{1.16}$$

Loss terms of this type have been discussed in Swan and Vincent (1977) and Swan (1980) in connection with cancer chemotherapy problems, where the level of anticancer drug replaces the radiation dosage.

However, since f(L) can be interpreted as being proportional to the fraction of cells that are well oxygenated an alternative approach is the following. After a radiation insult one may assume that this fraction of well exygenated cells is reduced by an appropriate amount, say v, so that, instead of (1.15),

$$\dot{L}(t) = Lf(L) - [vf(L)]L.$$

It seems reasonable to expect that v is some function v(D) of the radiation dose level D. For example, in the case of Gompertz growth

$$\dot{L}(t) = [1 - v(D)]\lambda L \, \ell n(\theta/L). \tag{1.17}$$

Looney et al. (1975) investigate changes in tumor growth rates for a solid tumor model (hepatoma 3924A). At a certain time (days after tumor inoculation) the tumor is irradiated with a single dose. The progress of the tumor is followed for a number of days after the radiation insult and tumor volumes are estimated. This work by Looney and coworkers is examined by Norton and Simon (1977a), who indicate that it is possible (in general) to represent the unperturbed tumor growth in terms of a Gompertz equation. To account for the tumor growth curves seen after a single irradiation insult they postulate that (in the present notation)

$$\dot{L}(t) = [1 - v(D,t)]\lambda L \,\ell n(\theta/L), \qquad (1.18)$$

where L(t) is the tumor volume at time t. The coefficient v(D,t) in the loss term is written as

$$v(D,t) = P(D)(t - 4)^{E(D)} \exp[(4 - t)/F(D)], \qquad (1.19)$$

in which the 4 indicates that the tumor was treated on day 4. The right-hand side of (1.19) is an unnormalized gamma distribution and was selected by Norton and Simon to provide the best graphical fit of the equation to the data. Certainly the fit appears to be reasonable. Their investigations suggested that E(D) = constant = 0.5215, F(D) = constant = 13.61 and

$$P(D) = K_1 \exp\{K_2/(D + K_3)\},$$

where K_1, K_2 and K_3 are numerical constants. However, when D = 0, P(0) is nonzero, which does not appear to be reasonable. If there is no radiation then there cannot be any loss term and v(0) should therefore be zero. A better choice is to set

$$P(D) = \frac{0.839570\ D}{D + 507.597} .$$

Related papers are by Norton and coworkers (1976, 1977b, 1978 and 1979) and Looney et al. (1977).

Norton and Simon claim that a tumor that grows according to a Gompertz equation may be most sensitive to treatment at the point of inflection of this sigmoid-type growth curve. Steel (1979) points out that one main argument against this claim is as follows. The Gompertz model predicts a point of inflection at a tumor size that is 0.37 of the asymptotic maximum tumor size θ. Calculated values of θ for tumors in animals are frequently in the range 10-100 g. This means that the Norton-Simon hypothesis leads to a maximum sensitivity being expected in mouse and rat tumors weighing at least a few grams. Direct experimental evidence contradicts this and indicates that within the dissectable range of tumor sizes "small is sensitive".

More recently Cox et al. (1980) present an interesting mathematical model of tumor growth. They derive the equation

$$\dot{L}(t) = \alpha L/(1 + \beta L),\ L(0) = L_o,$$

where α is the inherent growth rate of the tumor when all cells are in cycle and β is a parameter which gives a measure of the combination of cellular rate of secretion of a postulated inhibitory molecule, its volume of distribution and its rate of degradation or excretion. The quantity L is the number of viable cells in the tumor population. To account for cellular loss from the tumor during its growth a loss term proportional to L is introduced. This leads to the growth equation

$$\dot{L}(t) = \frac{\alpha}{1 + \beta L} - \gamma L, \; L(0) = L_o.$$

The solution of this equation increases to a shoulder and eventually approaches a horizontal asymptote. Cox and coworkers fitted this mathematical model to the data in the paper by Simpson-Herren and Lloyd (1970) and obtained estimates of α, β and γ.

Unfortunately there does not appear to be any experimental evidence in support of this or any other mathematical model.

Mathematical models should be used with extreme care and appreciation for the fact that they may contain artifacts that have no relevance for the problem in which they are being used. Several different mathematical models could be employed and it is often left to the whims of the investigator which one is used.

1.4 Spatial Distribution of the Radiation Dose

The actual spatial distribution of the radiation dose is one of the variables which is of importance during radiation treatment. One goal in radiation therapy is to try to choose an optimal dose distribution. To approach this problem Fischer (1969) describes a viable tumor by a cell density function, which measures the expected concentration of cells at any point in the tumor-bearing volume. His approach generates the corresponding cell density function after any particular treatment. This leads to information on the probability of cure of the tumor and the probability of recurrence in any region. Although Fischer's development is based on the use of the multi-target, single-hit survival function (2.1) with $k = 1/D_o$ and D_o being the mean lethal dose, the present exposition is broad enough to include any particular surviving function.

Introduce a cell density function $\rho(\xi,\eta,\zeta,t)$ where ξ,η,ζ denote the three spatial coordinates in a Cartesian frame. The expectation value of the number of cells in a unit volume is the same as this cell density function. For regions in which tumor cells are distributed sparingly $\rho(\xi,\eta,\zeta,t)$ can be less than unity. The total number of tumor cells at time t is given by

$$L(t) = \iiint \rho(\xi,\eta,\zeta,t)\,d\xi d\eta d\zeta,$$

where the integration is taken over the "tumor-bearing space", that is, the space containing tumor cells. To avoid the inclusion of regions more than once it is assumed that the cell density function is single-valued and, further, that is integrable. It is evident that if knowledge on the cell density function is available then this would give important information on the total cell number. However, it is not an easy matter to obtain details on the values of L(t). Some information on $\rho(\xi,\eta,\zeta,t)$ can be obtained from measurements of tumor size together with knowledge of the individual cell size.

Define P_c to be the probability of curing a tumor, that is, the probability that no cells survive the radiation treatment. Also, let $S(<1)$ denote that fraction of tumor cells which survive a single radiation insult. The expected number of survivors from the tumor cell population is $SL(t)$. The probability P_c given by the Poisson probability for zero events when $SL(t)$ events are expected is $P_c = \exp[-SL(t)]$ or, more generally,

$$P_c = \exp[-\iiint \rho(\xi,\eta,\zeta,t)S(\xi,\eta,\zeta)d\xi d\eta d\zeta],$$

where $S(\xi,\eta,\zeta)$ is the fraction of tumor cells at the point ξ,η,ζ which survive a single dose of radiation. In one sense the integrand in the last display produces a measure of the efficacy of the treatment at the point ξ,η,ζ.

Fischer (1969) suggested that an optimum treatment plan should provide for a dose distribution in space which can produce equal probabilities of complete tumor irradication throughout the tumor-bearing volume. For example, if recurrence of the tumor in any area is equally undesirable then it is unwise to decrease the probability of recurrence in a particular region, perhaps at the cost of treatment morbidity, far below that which is known to exist in other areas.

Assume that the probability of local control is uniform throughout the tumor. This means that the local control probability C is given by

$$\rho(\xi,\eta,\zeta,t)S(\xi,\eta,\zeta) = C, \tag{1.20}$$

where C is a constant; also

$$-\ln P_c = C\iiint d\xi d\eta d\zeta.$$

It is possible for $\rho(\xi,\eta,\zeta,t)$ to be less than C. This situation occurs in areas, usually at the periphery, where the original cell density is less than the acceptable post-treatment density for the main portion of the tumor. Since $S > 1$ is not allowed the condition (1.20) is violated in these areas. Fischer suggests that no radiation be given to these areas. Hence the final cure probability is of the form

$$P_c = \exp[-\iiint_{\rho>C} \rho(\xi,\eta,\zeta,t)S(\xi,\eta,\zeta)d\xi d\eta d\zeta - \iiint_{\rho<C} \rho(\xi,\eta,\zeta,t)d\xi d\eta d\zeta]$$

$$= \exp[-C\iiint_{\rho>C} d\xi d\eta d\zeta - \iiint_{\rho<C} \rho(\xi,\eta,\zeta,t)d\xi d\eta d\zeta]$$

where the integrals on the left are evaluated over the tumor-bearing volume with $\rho \equiv \rho(\xi,\eta,\zeta,t) > 0$ and the remaining integrals are taken over the remaining volume.

Fischer (1969) considers an illustrative example of a tumor which has an indefinite boundary. The outside contour is assumed to have cylindrical symmetry and is an approximation to a normal curve. For this tumor he takes the cell density function $\rho(r,\theta) = N_o \exp(-r^2)$ as being appropriate since all variations in the ζ direction, along the axis of the cylinder, can be considered to be suppressed, see Figure 1.1a. The treatment is assumed to be with parallel opposed fields and r,θ are cylindrical coordinates. If R is the boundary outside of which no radiation is given then, for C arbitrary, $C = N_o \exp(-R^2)$. Hence, the cure probability

$$P_c = \exp[-C \int_0^{2\pi}\int_0^R r\,dr\,d\theta - N_o \int_0^{2\pi}\int_R^{\infty} r\,e^{-r^2}\,dr\,d\theta]$$

$$= \exp\{-\pi\, C[1 + \ell n(N_o/C)]\}.$$

Thus, for $N_o = 10^8$ cells/cm^2 and an arbitrary choice of $C = 10^{-3}/\text{cm}^2$, the overall cure probability is 92 percent. (An error in Fischer's formula gives $P_c = 0.94$).

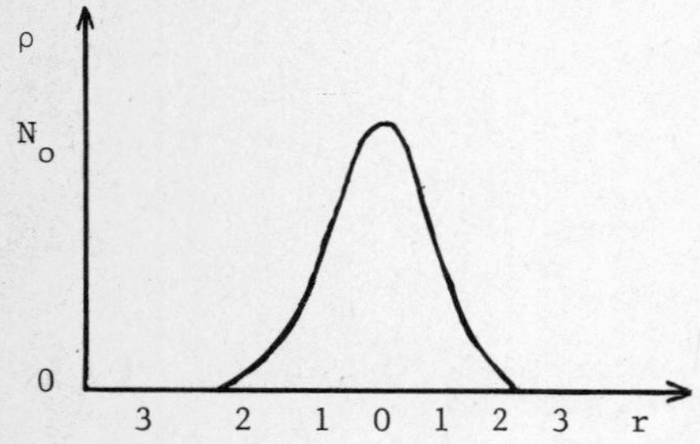

Figure 1.1a. Contour and cell density distribution $\rho = N_o \exp(-r^2)$ with $N_o = 10^8$ tumor cells/cm^2.

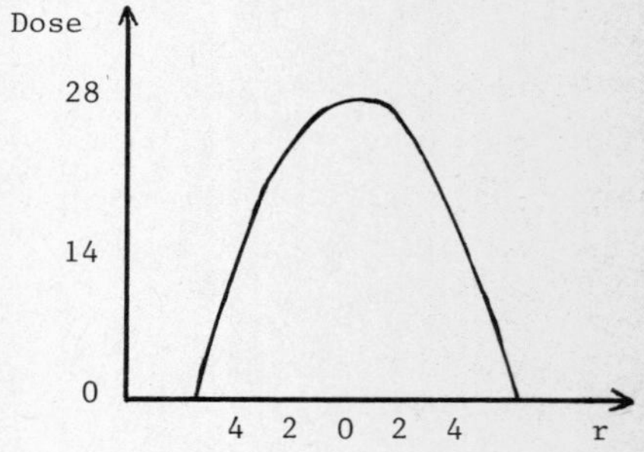

Figure 1.1b. Calculated dose distribution in units of D_o.

Assume, for example, that S is given by the survival expression (2.1) then, for $\exp(-D/D_o) \ll 1$, $S \approx n \exp(-D/D_o)$. With $D \equiv D(r)$, the result (1.20) can be rearranged to give

$$D(r) = [\ell n(n\, N_o/C) - r^2]D_o$$

$$= [(5.167)^2 - r^2]D_o;$$

and n is taken to have the value 4. The dose distribution D(r) is a parabola with greatest height of 26.7 D_o rads; see Figure 1.1b.

Fischer indicates that no radiation be given outside of the circle with radius 5.6 cm, where the probability before treatment of finding a tumor cell is less than $10^{-3}/\text{cm}^2$. From Figure 1.1a it is apparent that a simple physical examination would not reveal any portion of the tumor beyond 2 cm from the center. However Fig. 1.1b indicates that a dose of almost 9 percent of the central axis dose must be given in order to reduce the possibility of recurrence after treatment to the same level as will result at the tumor center. One conclusion from this example is that an ideal treatment could be achieved for this tumor model by using a custom made filter to produce the dose distribution given by the formula for D(r).

Instead of (2.1) use the exponential-quadratic survival expression (3.1) in the result (1.20) which can be rearranged to give the dose distribution D(r) in the form

$$D(r) = \frac{1}{2\beta}\left[\alpha^2 + 4\beta \ln \frac{N_o}{C} - 4\beta r^2\right]^{1/2} - \frac{\alpha}{2\beta} .$$

The general shape of the curve given by this expression is similar to the graph in Figure 1.1b. From Chadwick et al. (1976) the values $\alpha = 2 \times 10^{-3}$ rad^{-1} and $\beta = 4 \times 10^{-6}$ rad^{-2} are representative for irradiation of Chinese hamster ovary cells.

Chapter 2

SURVIVAL CURVES FROM STATISTICAL MODELS

2.1 Introduction

Figure 2.1 shows a number of different types of radiation and the energies associated with them. Electromagnetic radiation or non-ionizing radiation occurs for energies below that of X-rays and other ionizing radiations. Our knowledge of X-rays and gamma-rays begins with Roentgen's discoveries in 1895 and the Curies' isolation of radium in 1898. X-rays occur naturally in outer space and are the same nature as gamma-rays. On earth the production of X-rays is by electrical machines, such as the X-ray tube, in which a heating current is passed through a filament and at a sufficiently high temperature electrons boil off. Application of a high voltage across the tube guides these electrons to a target resulting in a violent impact that rays are produced from the disturbed atoms.

Light is comprised of various components - two of these are short wavelength ultraviolet radiation, and the radiation composed of physical particles such as electrons, neutrons, protons, alphas, and photons in the X-ray and gamma-ray energies. The noteworthy feature of these particles is that they are energetic enough to easily ionize one or more atoms in organisms, and this results in one or more chemical bonds being broken. Accordingly, then, irradiation may produce drastic effects on biological tissues; target organisms can be killed.

The physical mechanism of action of these ionizing radiations is that an electron is ejected and leaves behind an ionized atom or molecule. A unit of negative electrical charge has been lost from the atom which now has an unbalanced surplus of positive charge. It is usual for the dislodged electron to be caught on a neighboring atom, which thus acquires an unbalanced extra unit of negative charge. The word ion refers to these fragments - one electrically positive due to the removal of an electron, the other electrically negative through the addition of an extra one; the process itself is called ionization. Ejection of the outermost electron usually occurs because it is the one most weakly bound to its atom or molecule. Since this same outer electron is involved in chemical bonds, the bond is readily broken by the ionization.

The type of incident particle influences the ejection of electrons by two mechanisms. Electrically charged particles, such as electrons, protons, alphas, when flying past an atom or molecule, exert an electric force on the electrons, and consequently effect their ejection. It follows that the uncharged particles (X-rays, gamma-rays, and neutrons) have less of a direct mode of action. Briefly, when X-radiation impinges on a biological material energy is absorbed as a result of electrons set in motion by the photoelectric, Compton, and pair production processes. The physics of these processes is well understood; see, for example, Selman (1977). (Perhaps a more picturesque way of describing the collision process is to say that the photons act like billiard balls to strike the electrons and knock them out of

WAVELENGTH IN CM	TYPE OF RADIATION		FREQUENCY
100 000 000 000	10^{11}		10^{-1}
10 000 000 000	10^{10}	ELECTRICAL	10^{0}
1 000 000 000	10^{9}	WAVES	10^{1}
100 000 000	10^{8}		10^{2}
10 000 000	10^{7}		10^{3}
1 000 000	10^{6}		10^{4}
100 000	10^{5}		10^{5}
10 000	10^{4}	RADIO	10^{6}
1 000	10^{3}	WAVES	10^{7}
100	10^{2}		10^{8}
10	10^{1}		10^{9}
1 CENTIMETER	10^{0}		10^{10}
0.1	10^{-1}		10^{11}
0.01	10^{-2}		10^{12}
0.001	10^{-3}	INFRA RED	10^{13}
0.0001	10^{-4}		10^{14}
0.00001	10^{-5}	visible	10^{15}
0.000001	10^{-6}	ULTRA VIOLET	10^{16}
0.0000001	10^{-7}	ROENTGEN RAYS	10^{17}
0.00000001	10^{-8}		10^{18}
0.000000001	10^{-9}		10^{19}
0.0000000001	10^{-10}	GAMMA RAYS	10^{20}
0.00000000001	10^{-11}		10^{21}

Figure 2.1. The electromagnetic spectrum, showing wavelength and frequency of the different bands. As the frequency increases (from top to bottom) so does the energy associated with the radiation. Non-ionizing radiations are associated with electrical waves down through the ultraviolet. The Roentgen rays (X-rays), gamma rays and cosmic rays are ionizing radiations. This figure was generated from an old wall chart displayed in the Electrical Engineering building at the University of Arizona, Tucson.

their orbits.) It is possible for an inner electron to be ejected. If this should happen then the electrons outside the orbit of the ejected electron will cascade inward and ultimately the outermost bonding electron will fall into the inner orbit resulting in a broken bond; again there is ionization and the breaking of bonds.

The present Chapter, parts of which are strongly influenced by the treatment presented by Elkind and Whitmore (1967), is devoted to some of the classical statistical approaches for deriving survival curves. Some other empirical derivations of survival expressions are also produced.

2.2 The Target Model

The study of direct actions of radiation is necessary when some property of the biological substance is under investigation. For our purposes it is assumed that only direct effects of radiation occur.

Throughout the subsequent discussion it will be assumed that a single ionization will produce the effect being measured. This assumption is not true in general, since there are parts of any organism (or biological material) which may be damaged without affecting some of the properties of the organism.

It is reasonable to expect that the bigger the organism the greater is the probability that the line of flight of the incident particle will pass through it. Also, this probability is proportional to the projected cross section of the organism. Even though the line of flight (or track) passes through the organism an effect is created only if an ionization is produced within it.

The rate of energy loss along a track is expressed in the units electron volts per micron (ev/μ) and this is referred to as the linear energy transfer (LET). X-rays, gamma rays and fast electrons produce tracks of low LET, whereas protons, neutrons and alpha-particles give rise to tracks of high LET. It appears that in condensed media such as solids or liquids, the deposition of energy occurs in discrete randomly spaced events along a track.

An α particle has a high LET. If a cell is traversed by such a particle then the cell has a high probability of being destroyed, whether only one hit or many hits is required. Only a small number of cells are affected, however, since the range of an α particle is limited. On the other hand a single γ ray has the ability to pass through many cells. It will destroy those cells in which only a single hit is required; other cells will sustain damage.

This leads naturally to the consideration of relative biological effectiveness or RBE. One can conceive of a cell having a number of critical targets. In that event many γ rays need to pass through the cell before consequential damage occurs. There are variations in the LET and the number of critical targets per cell. As a consequence one anticipates that there is the possibility of considerable variation in the RBE of differing radiations. For example, assume that a dose of 100 rads from β particles was adequate to destroy some biological entity and 200 rads of X-rays were necessary for the destruction of a similar biological entity, then the β particles have twice the RBE of the X-rays.

The target model is based on direct actions of radiations together with the discreteness and randomness of events. For a list of many of the early papers which first discussed the target "theory" see references 6 to 12 on pages 50, 51 of Elkind and Whitmore (1967).

Just prior to this book going to the publisher the author found out about the paper by Ahnström and Ehrenberg (1980). The title of their paper indicates that its content is of relevance to the material in the present section.

Sparsely ionizing radiations, such as very high energy charged particles, X-rays, and gamma-rays, have low LET. Also, for such radiations, the probability of an ionization occuring within the biological material is directly proportional to its thickness, since the thicker the biological material the more likely it is that an ionization will take place before the incident particle has passed entirely through. Consequently the probability of producing an effect by radiation can be written as

p = probability that the line of flight goes through the biological material (or organism) x the probability that an ionization occurs within the biological material (or organism).

The first probability, as noted earlier in the third paragraph of this section, is proportional to the cross-sectional area A of the organism (or biological material), and the probability is proportional to its thickness ℓ. Thus the total probability is proportional to the product $A\ell$, which is a measure of the average volume of the organism. Low linear energy transfer particles therefore produce an effect which is proportional to the volume of the organism or biological material.

2.3 Single-hit-to-Kill Model

Consider a homogeneous population of cells. Let V denote the total cell volume of the population being exposed and let D be the density of active events produced in the population by the incident radiation. Here, D is the total number of active events per unit volume of cells and is proportional to the absorbed dose. There does not appear to be a consensus of opinion on what is meant by "active event". Let $\mathcal{D}$ denote the number of active events scored in the total cell volume, then $\mathcal{D} = VD$. Define the hit probability

$$\rho = v/V,$$

where v denotes the sensitive volume (or target) within a cell. Note that, when v equals the volume of a cell, ρ takes on its maximum value equal to the number of cells in the population, providing that only hits within a cell are effective.

Define $P(\rho,h,\mathcal{D})$ to be the net survival probability that a single cell in a homogeneous population will receive h hits when $\mathcal{D}$ active events are registered in the population. Assume that the probability of scoring the hth hit is independent of the (h - 1) hits already scored (i.e. no conditional probabilities allowed). This assumption reflects the situation that the probability of a hit depends primarily on the composition of the target cell and therefore is essentially independent of the dose. The probability that a cell will be hit h times is given by the product

$$\rho^h(1 - \rho)^{\mathcal{D}-h}({}_{\mathcal{D}}C_h).$$

Here, the first term is the probability that a cell will be hit h times. The second term is the probability that the remaining $\mathcal{D}$ - h active events will not be hits. Also the binomial coefficient

$$_{\mathcal{D}}C_h = \mathcal{D}!/[h!(\mathcal{D} - h)!] \geq 1,$$

and accounts for all the different ways of scoring h hits and $\mathcal{D}$ - h misses when $\mathcal{D}$ events are registered in the population. The net survival probability $P(\rho,h,\mathcal{D})$ corresponding to h hits is now given by

$$P(\rho,h,\mathcal{D}) = \rho^h(1 - \rho)^{\mathcal{D}-h}({}_{\mathcal{D}}C_h)H(h),$$

where H(h) represents the <u>hit-survival function</u> and is the probability that a cell may be able to survive with h hits. (For a discussion of hit-survival functions see Elkind and Whitemore (1967), pp. 18-20). It follows that, if $S(\rho,\mathcal{D})$ represents the total survival probability per cell,

$$S(\rho,\mathcal{D}) = \sum_{h=0}^{\mathcal{D}} P(\rho,h,\mathcal{D})$$

and depends only on the hit probability and the dose.

A simple application of this result is as follows. Assume that a cell survives if it does not receive a hit and is always inactivated if it receives one or more hits. Accordingly, express the hit-survival function as

$$H(h) = \begin{cases} 1, & \text{for } h = 0, \\ 0, & \text{for } h > 1, \end{cases}$$

then

$$S(\rho,\mathcal{D}) = P(\rho,0,\mathcal{D}) = (1 - \rho)^{\mathcal{D}} = \exp[-k(\rho)\mathcal{D}],$$

where $k(\rho) = \ln(1 - \rho)$. The derived form for $S(\rho,\mathcal{D})$ is referred to as <u>exponential survival</u>.

An alternative, more direct, way to derive this result is now shown. Let N_o denote the number of organisms (cells, etc.) initially present and let N be the number surviving after a single dose D. Now assume that the rate of change of N with D is given by

$$dN/dD = -kN.$$

In logarithmic form

$$\ln S = -kD.$$

The graph of the natural logarithm of the surviving fractions versus dose gives a straight line with negative slope. Let D_o be the dose corresponding to a survival fraction of e^{-1} ($\sim$37% of the original number of cells) then $k = 1/D_o$.

The following assumptions also apply to the single-hit-to-kill model:

(i) the degree of effect is not influenced by the dose rate $\phi(\equiv D/t)$,

(ii) experimental conditions during irradiation or immediately after are not important.

Applications of the single-hit-to-kill model to the calculation of the target size of large viruses underestimates the target volumes. Furthermore, the survival curves obtained from radiation experiments on these larger organisms do not conform to the shape of simple exponential decay.

2.4 Multitarget, Single-hit Survival

Frequently a number of targets are involved, such as a cell containing n nucleii one or more of which must be hit at least once to kill a cell. The survival function for this situation is now derived.

Assume that (i) there are n targets in each cell; (ii) each target has the same probability of being hit, which is independent of the number of targets hit; and (iii) one hit is adequate to inactivate each target.

From the developments in the previous section it is apparent that the exponential survival function gives

$$e^{-kD} = \text{percentage of surviving organisms}$$

$$\equiv \text{the probability of a target not being hit.}$$

Now the total probability of a target being hit or not being hit is unity. Hence, the probability of a target being hit is $1 - \exp(-kD)$ and the probability of all the n targets being hit is

$$(1 - e^{-kD})^n,$$

since the probability for each is the same. The survival function $S(k,n,D)$ is the probability of the unit surviving, that is, the probability that not all of the targets will be hit or

$$S(k,n,D) = 1 - (1 - e^{-kD})^n. \tag{2.1}$$

(The survival expression (2.1) is in widespread usage as a result of its historical importance. But the effects of repeated small radiation fractions, or of continuous irradiation at low dose rates in mammals, or in clinical radiation therapy provide situations in which the formula is inadequate. More discussion is given in Section 2.7.)

However, the probability that a cell will survive with r targets hit, and thus inactivated, namely $P(k,r,n,D)$, is given by the binomial distribution term for r hits and $n - r$ misses multiplied by the probability $P(r)$ that a cell will survive with r targets inactivated. Therefore

$$P(k,r,n,D) = (1 - e^{-kD})^r (e^{-kD})^{n-r} ({}_nC_r)P(r),$$

with ${}_nC_R = n!/[r!(n - r)!]$ denoting the number of different combinations of targets hit r times and missed n - r times. Assume that a cell will be killed only when at least m targets have been hit, $1 \leq m \leq n$, i.e. specify that

$$P(r) = \begin{cases} 1, & 0 \leq r \leq m-1, \\ 0, & r \geq m. \end{cases}$$

The survival function is

$$S(k,m,n,D) = \sum_{r=0}^{m-1} P(k,r,n,D) \tag{2.2}$$

$$= \sum_{r=0}^{m-1} \frac{n!}{r!(n - r)!} (1 - e^{-kD})^r (e^{-kD})^{n-r}.$$

When m = n this last result becomes equivalent to (2.1), i.e. S(k,m,n,D) = S(k,n,D).

The term multitarget, single-hit is identified with (2.1) or the more general survival function ($m < n$) in (2.2).

Also, the expression (2.2) is derived on the basis that there are n or more hits in a single target of size v.

Consider (2.1): If kD is large enough so that the second and higher powers of exp(-kD) may be neglected then binomial expansion of the right-hand side produces

$$S \equiv S(k,n,D) = n\, e^{-kD},$$

or, in logarithmic form

$$\ln S = \ln n - kD, \tag{2.3}$$

the right-hand side being linear in D. Elkind and Whitmore (1967, p. 60) consider as a measure of the reciprocal of the slope of this straight line the dose required to reduce survival by 1/e ($\approx$ 0.37) and denote it by $\tilde{D}_o$. They do this in order to distinguish it from the mean lethal dose (i.e. the average dose absorbed by each cell before it is killed) in multitarget, single-hit inactivation.

Survival curves, in general, have a shoulder region whose width can be specified by the dose at which the back extrapolate intersects the abscissa. Alper et al. (1960) refer to this dose as the quasi-threshold dose and it is denoted by $\tilde{D}_q$. The extrapolation number, $\tilde{n}$, refers to the ordinate intersected by the back extrapolate, when the zero dose survival is normalized to unity. It is an observed quantity whereas n is a theoretical parameter. These remarks lead to

$$\tilde{D}_q = \tilde{D}_o \ln \tilde{n}.$$

Note that the exponential survival curve and the exponential quadratic survival expression do not have shoulders.

2.5 Multitarget, Multihit Survival

It is a natural consequence of the mathematical results of the previous section that the expression

$$S = \exp(-k_1D)[1 - \{1 - \exp(-k_2D)\}^n] \tag{2.4}$$

gives the survival probability if cell killing can be caused independently by a one hit and multihit process. Here n is the extrapolation or target number. Expression (2.4) is often referred to as a two-component model; see, for example, Wideröe (1966, 1971, 1978).

The quantity $\exp(-k_1D)$ in (2.4) represents the contribution from irreversible cumulative radiation injury, which is proportional to the dosage level, but independent of radiation fractionation or other time factors. The term in square brackets is seen to be the right-hand side of (2.1), and is the formula for cellular surviving functions that incorporate an extrapolation number $n(>1)$.

The result (2.4) is a special case of the more general survival function

$$S = e^{-kD}[1 - \{1 - e^{-k_2D}\}^{n_1}][1 - \{1 - e^{-k_3D}\}^{n_2}]\ldots,$$

which was given as equation (2) in the paper by Bender and Wolff (1961). They refer to each term as representing the chance of survival from 1-hit, n_1-hit,... events.

2.6 Single-target, Multihit Survival

In contrast to the previous models the single-target multiple hit survival model considers a target which is hit one or more times. Assume that the probability of scoring a hit is w. Then for a given $\mathcal{D}$ the average number of hits per cell λ is given by

$$\lambda = w\mathcal{D}.$$

Application of the Poisson distribution indicates that the probability of receiving hits is

$$(\lambda^h/h!)e^{-\lambda}$$

and the net survival probability corresponding to this is

$$P(w,h,\mathcal{D}) = (w\mathcal{D})^h \exp(-w\mathcal{D})\ H(h)/h!$$

If the hit-survival function

$$H(h) = \begin{cases} 1, & 0 \leq h < m, \\ 0, & h \geq m, \end{cases}$$

then the single-target, multihit survival function is

$$\sum_{h=0}^{m-1} P(w,h,\mathcal{D}) = e^{-w\mathcal{D}} \sum_{h=0}^{m-1} \frac{(w\mathcal{D})^h}{h!} ,$$

or, in terms of D,

$$\sigma(k,D) = e^{-kD} \sum_{h=0}^{m-1} \frac{(kD)^h}{h!} , \qquad (2.5)$$

where k = wV.

The expression (2.5) requires at least one hit in each of n targets with each target of size v.

2.7 Properties of In Vitro Survival Curves

The multitarget, single-hit survival function (2.1) has zero slope at zero dose. Also, it requires the determination of two parameters when fitting to data. Hall (1975), from data on the survival of cultured CHO and V79 Chinese hamster cells exposed to ^{60}Co gamma rays, indicates that the simple multitarget, single-hit expression (2.1) does not fit to the data. However, he showed that the two-component model (2.4), with its greater flexibility (it has three parameters) could be fitted to the data for synchronized CHO and V79 Chinese hamster cells exposed to ^{60}Co gamma rays.

Several investigators, e.g. Dutreix et al. (1973) and Wambersie et al. (1974), have measured the repair of sublethal damage, after smaller and smaller doses, in cells in a number of different tissues. They concluded that the expression (2.1) did not fit to the data, whereas the form (2.4) appeared to be appropriate.

It is noteworthy that the above conclusion by Hall, Dutreix and coworkers is in agreement with earlier findings by Bender and Gooch (1962). The latter noted the fitting of the two component model (2.4) to survival data from the GH7A6 cell line and the other with the S-3 sub-line of HeLa cells was better than the simple multitarget single-hit model (2.1).

More recently Hethcote et al. (1976) examine isoeffect data in four planes and conclude that the two-component model (2.4), with its greater flexibility, provides a better fit to the survival data of Dutreix et al. (1973), Fowler and Stern (1963), and Douglas and Fowler (1975). Other support, from a different point of view, comes from Wideröe (1977, 1978). Accordingly, then, use of the survival function given by (2.4) is gaining more support.

Studies in recent years have focussed attention on the importance of the initial slope of the survival expression being non-zero. This area was the focus of a conference; see Alper (1975). However one has to be careful in dealing with mathematical models and interpretations of experiments based on them, when looking at initial slopes. For example (2.1), which is a commonly used survival function, has zero slope (for $n \geq 2$) at zero dose and so does the expression (3.1). Yet (3.1) is in a more tolerable agreement with experimental observations on the effects of radiation given in fractions or at low dose rates than is (2.1). Just because a mathematical expression for the survival function has a zero slope for zero dose should not, of itself, suggest rejection of the expression.

More serious objections to the various hit and target "models" of this Chapter are that they are probabilistic approaches based on the notion that there is a small number of sensitive targets per cell which require to be inactivated for cell death. These targets cannot adequately represent the dynamic states of real intracellular structure. At the intermediate to high dose range a number of the experimental curves can be adequately fitted to the corresponding mathematical formula. Because of the form of the latter expressions it would have been a surprise if the fit was not reasonable.

An empirical argument of Ginsberg and Jagger (1965) is a follows: $e^{-\alpha D}$ is that fraction of the total population that has escaped initial lethal damage, and thus $e^{-\alpha D}/S$ is that fraction of the surviving population which has escaped initial damage. The quantity $1 - e^{-\alpha D}/S$ represents that fraction of the surviving population that has sustained initial damage and subsequently recovered. Their data gives this fraction and is plotted against dose to reveal a curve which rises exponentially from zero and approaches a plateau at high doses. One way to express this mathematically is to write

$$1 - e^{-\alpha D}/S = A(1 - e^{-rD}),$$

or, upon rearrangement and writing $A = \rho/(1 + \rho)$,

$$S = (\rho + 1)/[\rho e^{(\alpha - r)D} + e^{\alpha D}]. \tag{2.6}$$

The slope of this survival curve is given by

$$\frac{d\,\ell n\,S}{dD} = -\alpha + \frac{\rho r e^{-rD}}{1 + \rho e^{-rD}}.$$

It is noteworthy that Ginsberg and Jagger (1965) show that their survival function provides a satisfactory description of their data, both qualitatively and quantitatively, and also takes into account the radiation response of the population at both high and low doses without requiring assumptions of different kinds of initial damage.

Because of the presence of the two exponential functions in the denominator of the expression for S it is not possible to express dS/dD as some function of S, so long as $\alpha \neq r$. However, if $\alpha = r$ then (2.6) becomes

$$S = (\rho + 1)/(\rho + e^{\alpha D}),$$

which satisfies the differential equation

$$dS/dD = -\alpha[1 - S\rho/(\rho + 1)]S. \tag{2.7}$$

With no motivation, Green and Burki (1974) postulated that the differential equation (2.7) represents the simplest characterization of cell population survival, which incorporates repair or recovery, with ρ being identified as a recovery parameter. (The coincidence between the empirical survival functions of Green and Burki and Ginsberg and Jagger is rather striking.) There is a good fit of the survival function to experimental data from the inactivation of E. coli WP2 hcr^+ and the ultraviolet inactivation of a thymine-deficient mutant E. coli BT^-. They compare their survival function with three other formulae and indicate that it is chosen more times than the others as giving the best fit to data.

No theoretical explanation appears to be available to explain why these empirical survival functions should fit so well to data. However there are some similarities with the low LET and high LET kinetic model of Section 4.6, although the latter does not allow for recovery.

A recent extensive theoretical discussion of hit and target models, of the type considered in this Chapter, is presented by Turner (1975). He gives a catalog of thirty-nine mathematical models. This compendium may be of interest to a number of investigators interested in the probabilistic approach to generate survival expressions.

Recently DeMott et al. (1979) report on experiments involving the irradiation of thyroid cells. They fit their experimental data to the multitarget single-hit survival curve given by (2.1) and the "α,β" survival expression (3.1). Their results indicate that the latter curve deviated more than the multitarget single-hit curve at seven of the nine data points, falling below the observed points and the target model line at both high and low doses. Accordingly they decided to use (2.1).

Barendsen et al. (1966) provide a number of experimentally derived survival expressions for the situation of different linear energy transfer.

Chapter 3
A MOLECULAR MODEL OF CELL SURVIVAL

3.1 Introduction

The models in the previous Chapter are of a statistical nature and give expressions for the survival probability as a function of the dose. By dramatic contrast the developments in this Chapter proceed from a molecular framework concerned with the production of breaks in double strand DNA (deoxyribonucleic acid) and cell survival. One result is that the parameters in the model have specific biological significance.

This model, presented by Chadwick and Leenhouts (1973), was conceived for the purpose of trying to provide a rational and quantitative explanation to various radiobiological effects. The basic result is contained in (3.1), which can be used to analyze dose-effect curves for synchronized cell populations. The extension to asynchronous cell populations presents no difficulties.

Although the Chadwick-Leenhouts model currently appears to receive a lot of attention, it is worthwhile noting the earlier related work by Neary (1965), Sinclair (1966) and Kellerer and Rossi (1971).

More recently , Chadwick and Leenhouts (1975) propose that the induction of mutations arises from DNA double-strand breaks. Furthermore, they suggest that the initial slope of a mutation or cancer induction curve may be more relevant to the determination of the radiation sensitivity at low doses than the initial slope of a survival curve.

This chapter contains the elements of the discussion of the original 1973 work by Chadwick and Leenhouts. Recently they have revised their original derivation and, for completeness, these modifications are also incorporated here.

A graph of the general survival expression (3.1) is in Fig. 3.1.

3.2 The Molecular Model

Chadwick and Leenhouts (1973) consider that, within the cell, there are critical molecules whose integrity determines the ability of the cell to reproduce. For the present purposes these critical molecules are assumed to be in the DNA double helix. Critical damage is assumed to be a double strand break in the DNA helix.

When a cell is irradiated the main effect is assumed to be one or more breaks in the molecular bonds in the strands of DNA. It is further assumed that some form of cellular recovery is possible. The extent of recovery depends on the nature of the primary radiobiological damage. Also, the repair processes are, for example, combinations of biochemical enzymatic repair processes, and the physical recombination processes and energy transfer.

Define

$P(D) \equiv$ number of broken bonds per unit mass,

N_o ≡ number of critical bonds per unit mass which will lead to a single break if damaged.

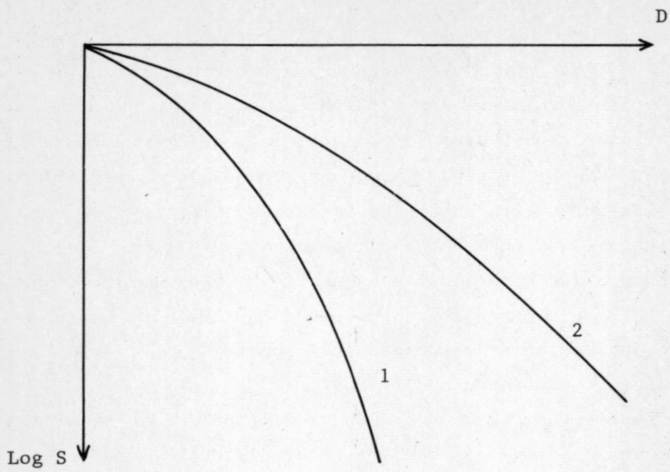

Fig. 3.1 Curve 1 is the general form of the survival curve given by (3.1). For comparison curve 2 is the general form of the survival curve for the multitarget single-hit relation (2.1). From Chadwick et al. (1976) representative values for Chinese hamster ovary cells give $\alpha = 2 \times 10^{-3}$ rad^{-1} and $\beta = 4 \times 10^{-6}$ rad^{-2}.

Assume that the rate of change of the number of broken bonds per unit mass is proportional to the difference between N_o and $P(D)$. It therefore follows that

$$dP(D)/dD = \rho[N_o - P(D)].$$

where ρ is the probability per bond per unit dose that the bond is broken. Note that this equation requires that the derivative $dP(D)/dD$ has meaning and exists. At zero dose it is assumed that there are no broken bonds per unit mass, i.e., $P(0) = 0$. Hence, for ρ constant ($\rho > 0$),

$$P(D) = N_o(1 - e^{-\rho D}).$$

Let r denote the proportion of broken bonds which are restituted or repaired, then $f = 1 - r$ represents that proportion of broken bonds which are not restituted or repaired. The average number of DNA single strand breaks is now given by

$$fN_o(1 - e^{-\rho D}),$$

where it is assumed that this expression is applicable to a set of irradiation conditions.

As a result of the action of radiation the DNA molecule may be broken in the manner following -

(i) both strands are broken as the result of one radiation event,

(ii) each strand is broken independently in different radiation events.

Consider the latter situation. For convenience let the DNA molecule consist of strands 1 and 2 with

n_1 ≡ number of critical bonds on strand 1 per cell,

n_2 ≡ number of critical bonds on strand 2 per cell, $n_1 \neq n_2$,

k ≡ probability per bond per unit dose that the bond is broken,

f_i ≡ proportion of broken bonds on strand i not restituted or repaired. Since there are two strands, $i = 1,2$.

If a proportion Δ of the dose D results in the mode of action (i) and $1-\Delta$ is the proportion giving rise to (ii), with Δ dependent on the linear energy transfer of the radiation, then the number of bonds broken and unrepaired is

$$f_1 n_1\{1 - \exp[-k(1 - \Delta)D]\},$$

for strand 1, and is

$$f_2 n_2\{1 - \exp[-k(1 - \Delta)D]\},$$

for strand 2. Consequently, if ε is the proportion of these broken bonds which combine to produce a double strand break (and so cause cell death), the average number of <u>double strand breaks</u> per cell is

$$\varepsilon n_1 n_2 f_1 f_2\{1 - \exp[-k(1 - \Delta)D]\}^2.$$

Chadwick and Leenhouts suggest that for two broken bonds to combine and cause a double strand break they need to be associated in time and space and ε is a measure of this association. They regard ε as being an average value for the single strand breaks and consider its value to be 1 for two-strand breaks which are opposite or near to each other, and $\varepsilon = 0$ for strand breaks which are widely separated.

For the first mode of action (i) let

n_o ≡ the number of "sites", where $n_o \leq n_1, n_2$,

k_o ≡ the probability per "site" per unit dose that the double strand is broken.

The average number of DNA double strand breaks formed by this mode of action is

$$n_o[1 - \exp(-k_o \Delta D)].$$

On combining the results for both modes of action, the average number of DNA double strand breaks per cell after a dose D is given by

$$a(D) \equiv n_o[1 - \exp(-k_o\Delta D)] + \varepsilon n_1 n_2 f_1 f_2\{1 - \exp[-k(1 - \Delta)D]\}^2.$$

To account for repair of DNA double strand breaks each expression in this last display is multiplied by the quantity f_o, which denotes the proportion of DNA double strand breaks not restituted or repaired. The probability for cell death per dose D, by Poisson theory, is now given by $E(D) = 1 - \exp[-pf_o a(D)]$, where p represents a proportionality factor connecting DNA double strand breaks with cell death. Now

$$pf_o a(D) = pf_o n_o \Delta D + pf_o \varepsilon n_1 n_2 f_1 f_2 k^2(1 - \Delta)^2 D^2 + O(k_o{}^2) + O(k^3).$$

That is, $pf_o a(D) = \alpha^* D + \beta^* D^2$, on neglect of the higher order terms, since k_o and k are small in comparison with unity. Here

$$\alpha^* = pf_o n_o k_o \Delta, \quad \beta^* = pf_o \varepsilon n_1 n_2 f_1 f_2 k^2(1 - \Delta)^2.$$

If it is now assumed that one of these DNA double strand breaks causes a loss of the reproductive ability of the cell then the probability that it survives is given by the quantity $1 - E(D)$. This leads to the survival function

$$S(D) = \exp(-\alpha^* D - \beta^* D^2), \tag{3.1}$$

which is an approximation to the more general expression

$$\exp(-\alpha^* D - \beta^* D^2 - \gamma^* D^3 - \dots). \tag{3.2}$$

One noteworthy feature of the graph of (3.1), see Fig 3.1, is that it has a nonzero slope at zero dose. The derivation of this form of the survival function applies to a synchronized cell population. During the cell cycle the coefficients α^* and β^* can be expected to vary. However, (3.1) can be used to fit the survival data of an asynchronous population of cells.

It is tempting to compare the part of (3.1), which just involves α^*, with the exponential survival function of Chapter 2. But this is not a valid comparison, since (3.1) accounts not only for the physico-chemical induction of breaks but also incorporates repair and restitution.

The mathematical form of (3.1) was given earlier by Kellerer and Rossi (1971) who presented the following derivation. Since the end effect of the radiation produces a lethal species within a cell (see Section 4.2) its concentration can be represented as a power series in terms of the dose D. In the Kellerer and Rossi notation this series is written in the form

$$E(D) = k_1 D + k_2 D^2 + \dots,$$

and in their description, E(D) represents the frequency of primary lesions. For a two-step inactivation process they deduce that

$$E(D) = g\psi D + \psi^2 D^2/2, \quad g << 1,$$

where g is the fraction of events which induces a double lesion at once, and ψ (they use the symbol ϕ) is the total frequency per unit dose of events affecting the undamaged site. They consider that a primary lesion requires a certain threshold of energy deposition in a single region, or site, within the cell. When the number of sites, N, is large then the probability of survival is

$$S(D) = [1 - E(D)]^N = 1 - NE(D) + \frac{N(N-1)}{2!}[E(D)]^2 - \ldots$$

$$\approx 1 - NE(D) + [NE(D)]^2/2! - \ldots$$

i.e. $$S(D) \approx \exp[-NE(D)],$$

which is of the form (3.1).

The expression (3.2) can be obtained purely on mathematical grounds as follows. From (A.3) the concentration of lethal species can be written as

$$x_n(D) = a_{n1}\, D + \sum_{j=1}^{n} a_{nj}\, a_{j1} \frac{D^2}{2!} + \ldots$$

Now assume that

$$a_{n1} = \alpha^*,$$

$$\sum_{j=1}^{n} a_{nj}\, a_{j1} = 2\beta^* - (\alpha^*)^2,$$

$$\sum_{j=1}^{n} \sum_{h=1}^{n} a_{nj}\, a_{jh}\, a_{h1} = 6\gamma^* - 6\alpha^*\beta^* + (\alpha^*)^3,$$

etc., then

$$x_n(D) = \alpha^* D + (\beta^* - \frac{\alpha^{*2}}{2!})\, D^2 + (\gamma^* - \alpha^*\beta^* + \frac{\alpha^{*3}}{3!})\, D^3 + \ldots$$

and the survival function

$$S(D) = 1 - x_n(D)$$

$$= \exp(-\alpha^* D - \beta^* D^2 - \gamma^* D^3 - \ldots).$$

This last result includes (3.1) and is a mathematical generalization of it.

3.3 Interpretations of the Molecular Model

The result (3.1) was derived by Chadwick and Leenhouts (1973) with the consideration that the two single strand breaks are to be regarded as separate entities, which, under certain conditions, would combine to produce a double strand break in the DNA molecule.

A revision of this interpretation of the process is presented by Leenhouts and Chadwick (1975). In this latter paper they consider the process to be in two separate steps to allow for the possibility that two different processes are involved in the induction of the two single strand breaks. They suggest that the first single strand break on an intact DNA molecule is the result of damage due to an OH radical formed about 8 Angströms from the DNA. Also, this first single strand break results from a similar process as that which causes the double strand break in one radiation event. As a consequence of this first single strand break the unbroken strand opposite to it appears to become more sensitive to breakage by a radical.

On setting $\alpha^* = p\alpha$ and $\beta^* = p\beta$ the result (3.1) can be expressed in the alternative form

$$S(D) = \exp[-p(\alpha D + \beta D^2)]. \qquad (3.3)$$

The quantity $\alpha D + \beta D^2$ is the mean number of DNA double strand breaks in a cell after it receives a dose D of irradiation. With the assumption that a DNA double strand break can lead to cell reproductive death with a probability p then (3.3) gives the probability that a cell survives the dosage D. Also, α denotes the probability that both strands are broken in the passage of one ionizing particle; β denotes the probability that two independently induced single strand breaks in opposite strands of the DNA occur close enough in time and space that a double strand break is created.

Leenhouts and Chadwick (1975) indicate that the works of Barendsen et al. (1965), Todd (1967) on T 1 cells, of Madhvanath (1971) on lymphocytes, and of Roux (1974), are in agreement with the molecular model--that the product $p\alpha$ in (3.3) should reflect the induction of DNA double strand breaks in one radiation event. Experiments in support of the interpretation of the product $p\beta$ are in progress.

Independent support for the Chadwick-Leenhouts molecular model has come from the work of Neufeld et al. (1974), Gillespie et al. (1975a, b) and Douglas and Fowler (1976). However, more recently, Wideröe (1977, 1978) presents experimental evidence that does not conform with the Chadwick-Leenhouts model.

The subject of DNA strand breaks and its relevancy to the lethality resulting from the exposure of mammaliam cells to ionizing radiations is controversial. A detailed synopsis of the principle findings is presented by Bronk (1976, pp. 298-306).

There are technical difficulties in measurements of single strand breaks and certainly of double strand breaks in mammalian DNA. Measurements, of improved precision, are reported by Dugle et al. (1976). Their principle finding is that double strand breaks are induced in proportion to the square of the absorbed dose in the range 10-50 krad. They did not observe any rejoining of double-strand breaks and suggest that, in mammalian cells, most double-strand breaks are not repairable, while all single-strand breaks are repaired, save those that are sufficiently close on complementary strands to constitute double-strand breaks. This experimental work lends support to the Chadwick-Leenhouts molecular model.

Recently Leenhouts and Chadwick (1978a) present an extensive review of their work in the area of analysis of DNA strand breaks. A novel feature is the presentation of their suggestions for the implications of their theory to such areas as radiological protection, chromosomal aberrations, somatic mutations, radiation-induced malignancy and hereditary effects.

The underlying basic assumption of the molecular theory of cell survival is that the DNA double strand break is the most critical radiation-induced molecular lesion. However the direct relation between DNA double-strand breaks and cell survival has not yet been established experimentally in eukaryotic cells.

The Chadwick-Leenhouts model, which led to (3.1), is used by Todd et al. (1978) to describe the survival of acutely radiated single cells. Also Fertil et al. (1978) indicate that a quadratic survival expression of the form (3.1) provides the best fit to their data.

It is evident that the whole matter of breaks in DNA and repair mechanisms will continue to develop. For recent representative work see Hanawalt et al. (1978) and Elkind (1979). See, also, Barendsen (1979) and Hagen et al. (1980).

The mathematical analysis in Section 3.2 implies that one should be able to take expressions from the hit and target "theories" of Chapter 2 and put them in the form of (3.1). Exercises of this sort do not of course make the "theories" any more correct than they were before but may be useful to those who prefer the probabilistic approach. For purposes of exposition one such exercise is now presented.

Assume that a break in the primary lesion can be produced at a finite number m of site-pairs, either by a single ionization track, or by the interaction of two independent ionization tracks, which each break one strand of the pair. Consider some typical site at which damage occurs. The quantity D/D_1 is the average expected number of events (each of which is capable of inactivating the site) produced by a single track and D/D_2 is the number of interacting events (each capable of breaking one strand of the pair). Define

$$p_1 = \text{probability of survival of a site due to the first mechanism}$$
$$= \exp(-D/D_1)$$
$$p_2 = \text{probability of survival of a site due to the second mechanism}$$
$$= 1 - [1 - \exp(-D/D_2)]^2.$$

If S denotes the overall survival then, with m denoting a fixed number of sites per cell,

$$S = p_1^m \, p_2^m .$$

Now a direct Taylor series expansion of $\exp(-D/D_2)$ gives

$$p_2 = 1 - x^2 + x^3 - 7x^4/12 + \ldots, \quad x = D/D_2,$$

$$\approx 1 - x^2,$$

on neglect of terms involving cubic and higher powers of D/D_2. Hence $p_2 \approx \exp(-x^2)$ and now

$$S \approx [\exp(-D/D_1)\,\exp(-D^2/D_2^{\,2})]^m$$

$$= \exp(-mD/D_1 - mD^2/D_2^{\,2}),$$

which is in the form of (3.1). This approach is based on Gilbert (1975) and Gilbert et al. (1980). The survival expression

$$S(D) = \exp(-mD/D_1)\,\{1 - [1 - \exp(-D/D_2)]^2\}^m$$

apparently gives as good a fit to survival data as does (2.4); see Hendley (1979).

Chapter 4
KINETIC MODELS OF BIOLOGICAL RADIATION RESPONSE

4.1 Introduction

The material presented in Chapter 2 consisted of statistical-type models. They are straightforward to construct, provide intuitive insights and are popular. However it was also pointed out that they are deficient in a number of ways. For example, no account is taken of the intermediate steps in the damaging process, there is no allowance for the recovery of the biological material during or after irradiation; dose-rate effects are ignored. A kinetic model was developed by Dienes (1966) which is a generalization of the previous models of Chapter 2 and does take into consideration intermediate steps, dose-rate and recovery effects. Some of his ideas are discussed in the present Chapter and it is shown how some of them reduce to the results of the "hit" and "target" models.

The kinetic model leads to a system of coupled ordinary differential equations from which the solutions are readily obtained.

One of the earliest papers which has some of the rudiments of the kinetic approach is by Swann and del Rosario (1931). They considered the situation when two impacts of an alpha particle with the sensitive element of the cell are necessary to cause death. The possibility of cell recovery after the first impact is allowed before the second impact takes place, so that there is no contributory effect from the first impact. Their kinetic equations (with a change in notation) are discussed in Section 4.5.

The paper by Swann and del Rosario (1931) is referred to by Kellerer and Hug (1963). In turn, Dienes (1966) refers to the Kellerer and Hug paper, and on pp. 179-181, he formulates and gives the mathematical solution to a slightly more general problem of dose-rate dependence with recovery.

The equation

$$dx(t)/dt = -I\alpha_t x(t) + R\beta_t[x_o - x(t - \tau)]$$

was derived by Sievert (1941). Here x denotes the concentration of some substance within a cell, I is an irradiation constant, x_o is an equilibrium value for x and R is a constant which measures the reaction of the cell to a departure from equilibrium. He introduced the concept of a "latent period" depending on radiosensitivity and the presence and speed of reconstitution of important reserves in the cell. Sievert thus wished to include the effects of cell recovery into his model. A noteworthy feature of his paper is that for certain parameter ranges he was able to give graphical representations of the solutions. Detailed mathematical properties of this time-lag equation are presented by Pinney (1950).

It appears that the first major contribution to the kinetic approach in biological radiation response occurs in the work of Kellerer and Hug (1963). Their work is very similar to that of Dienes (1966). Because of the breadth of topics covered and the somewhat more general nature of this latter paper it becomes the focal point of the present Chapter.

Before considering procedures which will aid in optimizing tumor radiation therapy it is essential to have tolerably good models of the biological response to irradiation. The Dienes approach is of considerable help in developing such models.

Applications of the Dienes kinetic approach is in Dienes (1971) which deals with general features of dose fractionation.

Recent years have been witness to the fascinating area of hyperthermia as a treatment for many types of tumors. There is also a symbiotic relationship between hyperthermia and irradiation in regard to cell kill. Recently Bronk (1976) has made good use of the kinetic approach in an attempt to understand various experimental results; see Section 4.9.

It is noteworthy that the kinetic approach has been of utility in some demographic investigations and provided insight into the interactions between basic population variables; Schweitzer and Dienes (1971).

4.2 Basic Postulates in the Dienes Model

Dienes (1966) postulates that on irradiation of the biological material a series of reactions takes place, these reactions remaining unspecified in the model, which leads to a final product that is lethal. For simplicity all the reactions are assumed to be first order. Mathematically, this means that the differential equations are all linear. Define x_i to be a species concentration then, symbolically, the kinetic process is described by

$$x_1 \underset{\alpha_{-1}}{\overset{\alpha_1}{\rightleftarrows}} x_2 \underset{\alpha_{-2}}{\overset{\alpha_2}{\rightleftarrows}} x_3 \cdots x_{n-1} \xrightarrow{\alpha_{n-1}} x_n. \tag{4.1}$$

The last species x_n is considered to be lethal to the organism. Define the radiation dose rate

$$\phi = D/t, \tag{4.2}$$

when D is the dose and t the time. One of the simplest assumptions is that the forward rate constants α_i, $i = 1,\ldots,n-1$, are each proportional to the dose rate with

$$\alpha_i = k_i\phi, \tag{4.3}$$

and

$$\alpha_i t = k_i\phi t = k_i D. \tag{4.4}$$

The backward rate constants α_{-i}, $i = 1,\dots,n-2$, are not considered to be influenced by radiations. It is also assumed that the species concentrations x_i are without dimension and are fractions (less than unity); each α_i has dimension $(\text{time})^{-1}$.

Instead of referring to x_i as a species one can think of it as a state with x_i being equivalent to the fraction of (biological) material present in state i. Also α_i can be thought of as a transition probability from state i to state i + 1.

A particular feature of the kinetic approach is that x_n is not given a precise definition. The main reason for this is that a specific experimental criterion for survival leads to a specific meaning for x_n. For example, x_n could be the state where a test for lethality occurs. If growth or proliferation is the experimental criterion for survival, then x_n is the fraction of nonviable cells.

Mathematically, it is convenient to write $x_i \equiv x_i(t)$, $x_{io} \equiv x_i(0)$ and $\dot{x}_i \equiv dx_i(t)/dt \equiv \dot{x}_i(t)$.

It is useful to bear in mind that the states are subdivisions of the whole population and are kept small in number in order to facilitate calculation and correspond with the very real limitations of experiment. Since the cell population can be divided into a very large number of experimentally distinguishable states it is desirable to minimize the number of states followed. This means that n is chosen to be as small as seems "reasonable". Each state may include a large variety of chemical states.

4.3 Low LET Kinetic Models with No Recovery

The first kinetic models that are now considered have the forward rate constants only and so are without recovery. Furthermore each model is assumed to be associated with low linear energy transfer (LET).

Model 1. Consider the scheme

$$x_1 \xrightarrow{\alpha_1} x_2 \xrightarrow{\alpha_2} x_3, \tag{4.5}$$

where x_3 corresponds to a lethal species and $\alpha_1 \neq \alpha_2$. The kinetic differential equations for this scheme are

$$\dot{x}_1 = -\alpha_1 x_1,\ x_1(0) = x_{10},$$

$$\dot{x}_2 = \alpha_1 x_1 - \alpha_2 x_2,\ x_2(0) = x_{20},$$

$$\dot{x}_3 = \alpha_2 x_2,\ x_3(0) = x_{30},$$

which are readily integrated to give

$$x_1(t) = x_{10} e^{-\alpha_1 t},$$

$$x_2(t) = [\alpha_1 x_{10}/(\alpha_2 - \alpha_1)](e^{-\alpha_1 t} - e^{-\alpha_2 t}) + x_{20}e^{-\alpha_2 t},$$

$$x_3(t) = x_{10} + x_{20} + x_{30} - x_{20}\, e^{-\alpha_2 t}$$

$$+ [x_{10}/(\alpha_2 - \alpha_1)](\alpha_1 e^{-\alpha_2 t} - \alpha_2 e^{-\alpha_1 t}).$$

Here, the initial concentrations of the various species at time, $t = 0$, are denoted by x_{i0}, $i = 1,2,3$. On writing the concentration of lethal species as a fraction of the total initial concentration of species present

$$x_3/(x_{10} + x_{20} + x_{30}),$$

then the surviving fraction S is given by

$$S = \frac{x_{10} + x_{20} + x_{30} - x_3}{x_{10} + x_{20} + x_{30}} = 1 - \frac{x_3}{x_{10} + x_{20} + x_{30}}.$$

At the initial time $t = 0$, there are no species concentrations x_2 and x_3; hence select $x_2(0) = x_3(0) = 0$. However, species 1 is present and it is reasonable to consider that it is of unit size initially; $x_1(0) = 1$. Hence

$$x_1(t) = e^{-\alpha_1 t},$$

$$x_2(t) = [\alpha_1/(\alpha_2 - \alpha_1)](e^{-\alpha_1 t} - e^{-\alpha_2 t}), \qquad (4.6)$$

$$x_3(t) = 1 + [1/(\alpha_2 - \alpha_1)](\alpha_1 e^{-\alpha_2 t} - \alpha_2 e^{-\alpha_1 t}),$$

with $x_1(t) + x_2(t) + x_3(t) = 1$. The surviving fraction

$$S = 1 - x_3(t) = (\alpha_2 e^{-\alpha_1 t} - \alpha_1 e^{-\alpha_2 t})/(\alpha_2 - \alpha_1),\ \alpha_2 \neq \alpha_1.$$

The definition (4.2) together with the assumptions (4.3), (4.4) indicate that the expressions for x_i, $i = 1,2,3$ can be written entirely in terms of the dose D and are independent of the dose rate.

For those readers who prefer to work with vector differential equation systems the mathematical descriptions appropriate to this situation are presented in Appendix 1.

It is straightforward to extend the discussion to include the scheme

$$x_1 \xrightarrow{\alpha_1} x_2 \xrightarrow{\alpha_2} x_3 \longrightarrow \dots\ x_{n-1} \xrightarrow{\alpha_{n-1}} x_n,$$

where x_n is a lethal concentration and $\alpha_1 \neq \alpha_2 \neq \ldots \alpha_{n-1}$. The solutions are given by the expressions

$$x_1(t) = e^{-\alpha_1 t},$$

$$x_m(t) = (\alpha_1\alpha_2 \ldots \alpha_{m-1})(-1)^{m+1} \left[\frac{\exp(-\alpha_1 t)}{(\alpha_1-\alpha_2)(\alpha_1-\alpha_3)\ldots(\alpha_1-\alpha_m)} + \frac{\exp(-\alpha_2 t)}{(\alpha_2-\alpha_1)(\alpha_2-\alpha_3)\ldots(\alpha_2-\alpha_m)} + \right.$$

$$\left. \ldots + \frac{\exp(-\alpha_m t)}{(\alpha_m-\alpha_1)(\alpha_m-\alpha_2)\ldots(\alpha_m-\alpha_{m-1})}\right], \quad m = 2,3,\ldots,n-1,$$

$$x_n(t) = \frac{\alpha_2\alpha_3\ldots\alpha_{n-1}(-1)^n}{(\alpha_1-\alpha_2)(\alpha_1-\alpha_3)\ldots(\alpha_1-\alpha_{n-1})}(1 - e^{-\alpha_1 t})$$

$$+ \frac{\alpha_1\alpha_3\ldots\alpha_{n-1}(-1)^n}{(\alpha_2-\alpha_1)(\alpha_2-\alpha_3)\ldots(\alpha_2-\alpha_{n-1})}(1 - e^{-\alpha_2 t}) + \ldots$$

$$+ \frac{\alpha_1\alpha_2\ldots\alpha_{n-2}(-1)^n}{(\alpha_{n-1}-\alpha_1)(\alpha_{n-1}-\alpha_2)\ldots(\alpha_{n-1}-\alpha_{n-2})}(1 - e^{-\alpha_{n-1} t}),$$

with $x_1(0) = 1$, $x_i(0) = 0$, $i = 2,\ldots,n$. The meaning of the notation involving the product of factors in the denominators of these results is that when one of these factors turns out to be zero then it is neglected and the product starts with the nonzero factor immediately to its left.

If assumption (4.3) is utilized, then, in terms of the radiation dose rate ϕ,

$$x_1 \xrightarrow{k_1\phi} x_2 \xrightarrow{k_2\phi} x_3 \longrightarrow \ldots \; x_{n-1} \xrightarrow{k_{n-1}\phi} x_n$$

with

$$\dot{x}_1 = -k_1\phi x_1,$$

$$\dot{x}_2 = k_1\phi x_1 - k_2\phi x_2,$$

$$\vdots$$

$$\dot{x}_{n-1} = k_{n-2}\phi x_{n-2} - k_{n-1}\phi x_{n-1},$$

$$\dot{x}_n = k_{n-1}\phi x_{n-1},$$

and $x_1(0) = 1$, $x_i(0) = 0$, $i = 2,3,\ldots,n$. The transition numbers k_i, $i = 1,\ldots,n-1$, represent an incremental fraction of the quantity x_i transferred from the state i to i + 1 by radiation damage per unit dose.

Also, it is interesting to show how the equations of this model correspond to the single-target multihit survival model of Chapter 2. This latter model requires that each probability of an effective hit be a constant and independent of previous hits. For the present kinetic model this is equivalent to the requirement that

$$\alpha_1 = \alpha_2 = \dots = \alpha_n = \alpha.$$

The basic equations for the case n = 2 are

$$\dot{x}_1 = -\alpha x_1,\ \dot{x}_2 = \alpha x_1 - \alpha x_2,\ \dot{x}_3 = \alpha x_2,$$

$$x_{10} = 1,\ x_{20} = x_{30} = 0,$$

with solution

$$x_1(t) = e^{-\alpha t},\ x_2(t) = \alpha t e^{-\alpha t},\ x_3(t) = 1 - (1 + \alpha t)e^{-\alpha t}.$$

For n hits,

$$1 - x_n = e^{-\alpha t}[1 + \alpha t + \frac{(\alpha t)^2}{2!} + \dots + \frac{(\alpha t)^{n-1}}{(n-1)!}], \qquad (4.7)$$

which is the expression (2.5) with $\alpha t = kD$.

The single-target multihit survival model therefore is a special case of the more general kinetic approach of Model 1.

Kellerer and Hug (1963) describe the kinetic scheme for n hits and from their vector differential equation system produce the survival function $S = 1 - x_n$. See Appendix 1.

<u>Model 2</u>. Consider the kinetic scheme

$$x_1 \xrightarrow{2\alpha} x_2 \xrightarrow{\alpha} x_3, \qquad (4.8)$$

where x_3 is a lethal concentration. Here there are two "targets". If the rate of hitting one target is α then the rate of hitting either target is 2α. The interpretation of x_2 is that it is a species containing a single target, since one target has already been destroyed, and the rate of hitting x_2 is α.

The differential equations corresponding to the scheme (4.8) are

$$\dot{x}_1 = -2\alpha x_1,\ \dot{x}_2 = 2\alpha x_1 - \alpha x_2,\ \dot{x}_3 = \alpha x_2,$$

$$x_{10} = 1,\ x_{20} = x_{30} = 0,$$

which have the solutions

$$x_1(t) = e^{-2\alpha t},\ x_2(t) = 2(e^{-\alpha t} - e^{-2\alpha t}),$$

$$x_3(t) = (1 - e^{-\alpha t})^2.$$

This leads to the survival function

$$S = 1 - (1 - e^{-\alpha t})^2,$$

For the more general kinetic scheme

$$x_1 \xrightarrow{m\alpha} x_2 \xrightarrow{(m-1)\alpha} x_3 \cdots x_n \xrightarrow{\alpha} x_{n+1} \qquad (4.9)$$

the differential equations are

$$\dot{x}_1 = -m\alpha x_1,$$

$$\dot{x}_2 = m\alpha x_1 - (m - 1)\alpha x_2,$$

$$\vdots$$

$$\dot{x}_n = 2\alpha x_{n-1} - \alpha x_n,$$

$$\dot{x}_{n+1} = \alpha x_n,$$

with the initial conditions $x_1(0) = 1$, $x_j(0) = 0$, $j = 2,\ldots,n + 1$. The solutions are

$$x_1(t) = e^{-m\alpha t},$$

$$x_j(t) = \frac{m(m - 1) \ldots (m - j + 2)}{(j - 1)!} e^{-(m - j + 1)\alpha t}(1 - e^{-\alpha t})^{j-1},$$

$$j = 2,\ldots,n + 1.$$

For the case when $m = n$ the survival function

$$S = 1 - x_{n+1} = 1 - (1 - e^{-\alpha t})^n,$$

which, for $\alpha t = kD$, is the same as the multitarget single hit survival function (2.1).

With the assumption that $\alpha t = kD$ then the survival function depends on the dose and dose-rate-dependent effects do not appear in S.

Before going on to an enlarged discussion of this second model there is one interesting point that should be noted.

Consider the schemes

$$x_1 \xrightarrow{3\alpha} x_2 \xrightarrow{2\alpha} x_3 \xrightarrow{\alpha} x_4,$$

and

$$x_1 \xrightarrow{\alpha} x_2 \xrightarrow{2\alpha} x_3 \xrightarrow{3\alpha} x_4.$$

The first of these is just (4.9) with m = n = 3 and the solutions for the concentrations are

$$x_1(t) = e^{-3\alpha t}, \; x_2(t) = 3(e^{-2\alpha t} - e^{-3\alpha t}),$$

$$x_3(t) = 3(e^{-\alpha t} - 2e^{-2\alpha t} + e^{-3\alpha t}), \; x_4(t) = (1 - e^{-\alpha t})^3.$$

However, the solutions for the second scheme are

$$x_1(t) = e^{-\alpha t}, \; x_2(t) = e^{-\alpha t} - e^{-2\alpha t},$$

$$x_3(t) = e^{-\alpha t} - 2e^{-2\alpha t} + e^{-3\alpha t}, \; x_4(t) = (1 - e^{-\alpha t})^3.$$

Although the intermediate concentrations x_1, x_2 and x_3 are distinct between the two schemes the final concentration x_4 is precisely the same for both of them. Therefore, each scheme has the same survival function. Accordingly, then, S versus t data is insufficient by itself to distinguish between the two schemes. Some additional piece of information, such as the concentration of one of the intermediates, is required in order to fix attention to one scheme.

The discussion of the previous paragraph carries over for the general schemes (4.9) and

$$x_1 \xrightarrow{\alpha} x_2 \xrightarrow{2\alpha} x_3 \ldots x_n \xrightarrow{m\alpha} x_{n+1}.$$

The final (lethal) concentration x_{n+1} is identical for each scheme but the intermediates are different.

4.4 Further Discussion of the Models.

It is worthwhile providing more insight into the kinetic schemes and the multi-target models. Introduce the following notation:

Let $x(n_1,n_2,\ldots,n_m)$ represent the species that has accumulated n_1 hits on target 1, n_2 on target 2, ... etc. For example, the following scheme represents a two-target one-hit process

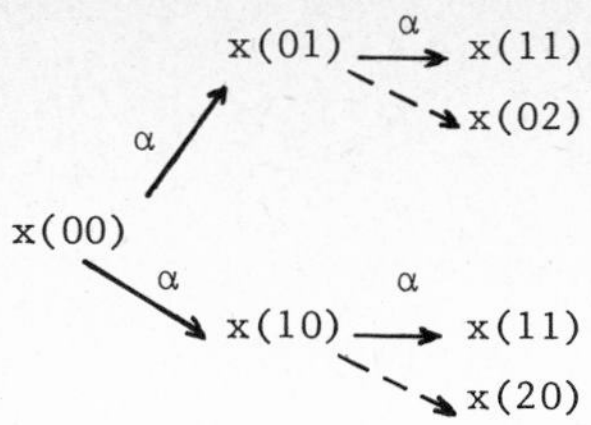
x(01)
α
x(11)
x(02)
α
x(00)
α
α
x(10)
x(11)
x(20)

(4.10)

Zirkle (1952) considers mechanisms of radiobiological action and, p. 338, presents a model of cellular biological action resulting in the inhibition of cell division in a yeast. He, p. 399, also presents a general model of the mechanism of cellular biological action. Each model commences with the normal state of the cell. As a result of radiation there is an energy transfer to relevant molecules and to irrelevant ones. This situation proceeds through each state until on the one hand the end effect is produced as the result of the activation of relevant molecules present whereas on the other the energy transfer is to irrelevant molecules. In the present case, the irrelevant portions are indicated by the presence of the dashed lines leading from x(01) and x(10). For this two-target one-hit process

$$dx(00)/dt = -2\alpha x(00), \quad x(00) = e^{-2\alpha t},$$

$$dx(01)/dt = \alpha x(00) - \alpha x(01), \quad x(01) = e^{-\alpha t} - e^{-2\alpha t},$$

$$dx(10)/dt = \alpha x(00) - \alpha x(10), \quad x(10) = e^{-\alpha t} - e^{-2\alpha t},$$

indicating that there is no distinction between x(01) and x(10). Also,

$$\frac{dx(11)}{dt} = \alpha x(01) + \alpha x(10), \quad x(11) = (1 - e^{-\alpha t})^2.$$

It therefore follows that the kinetic scheme (4.10) is equivalent to (4.8) with

$$x(00) \xrightarrow{2\alpha} x(01) \xrightarrow{\alpha} x(11),$$

and x(00) = 1, x(01) = x(11) = 0 at t = 0.

The kinetic sequence for the two target two-hit process is given by (4.11):

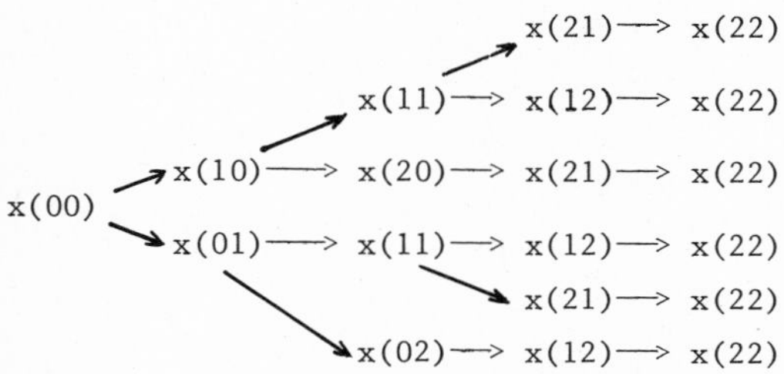
x(21) → x(22)
x(11) → x(12) → x(22)
x(10) → x(20) → x(21) → x(22)
x(00)
x(01) → x(11) → x(12) → x(22)
x(21) → x(22)
x(02) → x(12) → x(22)

(4.11)

Irrelevant reactions of the type $x(02) \dashrightarrow x(03)$ are omitted. Also, the forward rate constants for each step are assumed to be the same; each one being equal to α. For this scheme it is possible to deduce that

$$x(22) = [1 - (1 + \alpha t)e^{-\alpha t}]^2.$$

Simplification of the scheme (4.11) results in

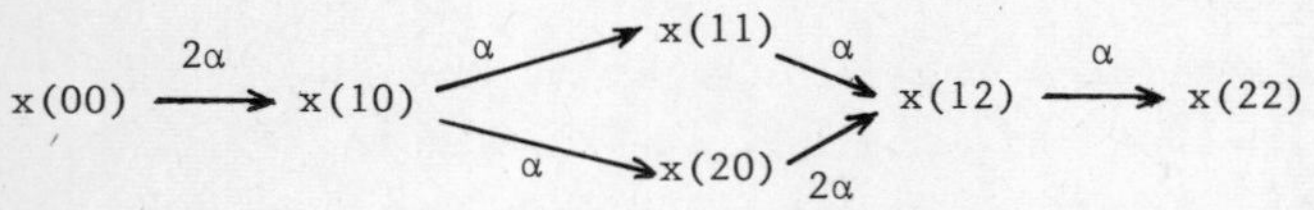

$$x(00) \xrightarrow{2\alpha} x(10) \begin{array}{c} \xrightarrow{\alpha} x(11) \xrightarrow{\alpha} \\ \xrightarrow{\alpha} x(20) \xrightarrow{2\alpha} \end{array} x(12) \xrightarrow{\alpha} x(22) \qquad (4.12)$$

whose validity can be directly verified by integration of the differential equations arising from (4.12)

Of course it is important to realize that (4.12) is not unique, and, for example, in its place the following scheme could be used

$$x(00) \xrightarrow{2\alpha} x(10) \begin{array}{c} \xrightarrow{\alpha} x(11) \xrightarrow{\alpha} \\ \xrightarrow{\alpha} x(20) \xrightarrow{2\alpha} \end{array} x(12) \xrightarrow{\alpha} x(22)$$

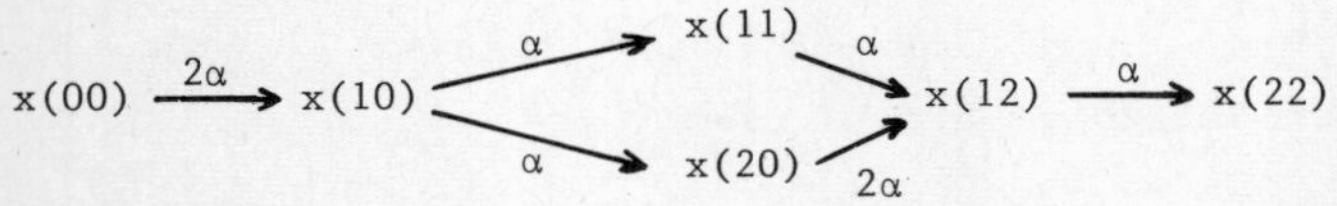

It therefore follows that there are kinetic equavalents of the multitarget multihit models which can be represented as sequences of branched kinetic steps.

One generalization of (4.12) is to allow for different rate constants as in the following scheme

$$x(00) \xrightarrow{2\alpha_1} x(10) \begin{array}{c} \xrightarrow{\alpha_2} x(11) \xrightarrow{2\alpha_3} \\ \xrightarrow{\alpha_2} x(20) \xrightarrow{\alpha_3} \end{array} x(12) \xrightarrow{\alpha_4} x(22)$$

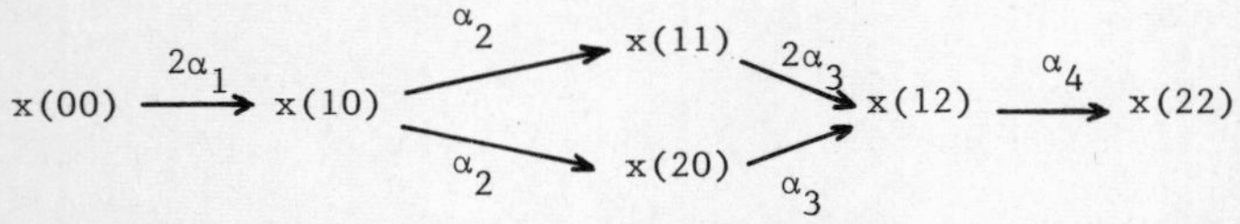

which is for a two-hit process with four independent rate constants.

The illustrative kinetic schemes of this and the previous section show that it is straightforward to construct expressions for the species concentrations. However there may be a non-uniqueness in the expressions for the intermediate concentrations, whereas the final concentration for a particular problem is unique. This non-uniqueness can be removed if some additional information, such as an intermediate measurement, is known.

4.5 Low LET Kinetic Models with Recovery

Each of the models previously considered in this Chapter is such that there is no provision for recovery of any of the species. In the present section a simple model which does allow for the recovery of an intermediate species is examined.

Consider a two-step process with the possibility of the middle species reverting to the first state:

$$x_1 \underset{\alpha_{-1}}{\overset{\alpha_1}{\rightleftarrows}} x_2 \xrightarrow{\alpha_2} x_3 \qquad (4.13)$$

This scheme can be interpreted as follows. The state with subscript 1 refers to a species in a cell which has suffered no collision with incident radiation, or which has recovered from a collision suffered. The state with subscript 2 refers to a species which has suffered one collision and has not yet recovered. Finally, the state with subscript 3 refers to a species which has suffered two collisions without recovery in between and is now a lethal species.

It is assumed that α_{-1} is independent of the radiation dose rate ϕ and that assumption (4.3) can be used. The differential equations are

$$\dot{x}_1 = -\alpha_1 x_1 + \alpha_{-1} x_2, \quad \dot{x}_2 = \alpha_1 x_1 - (\alpha_2 + \alpha_{-1}) x_2, \quad \dot{x}_3 = \alpha_2 x_2, \tag{4.14}$$

with prescribed initial conditions x_{10}, x_{20}, x_{30}. Substitution for x_2 from the first of these equations into the second gives a second order differential equation. After a little effort the solution to the system can be written in the form

$$x_1(t) = (Pe^{-at} + Qe^{-bt})/(b - a),$$

$$x_2(t) = [(\alpha_1 - a)Pe^{-at} + (\alpha_1 - b)Qe^{-bt}]/(b - a)\alpha_{-1},$$

$$x_3(t) = x_{10} + x_{20} + x_{30} - \alpha_2[(P/a)(\alpha_1 - a)e^{-at}$$

$$+ (Q/b)(\alpha_1 - b)e^{-bt}]/(b - a)\alpha_{-1},$$

where

$$P = (b - \alpha_1)x_{10} + \alpha_{-1}x_{20}, \quad Q = (\alpha_1 - a)x_{10} - \alpha_{-1}x_{20},$$

$$a = \{\alpha_1 + \alpha_2 + \alpha_{-1} + [(\alpha_2 + \alpha_{-1} - \alpha_1)^2 + 4\alpha_1\alpha_{-1}]^{1/2}\}/2, \tag{4.15}$$

$$b = \{\alpha_1 + \alpha_2 + \alpha_{-1} - [(\alpha_2 + \alpha_{-1} - \alpha_1)^2 + 4\alpha_1\alpha_{-1}]^{1/2}\}/2. \tag{4.16}$$

With $x_{10} = 1$, $x_{20} = x_{30} = 0$ the expressions for $x_i(t)$ simplify so that

$$x_1(t) = [(b - \alpha_1)e^{-at} + (\alpha_1 - a)e^{-bt}]/(b - a), \tag{4.17}$$

$$x_2(t) = \alpha_1(e^{-at} - e^{-bt})/(b - a), \tag{4.18}$$

$$x_3(t) = 1 - (be^{-at} - ae^{-bt})/(b - a). \tag{4.19}$$

The survival function is

$$S = (ae^{-bt} - be^{-at})/(a - b),$$

or, in terms of the dose D and radiation dose rate ϕ,

$$S(D) = (ae^{-bD/\phi} - be^{-aD/\phi})/(a - b). \tag{4.20}$$

Since $\alpha_1 > 0$, $\alpha_2 > 0$, $\alpha_{-1} > 0$, then $a > b > 0$ and $a/(a - b) > 1$. The size of the remaining coefficient $b/(a - b)$ can be checked in actual numerical examples.

Swann and del Rosario (1931) consider the situation when two impacts of an alpha particle with the sensitive element of a cell are necessary to cause its death. The possibility of a cell recovering after the first impact is allowed, and before the second, so that there is no contributory effect of the first impact. Their notation can be expressed in terms of the present symbols by defining

$$x_1 = n_o/\bar{n},\ x_2 = n_1/\bar{n},\ x_3 = n_2/\bar{n},\ \alpha_1 = N,\ \alpha_{-1} = \lambda,$$

and it is then straightforward to see that they have considered the scheme

$$x_1 \underset{\alpha_{-1}}{\overset{\alpha_1}{\rightleftarrows}} x_2 \xrightarrow{\alpha_1} x_3 .$$

That is, in the scheme (4.13) the rate constant α_2 is chosen to be the same as α_1.

Further examination of the scheme (4.13), which led to the equations (4.17) - (4.19) is now presented. With assumption (4.3) and $x_{20} = 0$ the survival function S can be expressed in terms of D and its graphs for various values of the rate constants and the dose-rate ϕ are given in Figure 4.1. Decrease of the dose-rate from a high value to a low one indicates that the chance of survival is improved. This comes about because the reverse reaction in (4.13) is of greater importance at a low rather than a high dose-rate and α_{-1} is not a function of ϕ.

The interesting feature of the scheme (4.13) is that dose-rate dependence can occur by the described kinetic mechanism even though the forward rate constants are just proportional to the dose-rate.

Also, the scheme (4.13) predicts recovery of the species x_1 if the irradiation is stopped. Complete recovery occurs when x_2 becomes zero.

Experimental evidence indicates that a biological system can recover its resistance to radiation in a nonsimple fashion. For example, the following scheme, Dienes (1966, p. 193),

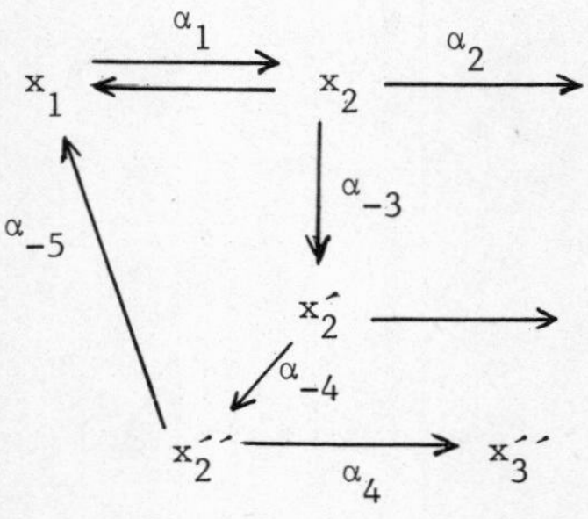

(4.21)

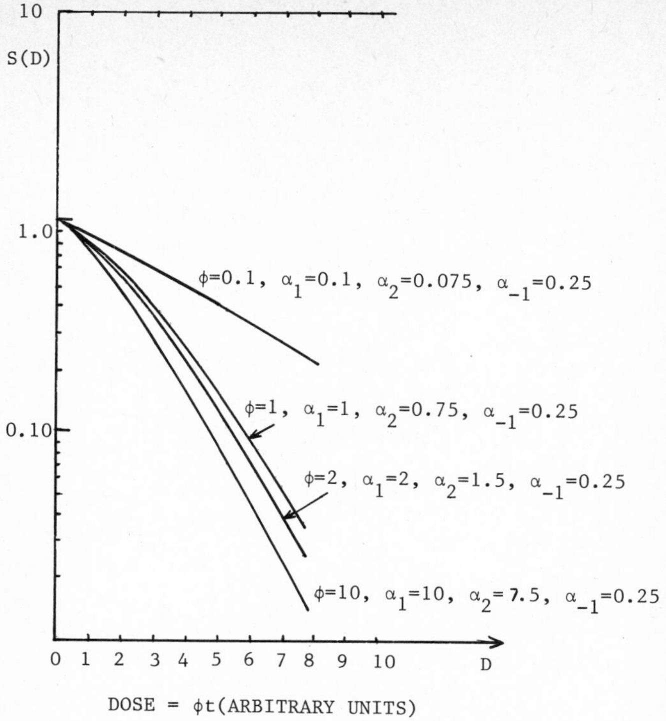

Figure 4.1 Dose-rate dependence arising from a thermally reversible reaction step. The fractional survival, S, is plotted against the dose for various values of the dose rate ϕ. (Dienes (1966), with permission).

with $\alpha_4 >> \alpha_3$ and $\alpha_3 < \alpha_2$ has x_2' as a relatively radiation-resistant species whereas x_2'' is a radiation-sensitive species. It is straightforward to construct the solutions to the scheme (4.21). For certain values of the rate constants Dienes shows that the recovery curves (with total irradiation time as ordinate and recovery time as abscissa) first have a maximum then follows a minimum and subsequently each curve increases to its respective saturation level for large recovery times.

4.6 Low LET and High LET Kinetic Model with No Recovery

Consider the scheme

$$x_1 \xrightarrow{(\beta+2\alpha)\kappa} x_2 \xrightarrow{(\beta+\alpha)\kappa} x_3 ,$$

where x_3 is a lethal species. The forward rate constant $\beta\kappa$ is assumed to represent the transition probability from state 1 to state 2 (and from state 2 to state 3) due to high linear energy transfer (LET). The other forward rate constants are assumed to be associated with low LET, as in Model 2 of Section 4.3. This scheme provides the kinetic equations

$$\dot{x}_1 = -(\beta + 2\alpha)\kappa x_1,\ \dot{x}_2 = (\beta + 2\alpha)\kappa x_1 - (\beta + \alpha)\kappa x_2,$$

$$\dot{x}_3 = (\beta + \alpha)\kappa x_2,\ x_{10} + x_{20} = 1,\ x_{30} = 0.$$

More specifically, it is reasonable to select

$$x_{10} = \alpha/(\alpha + \beta),\ x_{20} = \beta/(\alpha + \beta);$$

compare Model 2, Section 4.3, where $\beta \equiv 0$. Integration of the differential equations gives

$$x_1(t) = x_{10}\ e^{-(\beta + 2\alpha)\kappa t},$$

$$x_2(t) = x_{20}\ e^{-(\alpha + \beta)\kappa t} + (\beta\alpha^{-1} + 2)x_{10}e^{-\beta\kappa t}\ (e^{-\alpha\kappa t} - e^{-2\alpha\kappa t}),$$

$$x_3(t) = 1 - 2e^{-(\alpha + \beta)\kappa t} + e^{-(\beta + 2\alpha)\kappa t},$$

and the surviving fraction

$$S = 1 - x_3 = e^{-\beta\kappa t}[1 - (1 - e^{-\alpha\kappa t})^2].$$

This expression is formed as the product of $\exp(-\beta\kappa t)$, a dose-proportional cell killing action, with the nonlinear part $[1 - (1 - \exp(-\alpha\kappa t))^2]$. The quantity 2 may be thought of as representing the extrapolation number.

The above model for ionizing radiation is considered by Wideröe (1966, 1971, 1978) and referred to by him as "the two-component theory". (For ease in relating the mathematical expressions here to others in this Chapter the notation involving α and β is not the same as Wideröe's.)

4.7 Other Kinetic Schemes: Sparsely-ionizing Radiations

Previous kinetic schemes in this Chapter are of the type that the lethal species x_n is not directly produced as a consequence of the incident radiation but occurs as the end product of a chain of intermediate species concentrations. In the present section the kinetic scheme allows for the possibility of going directly from species x_1 to x_n with no recovery. This situation could represent DNA double-strand breakage. Also, the kinetic scheme can allow for the production of intermediate concentrations (for example, DNA single-strand breaks) which can be repaired by the cell. The simplest model is of the following type:

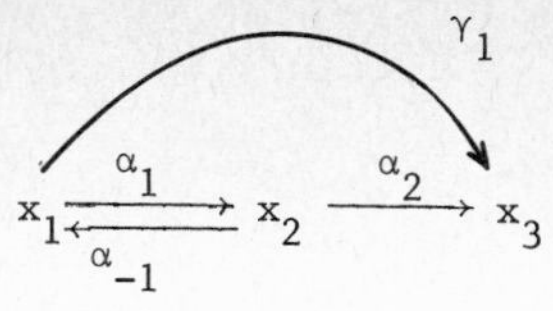

(4.22)

with x_3 being the lethal species. With a change in notation this is also the kinetic scheme of Kappos and Pohlit (1972), who refer to it as a "cybernetic model". The scheme (4.22) is the same as (4.13) excepting that there is the possibility of going directly from state 1 to state 3.

As in the scheme (4.13) the quantity α_{-1} is assumed to be independent of the radiation dose rate. The forward reaction rates α_1, α_2 are assumed to satisfy the relation (4.3); also $\gamma_1 = \Gamma_1\phi$, where Γ_1 is the radiation reaction rate constant for a radiation-induced transition from state 1 to state 3. Also, in the case of direct radiation effects α_1 and α_2 are constants pertaining to the essential molecule and should depend on the mean LET of the ionizing particles. The essential molecule (and several may exist in the cell) is the one primarily responsible for the radiation reaction. In this molecule can be tested the influence of radiation on the transport mechanisms or the reduction of protein synthesis, for example. The essential molecule is probably the DNA in the cell nucleus, but this is not an absolute fact.

In the first part of this section the survival curve for the scheme (4.22) is developed for the case of direct radiation effects. Thereafter the effects of sparsely-ionizing radiations are examined.

The differential equations for the scheme (4.22) are:

$$\left.\begin{aligned}&\dot{x}_1 = -(\alpha_1 + \gamma_1)x_1 + \alpha_{-1}x_2, \quad \dot{x}_2 = \alpha_1 x_1 - (\alpha_{-1} + \alpha_2)x_2,\\ &\dot{x}_3 = \gamma_1 x_1 + \alpha_2 x_2,\end{aligned}\right\} \qquad (4.23)$$

with the initial conditions $x_1(0) = 1$, $x_2(0) = x_3(0) = 0$. These equations possess the following solutions when α_1, α_{-1}, α_2 and γ_1 are constants:

$$x_1(t) = [(q - \alpha_1 - \gamma_1)e^{-pt} + (\alpha_1 + \gamma_1 - p)e^{-qt}]/(q - p),$$

$$x_2(t) = (\alpha_1 + \gamma_1 - p)(q - \alpha_1 - \gamma_1)(e^{-pt} - e^{-qt})/(q - p)\alpha_{-1},$$

$$x_3(t) = E(e^{-pt} - 1) + F(e^{-qt} - 1),$$

where

$$E = (q - \alpha_1 - \gamma_1)[\gamma_1 + (\alpha_2/\alpha_{-1})(\alpha_1 + \gamma_1 - p)]/(p^2 - pq), \qquad (4.24)$$

$$F = (\alpha_1 + \gamma_1 - p)[(\alpha_2/\alpha_{-1})(q - \alpha_1 - \gamma_1) - \gamma_1]/(q^2 - pq), \qquad (4.25)$$

$$p = (\alpha_1 + \gamma_1 + \alpha_2 + \alpha_{-1} + \Delta)/2, q = (\alpha_1 + \gamma_1 + \alpha_2 + \alpha_{-1} - \Delta)/2, \quad (4.26)$$

$$\Delta = [(\alpha_2 + \alpha_{-1} - \alpha_1 - \gamma_1)^2 + 4\alpha_1\alpha_{-1}]^{1/2} \geq 0.$$

When γ_1 is zero the solutions (4.24) - (4.26) reduce to the corresponding ones (4.17) - (4.19). The exponents p and q are each positive numbers. Hence both $x_1(t)$ and $x_2(t)$ approach zero as t becomes large whereas $x_3(t)$ tends to the constant limit - E - F, which reduces to the value unity, as required. The survival function is

$$S = 1 - E(e^{-pt} - 1) - F(e^{-qt} - 1)$$

and may be expressed in terms of the absorbed dose D by means of (4.2).

When the forward and backward reaction rates are not constants then the mathematical analysis of the equations usually has to give way to numerical solution. Kappos and Pohlit (1972) (in a different notation) consider the scheme (4.22). They are interested in the situation of sparsely ionizing radiations where indirect radiation effects play a predominant role in living cells. In this event it is anticipated that the forward reaction rates should be dependent on the absorbed dose, and mathematical expressions for these rates are now derived.

In the neighborhood of the essential molecule there originate radicals or molecular products which cause indirect radiation reactions and these must influence the forward rate parameters α_1 and α_2. This provides the suggestion that these parameters depend on the absorbed dose; now is the probability of a reaction between a radical and the essential molecule in the surroundings of the essential molecule, which can also react with the radicals. This concentration is high relative to the reactive agents, at low radiation dosage, and it seems reasonable to suggest that the corresponding reaction probability with the essential molecule is, therefore, a low value. As the absorbed dose increases there is a corresponding decrease in the concentration N_c of these molecules and this has the effect of increasing the probability for radiation reactions with the essential molecule. To a first approximation assume that there is a simple exponential decay of N_c with the absorbed dose D, that is, $dN_c/dD = -\upsilon N_c$. Also, assume that $\alpha_1 = \alpha_{1*}(1 - N_c/N_{co})$, where N_{co} is the value when there is no absorbed dose and α_{1*} is the value of the rate parameter when N_c is zero. This leads to the time- or absorbed dose-dependent rate parameter

$$\alpha_1 \equiv \alpha_1(t) = \alpha_{1*}(1 - e^{-\upsilon\phi t}) = \alpha_{1*}(1 - e^{-\upsilon D}).$$

The alternative assumption that there is a very fast repair process utilizing certain molecules also leads to the same dose dependence in α_1.

Assume that the probability for the transition from state 1 to state 2 is much higher than from state 1 to state 3. (There is some support for this assumption in experiments involving stationary diploid yeast cells; Kappos and Pohlit (1972), p. 62). Their experimental results also indicate that $\alpha_2 << \gamma_1$. Hence, it is reasonable to take γ_1 and α_2 as being constants. Kappos and Pohlit select $\gamma_1 = 0$, $\alpha_2 = 0$ and $\alpha_{-1} = 0$, and the equation for the species concentration x_1 is reduced to

$$\dot{x}_1 = -\alpha_{1*}(1 - e^{-\upsilon\phi t})x_1, \quad x_1(0) = 1.$$

This differential equation has the solution

$$\ell n\, x_1(t) = -\alpha_{1*}\left[t + \frac{e^{-\upsilon\phi t}}{\upsilon\phi} - \frac{1}{\upsilon\phi} \right],$$

and may be written in the following, alternative, form by means of (4.4)

$$\ell n \left[x_1\left(\frac{D}{\phi}\right) \right] = \frac{k_{1*}}{\upsilon} - k_{1*}D - \frac{k_{1*}}{\upsilon}\exp(-\upsilon D), \quad \phi k_{1*} = \alpha_{1*}. \qquad (4.27)$$

A graph of $\ell n[x_1(D/\phi)]$ as ordinate versus $k_{1*}D$ as abscissa for a particular k_{1*}/υ is readily generated and some examples of the theoretical dose-effect curves are shown in Fig. 4.2. (Note: to make the correspondence between the present notations and those used by Kappos and Pohlit identify $k_{1*} \equiv \eta^*_{AB}$, $\upsilon \equiv \eta_C$; η_{AB}/η_C in their Figure 2 should be η^*_{AB}/η_C.)

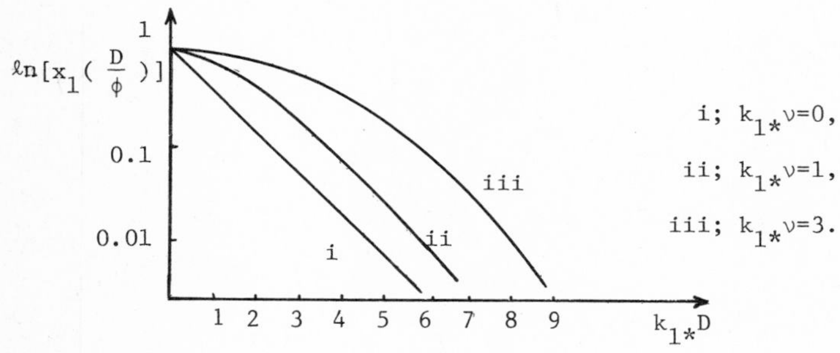

Figure 4.2 The theoretical dose-effect curves for the scheme (4.2) and solution (4.27). (Kappos and Pohlit (1972), with permission.)

Kappos and Pohlit compare the experimental values for X-ray irradiation of diploid yeast cells with the theoretical curves, Fig. 4.2, and indicate agreement for the curve with $k_{1*}/\upsilon = 2$. In turn, this supports the assumptions used in the development of the mathematical model that $\gamma_1 << \alpha_1$.

A split-dose experiment can be used to test the presence of a reverse reaction which is a recovery and replenishment of molecules after irradiation. For such an experiment Kappos and Pohlit suggest that the forward rate parameter from state 1 to state 2 is of the form

$$\alpha_1 = \alpha_{1*}\{1 - [1 - [1 - \exp(-\upsilon D_1)]\exp(-\varepsilon_c \Delta t)]\exp(-\upsilon D_2)\},$$

where D_1 is the first dose, D_2 is the second and separated by a time interval Δt, and ε_c^{-1} is a time constant associated with the decay of the competing molecules, N_c. Use of this form for α_1 leads to theoretical dose-effect curves which bear a close resemblance to experimentally-derived curves for diploid yeast cells under X-irradiation.

4.8 Kinetic Schemes with Age-specific Compartments in the Cell Cycle

As an aid to investigations of the progress of a cell through its cycle it is convenient to introduce divisions of it into a number of age-specific compartments. Each of the kinetic schemes developed so far in this Chapter have implicitly assumed that the cellular populations are within a single age class. In the present section a mathematical model is developed which allows for a description of the changes in time of cells in their cell cycle age-specific compartments after they have been irradiated. For the simpler kinetic models considered in previous sections the state is now identified with the damage class.

The approach will be to consider a particular kinetic scheme and convert it into a different notation which suggests generalizations to include the effects of radiation-induced injury and lethality. Thereafter, the general treatment is developed for a mathematical model which can be used to obtain an appropriate survival function.

Consider the scheme (4.22) in which α_1, α_2 and γ_1 are forward rate parameters. With assumption (4.3) as a basis define

$$\alpha_1 \equiv \varepsilon_1(1,2)\phi, \ \alpha_2 \equiv \varepsilon_1(2,3)\phi, \ \gamma_1 \equiv \varepsilon_1(1,3)\phi,$$

where the subscript 1 on the ε quantities is introduced here in anticipation of the subsequent developments of the present section to include age-specific concepts. The quantities $\varepsilon_1(1,2)$ and $\varepsilon_1(1,3)$ are interpreted as being the <u>efficiency</u> of the radiation in producing a transition from state 1 to state 2 and from state 1 to state 3, respectively. As before, ϕ is the radiation dose rate. Now define

$$r_1(2,1) \equiv \alpha_{-1}$$

to be the recovery rate from state 2 to state 1. For the situation of three damage classes,

$i = 1$, no damage (state 1 in scheme (4.22)),

$i = 2$, first damage class (state 2 in scheme (4.22)),

$i = 3$, lethal damage class (state 3 in scheme (4.22),

make the identifications

$$x_{1i}(t) \equiv x_1(t), \ i = 1,2,3.$$

The notation here is that the first subscript refers to that fraction of cells in the age-specific compartment with the label 1 and having damage of the ith class.

With these changes of notation the differential equation system (4.23) can be rewritten as

$$\dot{x}_{11}(t) = -[\varepsilon_1(1,2) + \varepsilon_1(1,3)]\phi x_{11}(t) + r_1(2,1)x_{12}(t),$$

$$\dot{x}_{12}(t) = \varepsilon_1(1,2)\phi x_{11}(t) - [r_1(2,1) + \varepsilon_1(2,3)\phi]x_{12}(t),$$

$$\dot{x}_{13}(t) = \varepsilon_1(1,3)\phi x_{11}(t) + \varepsilon_1(2,3)\phi x_{12}(t).$$

These are the equations for the scheme

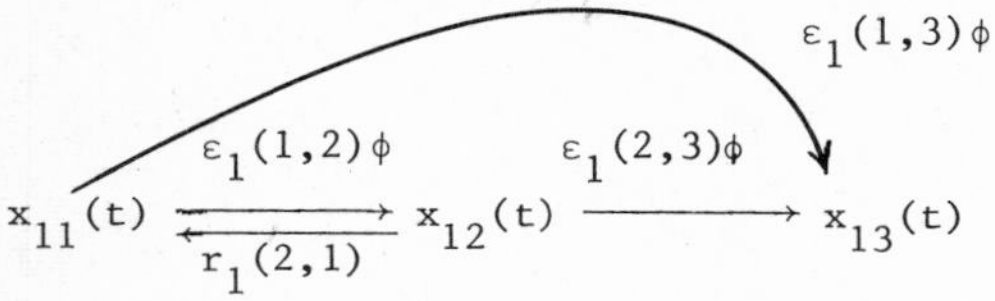

The structure of these equations may be seen more clearly in the matrix format

$$\begin{bmatrix} \dot{x}_{11}(t) \\ \dot{x}_{12}(t) \\ \dot{x}_{13}(t) \end{bmatrix} = \begin{bmatrix} -\varepsilon_1(1,2)\phi - \varepsilon_1(1,3)\phi & r_1(2,1) & 0 \\ \varepsilon_1(1,2)\phi & -r_1(2,1) - \varepsilon_1(2,3)\phi & 0 \\ \varepsilon_1(1,3)\phi & \varepsilon_1(2,3)\phi & 0 \end{bmatrix} \begin{bmatrix} x_{11}(t) \\ x_{12}(t) \\ x_{13}(t) \end{bmatrix}$$

with $x_{11}(0) = 1$, $x_{12}(0) = x_{13}(0) = 0$.

As an immediate extension consider the following situation:

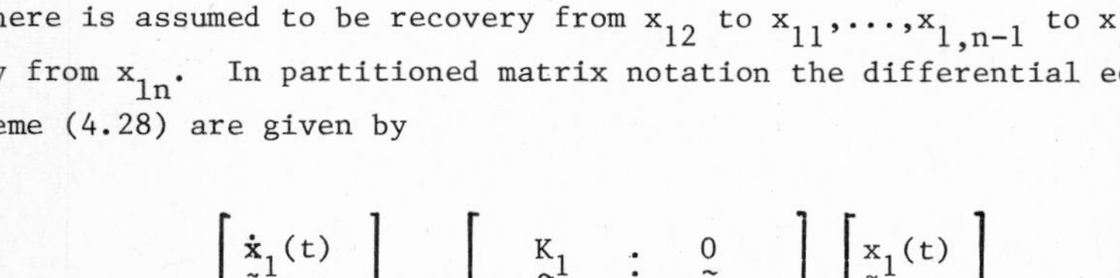

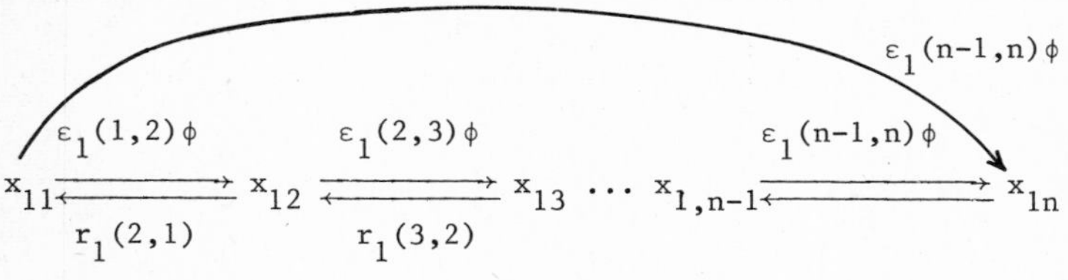

(4.28)

Here, there is assumed to be recovery from x_{12} to $x_{11}, \ldots, x_{1,n-1}$ to $x_{1,n-2}$, but no recovery from x_{1n}. In partitioned matrix notation the differential equations for the scheme (4.28) are given by

$$\begin{bmatrix} \dot{\underset{\sim}{x}}_1(t) \\ \dot{x}_{1n}(t) \end{bmatrix} = \left[\begin{array}{c:c} \underset{\sim}{K}_1 & \underset{\sim}{0} \\ \hdashline \underset{\sim}{\varepsilon}_1 & 0 \end{array}\right] \begin{bmatrix} \underset{\sim}{x}_1(t) \\ x_{1n}(t) \end{bmatrix}$$

where $\underset{\sim}{0}$ is a column vector with n-1 entries which are zeroes; the row vector

$$\underset{\sim}{\varepsilon}_1 = (\varepsilon_1(1,n)\phi,\ 0,\ldots,0,\ \varepsilon(n-1,n)\phi)$$

also has n-1 entries; also $\underset{\sim}{K}_1$ is an (n - 1)x(n - 1) tri-diagonal matrix of the form

$$\underset{\sim}{K}_1 = \begin{bmatrix} -\varepsilon(1,2)\phi - \varepsilon_1(1,n)\phi & r_1(2,1) & & & \bigcirc \\ \varepsilon_1(1,2)\phi & -\varepsilon_1(2,3)\phi - r(2,1) & r_1(3,2) & & \\ & \varepsilon_1(2,3)\phi & \ddots & \ddots & \\ & & \ddots & \ddots & r_1(n-1,n-2) \\ \bigcirc & & & \ddots & -\varepsilon_1(n-1,n)\phi - r_1(n-1,n-2) \\ & & & & \varepsilon_1(n-1,n)\phi \end{bmatrix}$$

Finally, the column vector

$$\underset{\sim}{x}_1(t) = [x_{11}(t), x_{12}(t), \ldots, x_{1,n-1}]^T,$$

where T denotes transpose. The initial conditions are

$$x_{11}(0) = 1,\ x_{1i}(0) = 0,\ i = 2,\ldots,n.$$

So far in this section the equations are concerned with a single age compartment. If the cell cycle is divided into m age compartments then it is apparent that the equations describing the transient behavior are given by

$$\begin{bmatrix} \dot{\underset{\sim}{x}}_j(t) \\ \\ \dot{\underset{\sim}{x}}_{jn}(t) \end{bmatrix} = \begin{bmatrix} \underset{\sim}{K}_j & \vdots & \underset{\sim}{0} \\ \cdots & \vdots & \cdots \\ \underset{\sim}{\varepsilon}_j & \vdots & 0 \end{bmatrix} \begin{bmatrix} \underset{\sim}{x}_j(t) \\ \\ x_{jn}(t) \end{bmatrix},\ j = 1,2,\ldots,m.$$

There are a number of factors which occur in the processes associated with radiation-induced injury and lethality at the cellular, systemic, and organismic levels. For example, these factors include

(i) the presence or absence of certain chemical substances prior to, during, and after radiation;

(ii) intracyclic differential sensitivity; see Mendelsohn (1975);

(iii) cell cycle kinetics;

(iv) the time at which a given endpoint is ascertained;

(v) the radiation quality;

(vi) the temporal distribution of the energy deposition events.

The above list is given by Scott (1977), who also introduces a general kinetic scheme, which uses a division of the cell cycle into a number of age-specific compartments. Extensions of the kinetic schemes to include these factors are possible and information on the transient behavior of the intermediate damage classes as well as the survival function can be found.

4.9 Thermal Potentiation of Cell Killing

Reports of tumor regression induced by hyperthermia have appeared in the literature since the treatments reported by Coley (1893). Bacterial toxins were used, however, and it was not clear whether the regression was due to their presence or to the fever. The advent of antibodies has resulted in an essential abandonment of the pathophysiology of therapeutic systemic hyperthermia; see Nauts et al. (1953). Scientific interest in the use of hyperthermia in the treatment of cancer languished for many years during the present century. Then Warren (1935) presented a report on whole body hyperthermia in 32 patients with far-advanced malignancies. Although no cures were obtained he suggested the need for more research in hyperthermia.

During the last decade there has been a dramatic renewal of interest in hyperthermia either by itself or in conjunction with X-irradiation and/or chemotherapy. See, for example, reviews by Cavaliere et al. (1967), Suit and Shwayder (1974), Gerner et al. (1975), Hahn et al. (1975), Miller et al. (1977), and Connor et al. (1977).

Earlier in this Chapter the kinetic schemes of Dienes (1966) were introduced, which allowed for a generalization of the historical hit and target models. Recently Bronk (1976) indicated an extension of the Dienes kinetic approach to include time-dependent phenomena such as rate of repair, dose-rate-dependent survival, effects of progress or delay in the cell cycle or sequential heat-radiation experiments. One significant feature of Bronk's paper is the use of the framework provided by the kinetic approach as a means of unifying the qualitative discussion of experiments involving the thermal potentiation of cell killing. His theoretical approach is now examined and is partly based on communications with the author.

Consider the kinetic scheme of Fig. 4.3. As before, ϕ represents the radiation dose rate. The K_i, $i = 1,2,\ldots,n-1$, are transition numbers which represent an incremental fraction of the quantity x_i transferred from the state i to i + 1 by radiation damage per unit dose. The transition numbers are known to depend on position or phase within the cell cycle and the temperature. It is surmised that K_i is probably a function of the metabolic state of the cell, but this remains to be shown. Bronk (1978) suggests that rates of change of state (e.g. $i \longrightarrow i + 1$) depend on the result

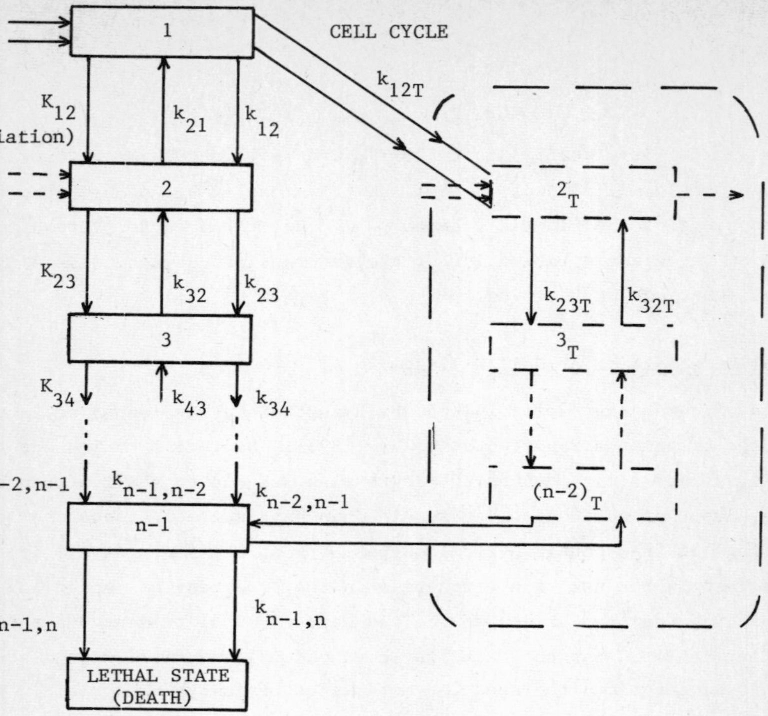

Figure 4.3 All parts of this combined diagram "may not be used in a logically consistent manner to discuss most combined heat-shock-radiation experiments"; Bronk (1978). State 1 represents undamaged cells which proliferate through the cell cycle, as indicated by the horizontal arrows. States 2 through n in the solid boxes represent various states of the damaged cell, which can return to the cycling states (1 and 2) through various states of intermediate damage. Bronk (1976), with permission.

of competitions among chemical reactions, each of which has a reaction rate which depends on environmental conditions such as temperature, pressure, etc. One can anticipate that environmental conditions will influence the cell's metabolic state. Terms in the kinetic equations involving the K_i's refer to radiation damage considered to be delivered over a short time period. The terms which involve the k_i's refer to fixing and recovery from damage and are expected to take place over a longer period of time. They, also, are considered to be dependent on the phases of the cell cycle, ambient temperature, and the medium. The connections between the states i -1, i and i + 1 are as follows:

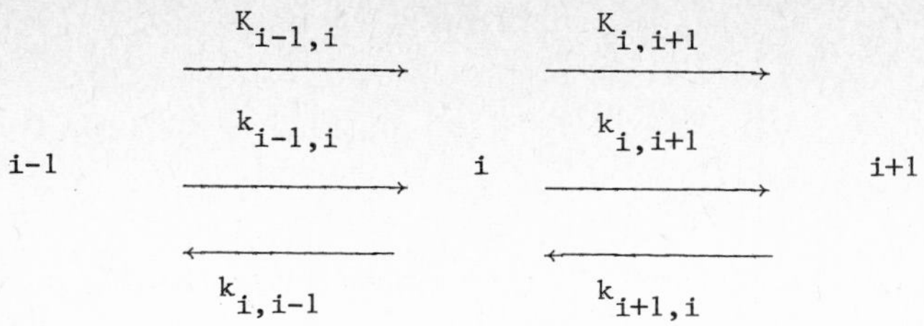

With x_i denoting, for example, the fraction of biological material present in state i then

$$\dot{x}_i(t) = -K_{i,i+1}\phi x_i - k_{i,k+1}\, x_i - k_{i,i-1}\, x_i$$

$$+ K_{i-1,i}\, \phi\, x_{i-1} + k_{i-1,i}\, x_{i-1} + k_{i+1,i} x_{i+1},$$

which includes the radiation damage terms (from arrows directed to the right) and recovery terms (from the arrows directed to the left). The fourth term on the right-hand side of this equation was inadvertently omitted during a retyping of Bronk's 1976 paper. The full system of kinetic equations is of the form

$$\dot{x}_1(t) = -(K_{12}\phi + k_{12})x_1(t) + k_{21}x_2(t),$$

$$\dot{x}_2(t) = (K_{12}\phi + k_{12})x_1(t) - (K_{23}\phi + k_{21} + k_{23})x_2(t) + k_{32}x_3(t),$$

$$\vdots$$

$$\dot{x}_{n-1}(t) = (K_{n-2,n-1}\phi + k_{n-2,n-1})x_{n-2}(t) - (K_{n-1,n}\phi + k_{n-1,n-2} + k_{n-1,n})x_{n-1}(t),$$

$$\dot{x}_n(t) = (K_{n-1,n}\phi + k_{n-1,n})x_{n-1}(t),$$

with appropriate initial conditions. By the manner of construction this is a tri-diagonal system of ordinary differential equations. There is no recovery from the nth state and x_n denotes a lethal species. These equations can be expected to apply in a situation of limiting reactions for transfer between states and over limited temperature ranges.

So far in this section the development is considered to be applicable to an experiment with radiation alone and refers specifically to that portion of Fig. 4.3 which is outside of the dashed portion. No initial distribution of the species x_i, $i = 1,\ldots,n$, has been specified and thus cells may be in any proportion in states 1 through n depending on previous radiation insult and recovery.

Now consider that portion of Fig. 4.3 which includes states 1, n-1 and n together with the part inside the dashed lines. This portion may be used for an experiment in which thermal shock (no ionizing radiation present) is applied with the k_{ijT} determining the rates of transfer from state i to state j at temperature T.

The representation of mixed thermal-radiation experiments is much more involved. To avoid ambiguities in interpretation an accurate representation of mixed-type experiments requires a two-index scheme in which $x_{i,j}(t)$ is defined to give that fraction of cells at time t in the ith state of radiation damage and the jth state of heat damage. This means that the transition rates in the kinetic equations will have four indices. Inclusion of effects depending on the phases of the cell cycle and change of metabolic state would require additional indices.

Further discussion of these points is given by Bronk (1976) in Section IV of his paper. He also presents details of the qualitative interpretation of a number of experiments in terms of parts of Fig. 4.3.

The interpretation of mixed thermal-radiation experiments is still in its infancy, and it is hoped as time progresses that detailed theoretical survival expressions will become available. These can then be used in some scheme which seeks to improve and perhaps optimize therapy based on some combination of hyperthermia and ionizing radiation.

Chapter 5

CELL SURVIVAL AFTER SUCCESSIVE RADIATION FRACTIONS

5.1 Introduction

In general, normal cells have a superior and rapid capability to repair sublethal damage than do tumor cells. One consequence of this feature is that radiation to a tumor is often given intermittently, so that the total exposure is split into a number of intervals in which there is no irradiation, and is called fractionated if the total time from the first to the last exposure is of the order of days or weeks and is referred to as pulsed irradiation when the overall time is much less than this.

Present mathematical models of the surviving fraction of tumor cells at the end of a number of fractions tend to be of an elementary nature. One of the simplest approaches is shown in Figure 5.1. At the times $0,\tau,\ldots$ it is assumed that there is an instantaneous decrease in the level of tumor cells as a result of the application of anticancer therapy (e.g. cytotoxic drug or radiation therapy). In the open time intervals $(0,\tau)$, $(\tau,2\tau)$, etc. the tumor population continues its growth. For the situation of Figure 5.1 it is also usually assumed that the growth characteristics of the cell populations after perturbation by the anticancer therapy are the same as they were prior to the perturbation, and this assumption is adhered to in the present Chapter.

The magnitude of the decrease in the level of the tumor cell population (or its surviving fraction) at the times $0,\tau,\ldots$ depends on the drug or radiation dosage.

Knowledge of the nature of the growth curve for the tumor cell populations under situations of free and perturbed growth would allow for a better understanding of the dosage levels to be applied and their timing could also be improved. These are two of the goals of optimization of human cancer radiotherapy and cancer chemotherapy.

In the remaining sections of this Chapter the derived results are for radiation therapy.

Normal tissues experience cell loss as a result of the radiation insult. It is assumed throughout this Chapter that, at each irradiation treatment, the normal cell population is instantaneously decreased. During the time interval to the next fraction the cells recover.

Section 5.2 presents the basic material for an understanding of the mathematical results used when dealing with the concept of an instantaneous decrease in the level of a cell population. It is shown how to derive the cellular level during exponential regrowth after a number of fractions of the same dose and equally spaced are given. This is the result (5.7)

The recovery of normal tissues after irradiation is of prime importance. In Section 5.3 a mathematical model is examined for the instantaneous normal cell kill followed by a logistic type of growth. The basic equation for normal cell recovery is (5.9). However it is important to stress that (5.9) is just one of a whole class

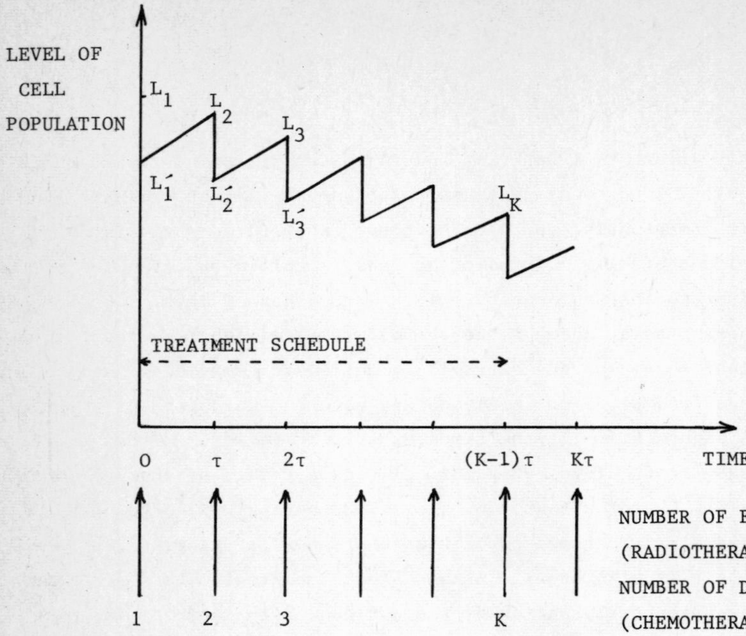

Figure 5.1 Instantaneous decrease of tumor population as a result of anticancer therapy. L_1, L_2, ... denote the cell population level immediately prior to the application of therapy, L_1',L_2',... denote the corresponding levels after therapy. The vertical lines at τ,2τ,... are included as a visual aid.

of mathematical equations which give essentially the same shape in the (N,t) plane. It is reasonable to use (5.9) but any other model which is biologically plausible can be used.

These two sections are preliminary to Section 5.4, which is the main contribution to the present Chapter. Section 5.4 presents a synopsis of some of the work by Cohen and coworkers. This work was developed as an aid to research workers and clinicians to enable them to compute cellular lethality in irradiated tissues when the dosage, number of fractions, treatment time and field-size or tumor-volume are known, and a set of acceptable values for the cellular radiosensitivity and repopulation parameters assumed. Their algebraic and numerical method of approach gives parameter values that are realistic and consistent with directly measured values. One use of these parameter values is in mathematical models which can permit the generation of iso-effect lines or tables.

Also, the availability of reasonable parameter values makes for more reasonable use of mathematical modeos, which can be developed in order to predict the outcome of a certain proposed course of treatment. Features such as the unscheduled interruption in the treatment scheme, the determination of therapeutic ratios and the development of treatment strategies that are superior to ones currently used can be examined via the mathematical models. This Chapter and the next illustrate some of these mathematical models.

Section 5.5 illustrates a model of the radiation therapy of a tumor containing variations in cell sensitivity to radiations at different phases of the cell cycle. The results of the model illustrate that continuous irradiation gives a relatively greater kill than does a fractionated course if there is a high target number in the resistant phase, if rapid proliferation is present, and if the proportion of time in the sensitive phase is large.

Section 5.6 presents some results in fractionated therapy.

5.2 Some Results in Connection with Instantaneous Cell Kill and Exponential Tumor Growth

Consider Figure 5.1 in the situation where there is a uniform schedule of fractionated irradiation - the first fraction is given on day zero, the second on day τ, the third on day 2τ and so on, with the Kth fraction being given on day $(K - 1)\tau$. Define $L_1, L_2, \ldots, L_K$ to respectively denote the levels of the cell population immediately prior to the administration of the 1st, 2nd,...,Kth fractions. Assume that with each fraction there is an instantaneous decrease in the level of the cell population. Now define $L_1', L_2', \ldots, L_K'$ to be the levels in the cell populations immediately after the fractions 1,2,... have been delivered.

The magnitude of the dosage at each treatment time is the same and, if it is assumed that there is a constant attenuation of the cell population whenever a fraction is given, then

$$L_i' = S\,L_i, \quad i = 1,2,\ldots, \tag{5.1}$$

where i is the number of fractions and S is the attenuation factor.

Assume that after the first fraction the tumor regrows exponentially according to the equation

$$\frac{dL}{dt} = \lambda L, \text{ or } L(t) = L(t_o)e^{\lambda(t-t_o)}. \tag{5.2}$$

Here, L(t) is some measure of the size of the tumor and could denote (for example) either the volume or the total number of tumor cells. The quantity λ is the growth or regeneration parameter, and is assumed here to be a constant. Now assume that there is exponential growth of the tumor after each successive fraction according to the relations in (5.2). Application of the expression for L(t) in (5.2) with the result (5.1) to the situation in Figure 5.1 indicates that

$$L_1' = SL_1,$$

$$L_2' = SL_2 = Se^{\lambda\tau}L_1' = S^2e^{\lambda\tau}L_1,$$

$$L_3' = SL_3 = Se^{\lambda(2\tau-\tau)}L_2' = S^3e^{2\lambda\tau}L_1,$$

$$\vdots$$

$$L_K' = SL_K = Se^{\lambda[(K-1)\tau - (K-2)\tau]}L_{K-1}' = S^Ke^{\lambda(K-1)\tau}L_1.$$

If the Kth fraction is the last one in the treatment schedule then L_K is the final level which contributes to L_K'. Hence the fraction of cells which survive the whole treatment schedule is given by

$$\frac{L_f}{L_1} = S^Ke^{\lambda(K-1)\tau}, \tag{5.3}$$

where L_f ($\equiv L_K'$) denotes the final level of the cell population immediately after the Kth fraction and a total time period of length $(K-1)\tau$.

The attenuation factor is denoted by the symbol S for the reason that it is identified as being the survival fraction after a single radiation dosage. Accordingly, then, the quantity S in (5.3) could be replaced by any one of the expressions (2.1), (2.2), (2.4), (2.5), (3.1) or (3.3). Wheldon and Kirk (1976) use the expression for S given by (2.1) in (5.3) with $\tau \equiv t$. However their subsequent analysis uses $\exp(\lambda K\tau)$ in order to allow for some mathematical simplicity. This simplified expression is also used by Wheldon et al. (1977), who use the expression for S given by (3.3). The substitution of (2.4) for S in (5.3) together with an appropriate interchange of symbols gives the result (1) of Cohen (1968) with $(K - 1)\tau = T$ days.

The relation (5.1) expresses the connection between values of the cell population level L(t) just before and just after a radiation dosage and does not of itself provide any more information. This means that it is not possible to deduce a unique mathematical form for the growth equation for L(t) from (5.1). To illustrate this point consider the following differential equation

$$\frac{1}{L}\frac{dL}{dt} = f(L) + \ln S\ \delta(t - \tau), \tag{5.4}$$

where f(L) is some well-defined function of $L \equiv L(t)$ and $\delta(\ )$ denotes the Dirac "delta-function". Integration of this equation between $\tau - \varepsilon$ and $\tau + \varepsilon$ produces

$$[\ln L(t)]_{\tau-\varepsilon}^{\tau+\varepsilon} = \int_{\tau-\varepsilon}^{\tau+\varepsilon} f(L(t))dt + \ln S.$$

Now let $\varepsilon \rightarrow 0$ and, for convenience, write $\tau_+ \equiv \tau + 0$, $\tau_- \equiv \tau - 0$. In the limit as

$\varepsilon \to 0$ there is no contribution from the integral and hence

$$[\ell n\ L(t)]_{\tau_-}^{\tau_+} = \ell n\ S, \qquad (5.5)$$

where the quantity on the left-hand side of this equation is to be interpreted as meaning "the change in the enclosed quantity in crossing τ". Note that (5.5) is just an alternative way of writing (5.1). Any differential equation of the form (5.4) is capable therefore of producing the relation (5.1). Conversely, given a relation like (5.1), then the differential equation for the quantity L(t) must be of the general form (5.4).

Consider the situation when $f(L)$ = constant, say λ, in (5.4). With $\tau = 0$ equation (5.4) now becomes

$$\frac{d\ \ell n\ L(t)}{dt} = \lambda + \ell n\ S\ \delta(t).$$

This equation indicates that for $t > 0$ growth is exponential with the condition (5.5), or (5.1), so that

$$L(t) = L(0_-)\ Se^{\lambda t} = L_1 Se^{\lambda t}.$$

It therefore follows that an alternative way of expressing the situation of K uniform fractionations given at the times 0, τ, 2τ,... with exponential growth in between them is by the equation

$$\frac{d}{dt}\ \ell n\ L(t) = \lambda + \ell n\ S \sum_{i=0}^{K-1} \delta(t - i\tau). \qquad (5.6)$$

Perhaps the easiest way to solve (5.6) is by the direct use of a Laplace transform and this gives (see Appendix 2)

$$L(t) = L(0_-)S^K e^{\lambda t} = L_1 S^K e^{\lambda t},\ t > (K - 1)\tau. \qquad (5.7)$$

Immediately after the Kth treatment, at time $t_+ = (K - 1)\tau + 0$, since $L_K' = L(t_+)$, the relations in (5.7) give $L_K' = S^K e^{\lambda(k-1)t} L_1$, as before, from which follows the result (5.3).

A similar derivation of the result (5.7) is given by Wheldon (1978).

If the dosages of radiation are not uniform but are given as $D_1, D_2, \ldots$ for the corresponding fractions 1,2,..., and if there is the assumption of exponential growth of the cell population after each fraction, then, instead of (5.3)

$$\frac{L_f}{L_1} = S(D_1)S(D_2)\ldots S(D_K)\ e^{\lambda(K-1)\tau}, \qquad (5.8)$$

when the Kth fraction is the last one in the treatment schedule.

5.3 Instantaneous Cell Kill Followed by Logistic Growth of Normal Tissue

In the previous section the simplest choice of the function f(L) in (5.4) was selected, namely f(L) = constant, and this led to the consideration of exponential growth of the tumor cell population. During a course of irradiation, in between fractions, the level N(t) of the normal cells tends to recover to its homeostatic level. Sacher and Trucco (1966) assumed that the regeneration of the irradiated normal cells could be approximately described by the logistic differential equation

$$\dot{N}(t) = hN(t)[c - N(t)], \tag{5.9}$$

where h and c are assumed to be constants. This equation gives the time-course of recovery of the normal cells after they have been perturbed by some external or internal disturbance. If the population is perturbed to the level N_o at time $t = t_o$ (with $N_o \gtrless c$) then the population level for time $t > t_o$ is given by the following solution of the logistic differential equation

$$N(t) = \frac{cN_o}{N_o + (c - N_o)\exp[-hc(t - t_o)]}, \tag{5.10}$$

with $N(t_o) = N_o$. Figure 5.2 shows the graphs of this solution when N_o is greater than, is equal to, or is less than the saturation level c.

Sacher and Trucco (1966, p. 238) refer to (5.9) as the recovery equation for normal tissues and constitutes a second-order kinetics model for the recovery process. The expression (5.10) is assumed to hold after a single irradiation of normal cells, with 1/h being the average population generation time. Because of accumulation in the irradiated tissues of injured cells, which are not replaced by regeneration, the restitution of normal structure and function is incomplete and this will affect the asymptotic level c. This is especially the case during the procedures of radiation fractionation.

Define $N_1', N_2', \ldots, N_K'$ to respectively denote the levels of the normal cell population immediately after the radiation fractions 1,2,... have been delivered. Assume that each fraction is responsible for an instantaneous decrease in the level of the normal cell population. After the respective fractions 1,2,... the normal tissue recovers to the levels $N_2, N_3, \ldots$, according to the assumption (5.9) For example, if the same dose of radiation is given at each fraction,

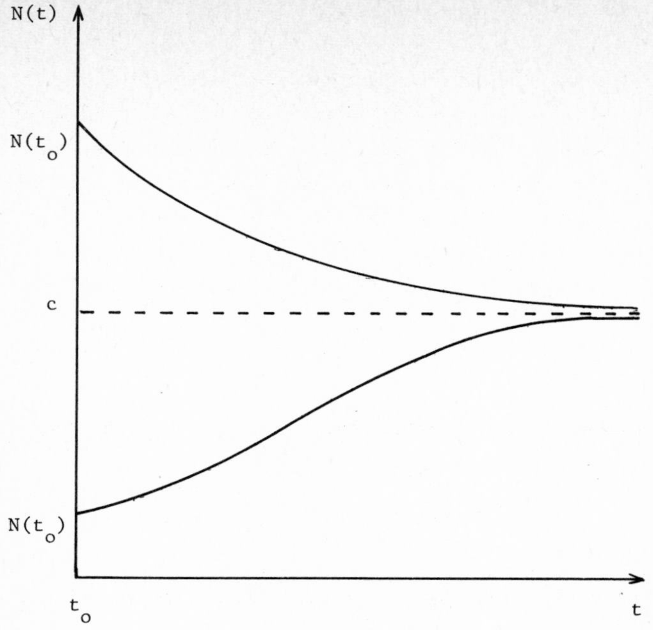

Figure 5.2 Graphic solutions of the logistic equation (5.9). Recovery of normal cells after a single irradiation insult reduced the population level to $N(t_o)$.

$$N'_1,$$

$$N'_2 = S_N N_2,$$

$$N'_3 = S_N N_3,$$

$$\vdots$$

$$N'_K = S_N N_K,$$

and the Kth fraction is the last one in the treatment schedule. The quantity S_N designates the surviving fraction of normal cells immediately after a single exposure. Also, for $N_i \equiv N(t_i)$, $i = 2,\ldots,K$,

$$N_i = cN'_{i-1} \; / \; \{N'_{i-1} + (c - N'_{i-1}) \exp[-hc(t_i - t_{i-1})\}.$$

This result is an application of the expression in (5.10).

Instead of using the somewhat complicated expressions for N_K and N'_K there is an alternative development which uses survival fractions. It is worthwhile examining this alternative approach.

As before, S_N represents that proportion of the normal cell population, immediately after a single exposure, which has survived the irradiation. Thereafter the normal cell population will recover. Its corresponding surviving fraction will also increase and without further perturbation will reach the homeostatic level of unity. After the radiation exposure one may assume that the survival fraction follows a sigmoidal type curve and, mathematically, the logistic curve is of this form. (Of course, other mathematical expressions can give similar geometrical behavior). Therefore, if $\alpha(\theta)$ represents the surviving fraction during the recovery phase,

$$d\alpha(\theta)/d\theta = [1 - \alpha(\theta)]\alpha(\theta),$$

with θ denoting the fraction of time that has elapsed since the exposure. The quantity θ may be expressed in the form

$$\theta = t/g,$$

where t is the time and g could represent the average normal cell population generation time. On writing $S(t) \equiv \alpha(t/g)$ then $\dot{S}(t) = S(t)[1 - S(t)]/g$ with

$$S(t) = S_o/[S_o + (1 - S_o) \exp(-t/g)], \tag{5.10a}$$

with $S(0) = S_o$. A derivation of this expression, similar to the above, is given by Cohen (1973b). His notation is different and he allows for the recovery level H to be different at the end of each subinterval just prior to the next radiation fraction; however in some numerical computations H is selected to be unity, Cohen and Scott (1968). See (5.13) and (6.27).

Now consider a uniform schedule of fractionated irradiation of the normal cell population in which an individual exposure of D rads is repeated K times at intervals of τ days. Immediately after the first exposure the surviving fraction of the normal cells is S_N, which is better expressed in the notation $S_N(1)$. Just prior to the second exposure the surviving fraction is given by the expression

$$S(\tau) = S_N/[S_N + (1 - S_N) \exp(-\tau/g)], \quad S_N \equiv S_N(1),$$

where $S(\tau)$ means $S(\tau_-)$; see Figure 5.3. Immediately after the second exposure the surviving fraction is

$$S_N(2) = S_N(1)S(\tau) = S_N(1) \cdot \frac{S_N(1)}{S_N(1) + [1 - S_N(1)]\exp(-\tau/g)} ;$$

also $S_N(2)$ is the same thing as $S(\tau_+)$. This quantity $S_N(2)$ is the initial condition for the solution of the logistic differential equation in the time interval $(\tau, 2\tau)$. Just prior to the third exposure the surviving fraction is given by

$$S(2\tau) = S(2\tau_{-}) = S_N(2)/(S_N(2) + [1 - S_n(2)]\exp\{-(2\tau - \tau)/g\}).$$

Hence, immediately after the third exposure the surviving fraction is

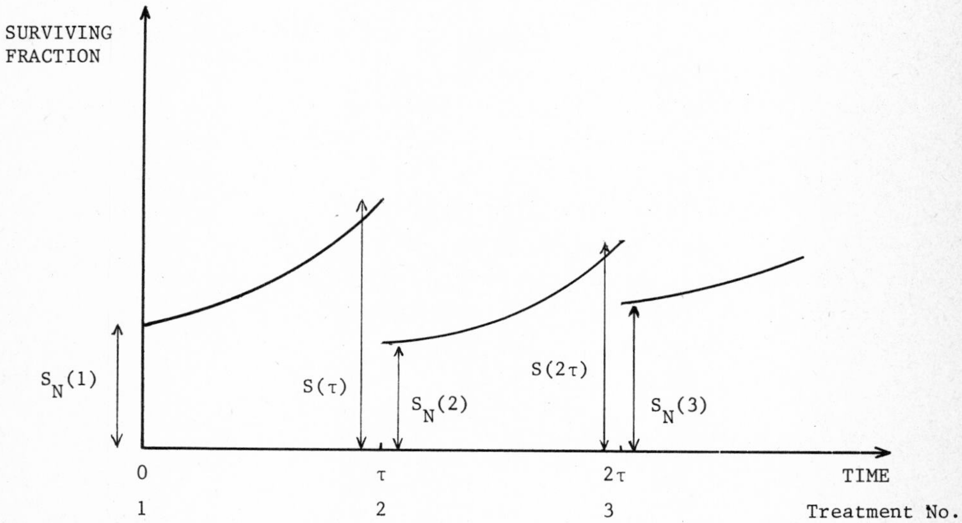

Figure 5.3 Geometrical representation of cellular surviving fractions after instantaneous cell death, under a uniform fractionation schedule. When cellular recovery is by logistic growth according to (5.10) the the surviving fraction immediately after the Kth treatment is given by (5.11).

$$S_N(3) = S_N(1)\, S(2\tau)$$

$$= S_N(1) \cdot \frac{S_N(1)}{S_N(1) + [1 - S_N(1)]e^{-\tau/g}} \cdot \frac{S_N(1)}{S_N(2) + [1 - S_N(2)]e^{-\tau/g}} .$$

It is evident that immediately after the Kth exposure the surviving fraction for the normal tissue is

$$S_N(K) = [S_N(1)]^K \prod_{i=1}^{K-1} \frac{1}{S_N(i) + [1 - S_N(i)]e^{-\tau/g}}$$

$$= \prod_{i=1}^{K-1} \frac{S_N(1)}{S_N(i) + [1 - S_N(i)]e^{-\tau/g}} . \qquad (5.11)$$

In this result the notation $S_N(1)$ represents a survival expression of the form (3.1) or some other appropriate expression. The result (5.11) in a different notation is given, for example, in Cohen and Scott (1968). In the next section the quantity g, which occurs in (5.11), is taken as the mean generation time for an unrestricted regenerating skin-cell population.

The mathematical result (5.11) for the surviving fraction for the normal tissue immediately after the Kth exposure is true when the cellular recovery is by logistic growth according to (5.10). Use of such a formula is consistent with the increase in the level of the normal tissue cell population due to repair or restitution, Andrews (1968, 1978a) following one day after irradiation of the tissue. During the first day (24 hr.) after irradiation a survival expression of the form (2.1) or (3.1), etc. is more appropriate. For example, see Figure 5.3,,

$$S_N(2) = S_N(1)\ S(\tau)$$

$$\equiv S_N(1)[1 - (1 - e^{-kD})^n],$$

where the multitarget single-hit survival expression (2.1) has been substituted for $S(\tau)$.

5.4 Cohen's Cell Population Kinetics Programs

Over the last decade Cohen and his coworkers have generated a number of computer programs for use in their analysis of fractionation schemes. Their early programs have been improved in terms of logic and scientific content. The latter information reflects better knowledge of cell survival data and cell kinetic parameters for a number of different tissue types. One of Cohen's objectives is to determine optimal fractionation schemes which can eventually be applied in human clinical radiology. The various algorithms allow research workers and clinicians to compute cellular lethality in irradiated tissues when the dosage, number of fractions, treatment time and field-size or tumor-volume are known, and a set of acceptable values for cellular radio sensitivity and repopulation parameters is available. The general outline and content of some of these programs are examined in the present section.

For ease of identification with some of Cohen's notation write the survival probability after a dose D rads in the form (c.f. (2.4))

$$S(D) = \exp(-JD)[1 - \{1 - \exp(-k_2D)\}^n] \qquad (5.12)$$

$$\simeq n \exp[-(J + k_2)D],$$

on expansion of $\{ \}^n$ by the binomial theorem. Here,

$J \equiv$ a single-hit radiosensitivity constant, defining the initial slope of the cellular lethality curve,
$k_2 \equiv$ the multitarget radiosensitivity constant,
$D_o = 1/(J + k_2) \equiv$ mean cellular lethal dose,
$n \equiv$ extrapolation number.

(Instead of k_2 Cohen uses K; however we have consistently used K to represent total number of fractions.) Cohen also introduces the following quantities:

$G \equiv$ the number of available cell divisions (cell-cycles). This is a repopulation limiting factor and reflects the assumption that there is not an indefinite regrowth of tissue,
$Y \equiv$ field-size dependent exponent which corrects the effect of a given treatment for the influence of field size of both normal tissues and tumors.

For example, if Z is a (linear) measure of the field diameter, which in turn is proportional to the treated tumor volume, then the surviving cell population is proportional to Z^Y. Cohen (1971) indicates that Y must be positive for tumors, and, if the number of cells is proportional to the tumor volume, it should have a value of 3 approximately. On the other hand Y values are negative for normal tissues, since larger fields generally react to smaller doses. It is uncertain what this relationship means physically. Introduce (However, see the discussion concerning (5.14).)

$$Q = \log S,$$

with S denoting the cellular surviving fraction. Define the equivalent single dose D_1 by

$$D_1 = D_o \, \ell n(n/S),$$

which is just the result (2.3) with $k = 1/D_o$. Substitution of the expression for S(D) into (5.3) gives the fraction of cells which survive the whole treatment schedule.

In his 1968 paper Cohen takes the natural logarithm of this cellular surviving fraction and denotes the result by the symbol Q. He increases the extrapolation number in integer steps while the remaining parameters J, k_2 and λ (the growth rate) are adjusted in a sequential manner. The effect of doing all this results in a system of m equations. It is straightforward to determine from this system the quantity

$$q = \sum_{i=1}^{m} Q_i^2 - \left[\frac{1}{m} \sum_{i=1}^{m} Q_i \right]^2 .$$

By means of a computer program, see Cohen (1968, p. 524) for a flow chart, "best fitting" values of J, k_2, λ, n and Q are obtained for those solutions in which the quantity q and the coefficient of variation lie beneath specified limits. It is interesting that there are no solutions with zero or minimal values of J or k_2, which lends support to the usage of the two component survival equation. The analysis estimates the following parameter values corresponding to 200 kVp X-rays:

normal skin cells: $J = 0.004\ \text{rad}^{-1}$, $k_2 = 0.007\ \text{rad}^{-1}$, $n = 27$, $\lambda = (5\ \text{days})^{-1}$,

tumor cells: $J = 0.004\ \text{rad}^{-1}$, $k_2 = 0.005\ \text{rad}^{-1}$, $n = 25$, $\lambda = (20\ \text{days})^{-1}$.

The main conclusions of the study are (i) that human skin can tolerate a dose of ionizing radiation which is of sufficient size to reduce the cell population to a small fraction, between 10^{-5} and 10^{-7} of its normal level, and (ii) that there is an apparent cure of epidermoid cancers when the surviving fraction is reduced to between 10^{-8} and 10^{-10}.

Cohen and Scott (1968) consider the effect of a uniform radiation schedule on normal tissue, using an expression like (5.11), and on the growth of a tumor using the result (5.3). In each case appropriate parameter values are assigned and the multitarget, single-hit survival expression (2.1) is used. The quantity g ($\equiv \lambda^{-1}$), see (5.11), is the mean generation time for an unrestricted regenerating skin-cell population. From the numerical calculation of $S_N(K)$ to the tolerance levels for small, medium and large fields, for a given fixed value of τ, the iso-effect curves can be determined. The main reason for doing this is that the computed iso-effect curves may suggest new fractionation schemes of practical importance. It is interesting that the computed iso-effect curves for normal tissue agree quite well with empirical dose-time combinations based on skin tolerance data; see Cohen (1968). There is also a close correspondence between the computed iso-effect curves for epidermoid cancer and the observed tumor-lethal dosage levels. They also introduce skin tolerance limits in terms of the cellular surviving fraction S (see Table 5.1).

When there are four days between treatments the tolerance limits of the normal tissue are lower than those for daily treatments. This suggests that the model is probably not valid for intervals of this length and longer. Some estimate of the

	small fields (<75 cm^2)	medium fields (75-150 cm^2)	large fields (>150 cm^2)
S	$\leq 10^{-7}$	$\leq 2 \times 10^{-6}$	$\leq 4 \times 10^{-5}$

Table 5.1 Skin tolerance limits.

effects of continuous irradiation can be made by progressively shortening the interval between treatments.

By comparing the survival fraction of normal cells $S_N(i)$ for constant surviving fraction of tumor cells $S_T(i)$, or vice versa, it is possible to assess the relative efficacies of different treatments. For the treatment that produces a lower $S_T(i)$ for constant $S_N(i)$ a higher cure-rate is expected. However, a treatment that yields a larger $S_N(i)$ for constant $S_T(i)$ results in fewer complications.

In a subsequent paper Cohen (1971) examines fractionated radiation therapy based on the survival expression (5.11). His analysis utilizes four separate data sets for skin tolerance, lung fibrosis, radiation damage to the central nervous system, and irreparable injury to the intestinal tract. Within each data set there is a list of a number of different fractionation schemes and each of those is associated with a given number of patients exposed, and a proportion of them indicates the particular reaction under study. The input variables for each treatment scheme are the dose level D, the number of fractions K, the overall treatment time T, the equivalent field diameter Z, the number M_1 of cases reacting and the number M_2 of cases not reacting, in each entry.

Earlier calculations by Cohen are based on the use of (5.11) in which the asymptotic level reached after each fraction is taken to be unity. In the present case this level is denoted by the symbol H and is not necessarily taken to be unity. Since H can be expected to vary after recovery and before each successive fraction, it is reasonable to let it depend on the fraction number. Hence (5.11) takes the modified form

$$S_N(K) = \prod_{i=0}^{K-1} \frac{S_N(1)\, H(i)}{S_N(i) + [H(i) - S_N(i)]\exp\{-H(i)\tau/g\}}, \tag{5.13}$$

with $S_N(0) = 1$ and $H(0) = 1$. However it is not evident how to select the structural form or magnitude of H(i). Cohen (1971) suggests that

$$H(i) = (\exp G) \prod_{j=1}^{i} S_N(j),$$

and this expression is used in conjunction with the previous displayed formula for the determination of the final cellular survival fraction after K radiation fractions with $S_N(1)$ denoting the two component model (2.4). (This form for the asymptotic level H(i) is used by Cohen in subsequent papers. However, Cohen (1978b) and Cohen and Moulder (1978) suggest that a more realistic representation is given by

$$H(i) = \min\,[1,\ 2^G \prod_{j=1}^{i} (1/\rho_j)],$$

where

$$\rho_j = H(j)/\{S_N(j) + [H(j) - S_N(j)]\exp(-\tau/g)\}.$$

But more work is required to determine a satisfactory form for H(i).) The difference R between $S_N(K)$ and the appropriate tolerance limit from Table 5.1 can be computed and a sum of squares can be formed in the manner

$$\sum_i C_i R_i^{\,2},$$

where each coefficient C_i is chosen according to the rule

$$C_i = \begin{cases} M_{1i}, & \text{if } R_i > 0, \\ M_{2i}, & \text{if } R_i < 0. \end{cases}$$

By proceeding to reduce the "sum of squares" it is possible by this means to obtain "best-fitting" numerical values of the seven parameters G, J, k_2, λ, n, Q = log S, and Y. These are given in Table II, p. 423 of Cohen (1971); note that his symbol L ≡ growth constant, λ. Other numerical values for parameters, such as the mean cellular lethal dose D_o, are also given in his Table II. Some of the parameter values are given in Table 5.2.

Parameters	Skin	Nerve	Lung	Gut
J rad^{-1}	0.0025	0.0022	0.0035	0.0026
k_2 rad^{-1}	0.0044	0.0049	0.0054	0.0047
λ day^{-1}	0.32	0.09	0.16	0.13
n	11	15	12	21
G cycles	6	18	16	18
Y	-0.36	-	-	-
Q	-4.1	-4.0	-3.0	-3.7

Table 5.2 Best fit parameter values for cell population kinetic model used in fractionated therapy; Cohen (1971), with permission.

The results in Table 5.2 indicate that the mean cellular lethal dose (=1/(J+K)) is of the order of 130 ± 15 rads. Also, J/K is approximately 1/2 and this suggests that one-third of the effect is due to irreparable damage (single-hit component in

(2.4)). Although the values of the extrapolation numbers are large they do lie well within the experimentally observed range. The computed λ values imply regenerative doubling times between two and eight days, which are compatible with experimental data on the cycle time for regenerating squamous epithelium.

The nature of the process involved in the determination of the parameters suffers from the deficiency that any group of them which produces a statistically acceptable fit with a given set of data will, in all probability, generate the identical iso-effect function. A probit analysis shows that median log-surviving fractions at which level fifty percent of cases would react lie consistently between -3 and -4. (Probit analysis of statistical data has been utilized during the first half of this century. However, more current attention is placed on the use of logistic regression models; see, e.g., Fischer and Fischer (1977)).

Figure 5.4 is taken from Cohen (1973a) and illustrates the potential for delivering an optimal dosage to the tumor. This illustrative example concerns the repeated irradiation of normal skin and mammary carcinoma.

There is an initial rapid regeneration of the depleted skin cell population to regain its homeostatic level. This produces a differential effect (divergence of the two curves). As irreparable effects accumulate there is a progressive loss of regenerative capacity and the two curves gradually approach each other as the treatment continues. Visually it is evident that an optimal therapeutic ratio exists at some intermediate number of fractions. Also, the iso-effect curves are non-linear and possess different curvatures. Their relative configurations indicate that there is a well-defined zone of intermediate times in which normal tissue tolerance exceeds the tumor lethal dose.

Implementation of a procedure to select the greatest value of the therapeutic ratio is hampered, in practice, by statistical uncertainties. For example the iso-effect curves for normal tissues and tumors represent loci of median values within a distribution of dose-response levels, and consequently there is the need to compare two probabilities. Cohen's treatment of the determination of these probabilities logically follows the work of Prewitt (1972) and Moore and Mendelsohn (1972) and is discussed in detail later in Section 8.2.

Cohen (1975) presents details on six computer programs for practical use in radiation therapy. These programs have as their basis the cell population kinetics models considered earlier in this section. They are also used in conjunction with a subprogram, CELKIL, which simulates a course of fractionated radiation therapy and determines the absolute log-surviving-fraction given the total dose, number of fractions, total time, field size and six parameters. The subprogram CELKIL has been updated and a newer version was published by Cohen (1978a); see below. Also in 1975 Cohen and Redpath updated the method for the determination of parameters for use with the single-hit multitarget cellular lethality model. Their work was published in Cohen and Redpath (1977); see Cohen (1978a), and the discussion later in this

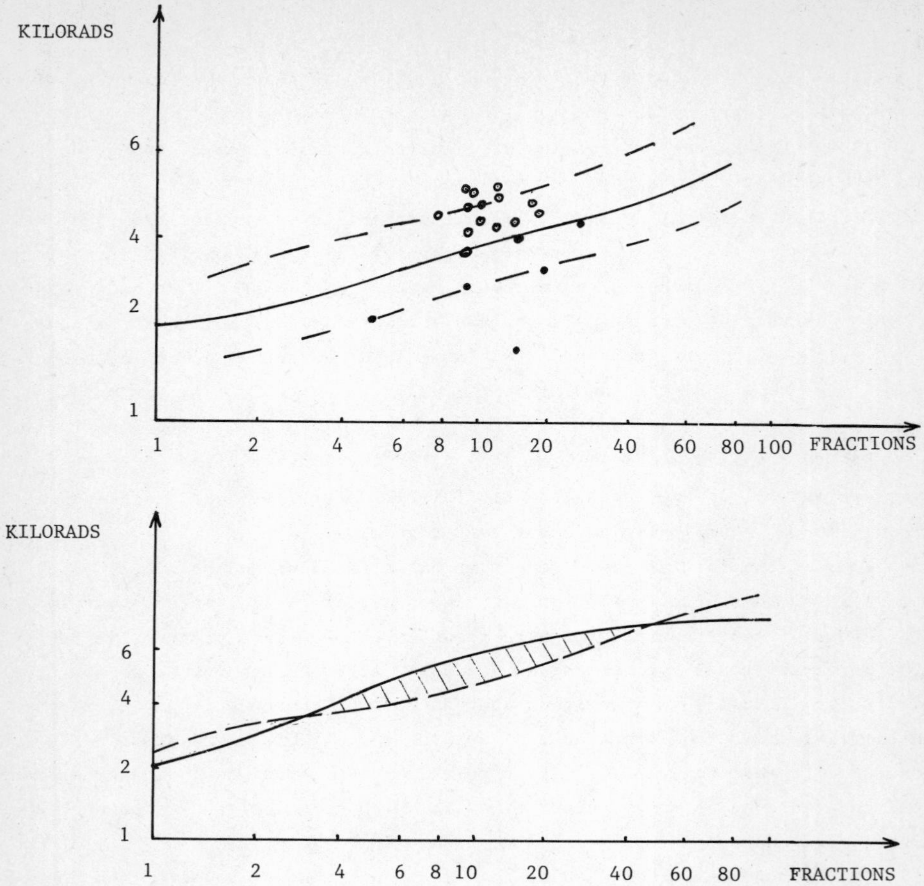

Figure 5.4 Computer-generated iso-effect curves for mammary carcinoma (Q = log S = -6, heavy line; plus or minus one standard deviation, broken lines). Open circles represent curves, solid circles recurrences, following irradiation of skin nodules in a series of patients (upper diagram). The lower graph illustrates the same function (broken line) superimposed on a similar iso-effect curve for normal skin (solid line). Therapeutic ratios are acceptable in zone centered around 20 fractions. Cohen (1973a), with permission.

section.

So far in the present section there have been two different expressions for the symbol Q. These different values for Q have been used in the eralier published work by Cohen up to and including Cohen (1973). Cohen (1975) introduced

$$Q = -\log S, \tag{5.14}$$

and referred to Q as being a standard biological measure of radiation effect. The value of Q given by (5.14) is the one that will subsequently be used in the various computer programs. The logarithm is taken to the base 10.

Cohen (1978a) considers the single-hit multitarget expression (5.12) with U representing the average radiation dose per fraction; his U has the same interpretation as the symbol D in (5.12). Instead of τ (see Figure 5.3) in the computer program (described below) use

$$V = \frac{\text{total treatment time, T}}{\text{number of equal fractions, K}} \text{ (days)}.$$

Figure 5.5 shows the version of the subprogram CELKIL for use with (5.12). The symbol N denotes the extrapolation number n and L (a regeneration rate constant, day^{-1}) denotes the reciprocal of the quantity g in (5.12). An array of six parameters ($P_1=D_o$, $P_2=N$, $P_3=L$, $P_4=k_2/J$, $P_5=G$, and $P_6=Y$) is designated by P. The subprogram is called by a statement of the type

```
Q = CELKIL (P,D,(T-1)/(K-1),Z,INT(K),$),
```

with $ being a logical variable (true for tumors, false for normal tissues). Line 0001 (Figure 5.5) contains the array P and the arguments in the subprogram. The recursive product in (5.13) is handled via the statements in lines 0020 and 0025. In the computer program of Cohen (1978a) the repopulation limit G is selected as G = $\exp(P_5)$. However, in a more recent version Cohen (1979) has $G = 2^{P_5}$, since it was felt that the number of cell divisions was an easier concept to appreciate than mean cell cycle times; see Figure 5.5. Initially $G = 2^{P_5}$ and diminishes successively with each fraction. Also H is correspondingly reduced when G < 1 in normal tissue, but that both G and H are unaltered for tumors.

Instead of (5.12) it is possible to use the exponential quadratic survival function (3.1). Cohen (1978a) defines an effective D_o for this model as

$$D_o = [\alpha^* + (\beta^*)^{1/2}]^{-1}.$$

An option to use (3.1) with this expression for D_o is available in CELKIL.

A considerably more detailed version of the subprogram (available from Dr. Cohen) is needed to take into consideration a split course of irregularly fractionated procedures, alternating-field fractionation schemes, variation in relative biological effectiveness and oxygen enhancement ratios. The presence of radiation-resistant components of the tumor cell population introduce additional complexities into the subprogram. (The next section examines a model of radiation therapy with resistant and sensitive cell populations. Section 6.4 contains a model involving hypoxic cells.)

```
      FUNCTION CELKIL (P,U,V,Z,N,T)
C     * CELKIL (VERSION 1) COMPUTES LOG(S) GIVEN FRACTIONS (N), DOSE/FR (U),
C     *AV. INTV(V) & SIZE(Z). LOGICAL T=TUMOR, .NOT.T=NORMAL TISSUES.
C     *P: 1=D/0; 2 =EXTR.N;3=REGEN.L;4=RATIO K/J;5=ASYMP.G:6=SIZE-EXP.Y.
C     *EXPONENTIAL-QUADRATIC OPTION WHEN P(2)<0;J=ALPHA,K=SQRT(BETA)

      REAL P(6), UJ*8, UK*8
      LOGICAL*1 T
      CELKIL = 20
      IF (P(1).LE.0.) RETURN
      S = 1
      H = 1
      G = 2.**P(5)
      Y = -U

C     *ADJUSTMENT FOR FIELD-SIZE (Y) OR TUMOR-VOLUME (S).

      IF(Z.LE.0.OR.P(6).LE.0.) GO TO 1
      IF(T) S=Z**P(6)
      IF(.NOT.T) Y=Y*(0.1(Z)**P(6)

C     *S1=SURVIVAL FOR 1 FRACTION: R1=REGENERATION OVER 1 INTERVAL.

    1 UJ = Y/(P(1) + P(1)*P(4))
      UK = UJ*P(4)
      IF(UK+UK*DMAX1 (1.D+0,P(2)*UK).LT.-5.D+1) RETURN
      IF(P(2).GT.0.) S1=DEXP(UJ)*(1.-(1.-DEXP(*K))**P(2))    MULTAR
      IF(P(2).LT.0.) S1=DEXP(UJ-UK*UK)                       EXPQAD
      IF(T)H=S+G
      R1 = EXP(-P(3)*V/H)

C     * RECURSIVE LOGISTIC REGENERATION FUNCTION: R2 = REPOPULATION

      DO 3 J=1,N
      IF(S.LT.1.E-20) RETURN
      R2=H/ (S+(H-S)*R1**H)
      IF(G.LT.1.) H=AMAX1(G,S)
      IF(.NOT.T)G=G/R2
    3 S = S*S1*R2
      CELKIL = -ALOG10(S)
      RETURN
      END
```

Figure 5.5 Subprogram CELKIL; Cohen (1978a; revised 1979)

More recently Cohen (1978c) gives a summary of his computer program RAD3, which can be used to derive estimates of cell population kinetic parameters from clinical statistical data. These parameters (introduced earlier in this section) are the mean cellular lethal dose, the extrapolation number, the ratio of sublethal to irreparable events, the regeneration rates, the repopulation limit (cell cycles) and a field-size or tumor-volume factor. For applications see Cohen and Moulder (1978) and Redpath et al. (1978).

5.5 A Model of Radiation Therapy with Resistant and Sensitive Cell Populations

Previous analyses of the use of formulae like (5.7) assumed that the total tumor cell population was susceptible to irreparable damage after being irradiated. In the present section two separate cellular populations are considered to account for the variations in cell sensitivity to radiations at different phases of the cell cycle. Differential equations are written for the two different populations and it is shown how to relate their solutions to continuous or fractionated radiation therapy.

The material in this section is based on the work of Brown et al. (1974). Although their approach and results involve the use of the survival function (2.4) the present development is constructed in such a manner that only when it becomes necessary to use an appropriate survival function is it introduced. In this way it is hoped that the structure of the approach will be evident.

There are a number of results from experiments which note a varying sensitivity during the cell cycle; see, for example, Whitemore et al. (1965) and Mauro and Madoc-Jones (1969). One way to approximate this variation is to regard the cell cycle as consisting of just two phases, one of which consists of radiation-sensitive cells and the other with cells which are much less sensitive to radiation (sometimes referred to as "radiation resistant"); see Figure 5.6.

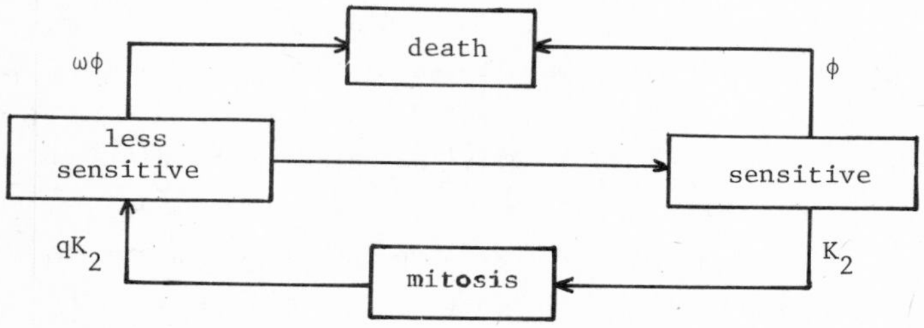

Figure 5.6 K_1 is the rate of progression of less sensitive, "radiation-resistant", cells to sensitive cells, ϕ is the radiation dose rate, and ω is the fraction of the irradiation dosage which does irreparable damage. From the sensitive to the less sensitive "compartment" it is assumed that the cells undergo mitosis thereby increasing the clonogenic cell number by a factor q.

In connection with Figure 5.6 introduce the following notations:

Let

$R^*(t) \equiv$ the number of cells in the less sensitive phase at time t,

$N^*(t) \equiv$ the number of cells in the sensitive phase at time t.

At time $t = 0$ the initial sizes of these populations are respectively denoted by $R^*(0)$ and $N^*(0)$. For convenience in talking about surviving proportions introduce the normalized quantities $R(t)$, $N(t)$ defined by

$$R(t) = \frac{R^*(t)}{R^*(0) + N^*(0)}, \quad N(t) = \frac{N^*(t)}{R^*(0) + N^*(0)} .$$

Define

$T \equiv$ average cell cycle time,

$K_1 \equiv 1/$(proportion of cells in the less sensitive phase of the cell cycle $\times$ T),

$K_2 \equiv 1/$(proportion of cells in the sensitive phase of the cell cycle $\times$ T).

If it is assumed (for simplicity) that K_1 and K_2 are constants then it is appropriate to take

$$K_1 = 1/R(0)T, \quad K_2 = 1/N(0)T.$$

During a short time interval of length dt a proportion $K_1 dt$ of the cells in the less sensitive phase are assumed to enter the sensitive phase and during the same time interval a proportion $K_2 dt$ leave the sensitive phase. This latter proportion enter mitosis and then proceed directly into the resistant phase. This sequence is assumed to be arbitrary.

Now introduce the quantity

$$q \equiv \text{average cellular proliferation rate.}$$

When cells undergo mitosis they are assumed to be replaced by an average of q daughter cells. Here q represents the average number of cells added to the tissue for each cell completing the cycle. A value of 1 for q indicates that the tissue is not growing, whereas $q = 2$ implies that all cells reproduce and there is no loss of any cell from the tissue. The parameter q accounts for the fact that the growth fraction is less than unity and that there is natural mortality in the tumor. A value of q in the range 1.0 to 1.1 appears to be reasonable in view of the (usual) discrepancy between untreated tumor doubling times and cell cycle times.

At low dose rates cell killing is represented by the rate ϕ from the sensitive population and $\omega\phi$ from the resistant cells, where

$\omega \equiv$ fraction of irradiation dosage which does irreparable damage to the less sensitive cells,

$\phi \equiv$ radiation dose rate.

Under continuous irradiation the kinetic equations for the two cellular populations are given by

$$\dot{R}(t) = -(K_1 + \omega\phi)R + qK_2N, \quad \dot{N}(t) = K_1R - (K_2 + \phi)N,$$

with the initial conditions

$$R(0) = 1/K_1T, \; N(0) = 1/K_2T.$$

When the coefficients in the differential equation system are constants then the solution is of the form

$$R(t) = c_1 \exp[(-A + W)t] + c_2 \exp[-(A + W)t], \tag{5.15}$$

$$N(t) = d_1 \exp[(-A + W)t] + d_2 \exp[-(A + W)t], \tag{5.16}$$

where

$$d_2 = \frac{1}{2qK_1K_2WT}(K_1 + \omega\phi - A - W)(K_1 + \omega\phi - A + W - qK_1),\ d_1 = -d_2 + 1/K_2T,$$

$$c_1 = qK_2d_1/(K_1 + \omega\phi - A + W),\ c_2 = -c_1 + 1/K_1T,$$

$$A = (K_1 + K_2 + \phi + \omega\phi)/2$$

$$B = K_1\phi + K_1K_2(1 - q) + \omega\phi(K_2 + \phi).$$

It is easy to check that $A^2 - B > 0$, and hence $W > 0$.

If $B < 0$ then $W > A$ and the populations $R(t)$ and $N(t)$ increase indefinitely as t increases; see the phase diagram, Figure 5.7.

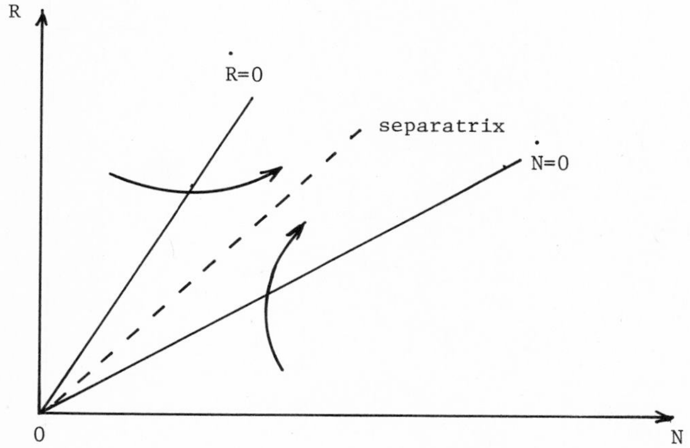

Figure 5.7 Case $B < 0$ (see text for definition of B). Arrows show direction of increase of time.

If $B > 0$ then $W < A$ and the populations $R(t)$ and $N(t)$ decrease monotonically as time increases; see the phase diagram Fig. 5.8.

The fraction of cells surviving a continuous treatment which terminates at the time t_f is given by

$$S(t_f) = R(t_f) + N(t_f).$$

Variations in q (the mean number of cells added to the tissue for each cell completing

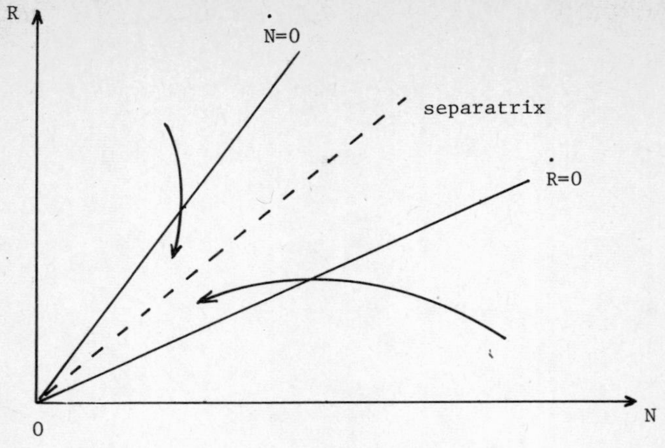

Figure 5.8 Case B > 0 (see text).

the cycle) and t_f allow for the determination of graphs of log $S(t_f)$ versus q; Brown et al. (1974, Fig. 2).

Brown et al.(1974) also consider fractionated irradiation. They set the dose rate equal to zero in the formulae (5.15), (5.16) for continuous irradiation during the time between fractions. Immediately after irradiation

$$R(t_+) = SR(t_-),\ N(t_+) = e^{-D} N(t_-), \tag{5.17}$$

where it is assumed that the multitarget, multihit survival expression (2.4) is used in the first of these equations in the form

$$S = e^{-\omega D}[1 - (1 - e^{-(1-\omega)D})^n].$$

Here ω denotes that proportion of resistant cells which are susceptible to one target killing; $1 - \omega$ represents multi-hit killing. The dose D is in units of D_o. The effect of proliferation rate q on a standard course of treatment by fractionated irradiation can also be determined; Brown et al. (1974, Fig. 3). A comparison of the graphs in the two situations described here indicates that

(i) the efficacy of treatment by continuous irradiation is not altered by very much even if q undergoes a dramatic change;

(ii) there is a significant change in the efficacy of treatment for the fractionated course in which the surviving fraction changes by at least a factor of 100 as q goes from 1 to 2.

When continuous low rate treatment is used the total dose can be delivered in a much shorter time than the case when two high dose fractions per cycle time are given. The above observations are what the mathematical model predicts for the effect of irradiation response of the proliferation rate, q.

When the surviving fraction as a function of the total dose delivered for continuous irradiation is compared to the corresponding result for fractionated irradiation then the continuous irradiation at a lower dose rate produces a lower surviving fraction. This may be explained as follows: The increase in total treatment time with the consequent increase in exposure in the sensitive phase outweighs the effect of proliferation during the incremental time period.

Continuous irradiation gives a relatively greater cell kill than does a fractionated course (as might have been anticipated without the mathematical model) under the conditions that

(a) there is a high target number on the resistant phase;

(b) rapid proliferation (q large) is evident;

(c) the proportion of time in the sensitive phase is large.

Courses of fractionated irradiation are relatively more destructive if

(i) there is a low target number in the resistant phase;

(ii) the proportion of the cell cycle that is in the sensitive phase is small.

5.6 Dose Fractionation and General Survival Curves

Figure 5.3 presents a geometrical representation of cellular surviving fractions after instantaneous cell death when a uniform fractionation schedule is implemented. If the doses are not uniform then

$$S_N(2) = S_N(1)S(\tau),\ S_N(3) = S_N(2)S(2\tau) = S_N(1)S(\tau)S(2\tau)$$

$$S_N(4) = S_N(3)S(3\tau) \text{ etc.},$$

where the suffix N refers to normal cells. However it is apparent that these equations can be applied to other cellular populations. Introduce

S_K = surviving fraction after application of a total dose C in K fractions,

$C = D_1 + D_2 + \ldots + D_K$,

then $S_K = S(1)S(\tau)S(2\tau)\ldots S[(K-1)\tau]$. Also $S(1)$, $S(\tau)$, etc. can refer to any particular expression and do not specifically mean the solution of a logistic equation as in Section 5.3. An alternative way of writing this last equation is as follows:

$$S_K = S(D_1)S(D_2)\ \ldots\ S(D_K) = \prod_{i=1}^{K} S(D_i), \tag{5.18}$$

where $S(D_i)$, $i = 1,\ldots,K$, can be interpreted as the surviving fraction as a function of the dose D_i in one exposure.

From the definition of C,

$$D_K = C - \sum_{i=1}^{K-1} D_i.$$

Define the recovery ratio z by

$$z \equiv S_K/S(C).$$

Then it follows that

$$z = \{S(D_1)S(D_2)\ldots S[C - (D_1 + D_2 + \ldots + D_{K-1})]\}/S(C).$$

One can now prove that the maximum z occurs for equal-dose fractions. Denote the maximum of z by z_{max}. Since S(C) and C are constants for any given experiment

$$S(C)\frac{\partial z}{\partial D_n} = S(D_1)\ \ldots\ \frac{dS(D_n)}{dD_n}\ \ldots\ S[C - (D_1 + \ldots + D_{K-1})]$$

$$+ S(D_1)\ldots\ S(D_n)\ldots\ \frac{d}{dD_n} S[C - (D_1 + \ldots + D_n + \ldots + D_{K-1})](-1)$$

for each value of $n = 1,2,\ldots,D=1$. When $\partial z/\partial D_n = 0$ then

$$\frac{1}{S(D_n)}\ \frac{dS(D_n)}{dD_n} = \frac{1}{S[C - (D_1 + \ldots + D_{K-1})]}\ \frac{d}{dD_n} S[C - (D_1 + \ldots + D_{K-1})].$$

Assume that the functions in this equation are single-valued; then it is possible to equate their arguments and obtain

$$D_n = C - (D_1 + \ldots + D_{K-1}),\ n = 1,2,\ldots,K-1,$$

which indicates that

$$D_1 = D_2 = \ldots = D_{K-1} = C/K.$$

These results can now be used in the definition of C to show that $D_K = C/K$. It follows that the equal doses give $z = [S(C/K)]^K/S(C)$.

To demonstrate that, in fact, the equal doses maximize the recovery ratio one may proceed as follows: If $x_1,\ldots,x_K$ are elements in a Euclidean space and f(x) is a concave function then

$$\frac{1}{K}\sum_{i=1}^{K} f(x_i) \leq f\left(\frac{1}{K}\sum_{i=1}^{K} x_i\right).$$

Now set $f(x) = \ell n\ F(x)$, where $\ell n\ F(x)$ is also a concave function, then

$$\prod_{i=1}^{K} F(x_i) \leq \left[F\left(\frac{1}{K}\sum_{i=1}^{K} x_i\right)\right]^K.$$

In this last result make the identifications $S \equiv F$ and $D \equiv x$ then

$$\prod_{i=1}^{K} S(D_i) \leq \left[S\left(\frac{C}{K}\right)\right]^K.$$

Hence

$$z = \frac{S_K}{S(C)} \leq \frac{[S(C/K)]^K}{S(C)} = z_{max},$$

and therefore the maximum of z occurs for equal-dose fractions.

The requirements of single-valuedness and concavity of the survival curves are satisfied by all such curves known to the author.

The main result in this Section, that equal-dose fractions maximize the recovery ratio, was given by Dienes (1971).

Chapter 6

OPTIMIZATION MODELS IN SOLID TUMOR RADIOTHERAPY

6.1 Introduction

A well-behaved mathematical function like $y = x^2$ is positive for all values of x save at x = 0, where it is zero. The graph of this function is u-shaped with a single minimum at the origin. The minimum value can easily be determined by direct substitution of values of x, from a suitably chosen finite interval size, and comparing the sizes in the resulting values of y. Even when the given function is of a more general and complicated structure, $y = f(x)$, the same type of numerical approach can be applied in general, so long as the domain of x is finite. While this approach may be expensive in terms of computer time nevertheless the method can be used to ascertain the location of local minima or maxima, if any exist, of the prescribed function. The problem of the determination of such local extrema of one-dimensional functions has been examined by many people and numerical techniques for systematically dealing with these problems can be found in a number of text books; e.g. Cooper and Steinberg (1970), Gottfried and Weisman (1973) and Daniels (1978). A recent account and comparison of many methods are given in the report by Garg (1977). These references also include material on the location of a minimum of a function of more than one variable.

For some functions it may be possible to use analytical techniques from differential calculus to locate the local extrema of the function.

Other problems involve the minimization of a function of one or more variables when there exists a constraining relation between the variables. Problems of this type occur in the optimization of human cancer radiotherapy and are examined in this Chapter.

An expression for the surviving fraction of cells after a fractionated course of irradiation was given in the previous Chapter by the result (5.3). During a particular fractionation regime this expression does not provide for some measure of radiation damage to both normal and tumor tissue. Ellis and coworkers introduced the concept of normal connective tissue tolerance--the practical upper limit of any radiation schedule. The Ellis result is based on radiation effects on skin and so is not applicable for other tissues. More recently Kirk et al. (1971) suggested that the Ellis relation could be applied to any radiation effect on normal tissue up to, and including, tolerance. This cumulative radiation effect (CRE), see Kirk (1978) and McKenzie (1979), is designated by the symbol R_F, and is empirically related to the dose per fraction D, the treatment number K, and the time between fractions τ, by the equation

$$R_F = DK^a \tau^{-b},$$

where a and b are dimensionless constants.

Elimination of the fraction number K between this Kirk CRE-equation and (5.3) gives the surviving fraction of tumor cells immediately after the Kth fraction as

$$Y = S^{(R_F/D)^{1/a}\tau^{b/a}} \exp[\{\left(\frac{R_F}{D}\right)^{1/a} \tau^{(1+b/a)} - \tau\}\lambda].$$

The function Y depends on the two variables D and τ and parameters R_F, a, b and λ. With the availability of this mathematical equation it is now possible to ask the following question: What are the values of D and τ (if any exist) such that the surviving fraction of tumor cells is minimized as a result of a fractionated course of irradiation? This problem is analyzed and solved in Section 6.2 when the multitarget single-hit survival expression (2.1) is used. It is concluded, within the limits of the empirical and mathematical expressions used, that the results of minimizing the cumulative surviving fraction Y produce "optimal" schedules which show considerable improvement over those conventional schedules in current usage.

The molecular theory of single and double strand breaks in chromosomal DNA gives the survival expression (3.1). This expression can be used in the minimization of the cumulative surviving fraction Y and this analysis is produced in Section 6.3. The interesting conclusion is that a new "W-schedule" is of benefit for slow or fast growing tumors. A comparison between the W-schedule and a conventional one, when there is a 10 day tumor doubling time, shows no difference.

It is evident that only the simplest of tumor models are utilized in Sections 6.2 and 6.3. A model which tries to account for a significant fraction of the total tumor cell population to consist of hypoxic cells is developed in Section 6.4 This tumor model, due to Fischer (1971a), involves four sub-populations--live-anoxic, dead-anoxic, live-oxygenated and dead-oxygenated cells. Formulae are presented for these four levels for the three phases--(i) after irradiation, (ii) after reproduction, and (iii) after reoxygenation. A sample calculation of these levels is included for illustration.

A simplification of the Fischer tumor model to include just the live-oxygenated and live-hypoxic cells was introduced by Hethcote and Waltman (1973). They formulated a multistage optimal control problem. The solution of this problem has as its objective the determination of radiation fractions for a full course of radiation therapy, which will result in the decrease in the size of a tumor consisting of a total of 10^{10} cells to a situation of less than one cell remaining. First, an appropriate mathematical framework is set up, which allows for the determination of the total tumor cell population after a single dose of irradiation; this leads to the basic state equation (6.19). However the irradiation dosage level occurs in this equation and is not known beforehand. During the recovery period, prior to the next irradiation, the cellular population is assumed to have an exponential growth. It is desired to maximize the surviving fraction of normal cells. The particular statement (6.22) is referred to as a performance criterion. For any given problem there may be one or more possible criteria. The situation of several criteria is examined in Section 6.6.

The mathematical problem contained in (6.19) - (6.23) is in the category of optimal control for discrete systems; e.g. Bryson and Ho (1969), Sage and White (1977). Some problems can be solved completely by analytic means, whereas others need to be approached via numerical procedures. In the latter situation a number of methods are available, some of which work. Various numerical approaches are in the above books and a detailed synopsis with particular examples is given in Chapter 7.

The dynamic programming method of solution of (6.19) - (6.23) was considered by Hethcote and Waltman (1973), and is discussed in Section 6.5. In this method the number of fractions is fixed in advance. At each value of the stage number $i(=1,\ldots,K)$ a selection of values is made for the radiation levels $D(i)$, the controls. This selection is made by guessing ranges in which the control values may lie.

The full equations of the Fischer tumor model are considered in Section 6.6. A conjugate gradient algorithm is introduced to determine the levels $D(i)$ when a cost function comprising four separate "payoff" levels is minimized.

Section 6.7 deals with an extension of the Hethcote and Waltman work to include effects of irradiation on the cell cycle.

6.2 Optimal Radiotherapy of Tumor Cells Based on Cumulative Radiation Effect and a Multitarget, Single-hit Survival Function

The selection of the most beneficial form of radiological treatment for a particular lesion depends on a number of factors. One of these is the provision of some measure of radiation damage to both normal and tumor tissue during a particular treatment regime.

In a series of papers Ellis and his coworkers presented an empirical approach to the rationalization of fractionated treatment regimes. This approach (see, e.g. Ellis (1969, 1971, 1974)) results in the expression

$$\mathrm{NSD} = (\text{Total Dose})K^{-0.24}\,T^{-0.11},$$

where the total dose is in rads, K is the number of fractions and T is the total treatment time. The quantity designated by NSD is a single number, which denotes the normal connective tissue tolerance, and can be used to designate any course of radiation that reaches that tolerance--the practical upper limit of any radiation schedule. The Ellis formula is suggested by the following discussion. Logarithmic plots of the clinical data (total radiation dosage on normal tissues as ordinate, number of fractions as abscissa) produce linear graphs with positive slope of magnitude 0.33. A quarter of a century earlier Strandqvist (1944) had derived a slope value of 0.22 for both skin reactions and for the cure of squamous cell carcinoma. What Ellis did was to use the Strandqvist value to be representative of all tumors to estimate the effect of fraction number only. He used the assumption that compensatory proliferation did not play any role in the response of the tumor. Subtraction of the value 0.22 for tumors from the 0.33 for normal tissues gives 0.11. The value 0.24 occurs because of a change from six to five fractions per week. Ellis concluded that

$$\text{Total Dose} = (\text{constant})\ (\text{time})^{0.11}\ (\text{fraction number})^{0.24},$$

which can be rearranged into the NSD form given earlier.

But it is apparent that the Ellis result is based on radiation effects on skin and so is not applicable for other tissues. For D = 6000 rads, K = 30 fractions and T = 37 days then NSD = 1800 rets. Any other scheme that gives 1800 rets should have the same effect on normal tissue.

No volume effects are taken into account. If one compares various doses then there are difficulties in interpretations. In general the "NSD formula" is adequate, although the most serious inadequacies appear to be for two fractions per week, with the formula suggesting doses which are too high; see, e.g. Bates (1975).

However, Kirk et al. (1971) took the point of view that the Ellis relation could be applied to any radiation effect on normal tissue up to, and including, tolerance and wrote it in the form

$$\text{Total Dose} = R_F K^{0.24}\ T^{0.11}.$$

The factor R_F is regarded as being a (positive) constant of proportionality. They suggested that, as R_F takes on different values, this equation represents the iso-effect curves of a variety of radiation effects with the value of R_F increasing as the severity of the effect. Also R_F is essentially a measure of the accumulated biological effect of successive doses of radiation and for this reason Kirk et al. (1971) proposed that it be termed the CRE (Cumulative Radiation Effect). For a more extensive treatment the reader is referred to the recent book, Kirk (1978).

In practice the differences between the NSD- and CRE-formula do not appear to be of great consequence. Because of author preference the latter formula is used.

Consider a uniform schedule of treatment (repetitive application of fractions of equal radiation dosages D at equal time intervals τ over a specified treatment time). The total dose is equal to the product KD, and the total time (inclusive of the first and last days of treatment) is then $T = K\tau$. With these results, the Kirk CRE-formula becomes

$$R_F = DK^a\ \tau^{-b}, \tag{6.1}$$

where a = 0.65 and b = 0.11. In treatment schedules K is in the range 4 to 60.

This last displayed empirical formula is used in the derivation of every result in the remainder of this Chapter. It is used in survival fraction expressions like (5.3) to eliminate the fraction number K to yield a relation in which the time between fractions τ and the dose per fraction D are regarded as being the key variables for the minimization of the tumor cell surviving fraction.

Consider the following theoretical situation. On day zero a growing tumor receives a single radiation insult. This same fraction of radiation is delivered a further K - 1 times. Then, see Fig. 5.1, under the assumptions of instantaneous cell kill and exponential growth after each fraction the result (5.3) was obtained:

$$\frac{L_f}{L_1} = S^K \, e^{(K-1)\lambda\tau}, \qquad (6.2)$$

where L_f represents the final level of the cell population immediately after the Kth fraction and a total time period of length $(K-1)\tau$, τ being the time between fractions. (If the first day of treatment is included then the time period is of length $K\tau$.)

If the tumor cell has n nuclei one or more of which must be hit at least once to kill the cell then the survival function (2.1) can be used in (6.2) so that

$$\frac{L_f}{L_1} = \left[1 - (1 - e^{-D/D_o})^n\right] e^{(K-1)\lambda\tau},$$

with D_o being the mean lethal dose and n is the extrapolation number. Elimination of the fraction number K between the final surviving fraction and the Kirk CRE-formula (6.1) yields

$$Y(D,\tau) = [1 - (1 - e^{-D/D_o})^n]^{(R_f/D)^{1/a}\tau^{b/a}} \exp\left[\left\{\left(\frac{R_f}{D}\right)^{1/a} \tau^{(1+b/a)} - \tau\right\}\lambda\right], \quad (6.3)$$

where, for convenience, $L_f/L_1 \equiv Y(D,\tau) = Y$ and gives the final surviving fraction of tumor cells explicitly as a function of the dose per fraction and the interval between fractions.

At this point the objective of the analysis is to minimize the surviving fraction $Y(D,\tau)$. This problem can be solved mathematically and some of the details are presented in the following paragraphs. The first report on the present mathematical model was given by Kirk and Wheldon (1974) and a summary of their main conclusions occurred in Wheldon and Kirk (1975); a more extended treatment is given by Wheldon and Kirk (1976). These papers consider a simplified problem in which, see (5.13), K - 1 is replaced with K. In the present description this is not done and various complications arise. However, it is shown below how to reduce the problem and obtain the results in Wheldon and Kirk (1976).

The expression (6.3) involves (i) the parameters a, b, and R_f which refer to radiation damage to normal connective tissue, (ii) the parameters n, D_o and λ which refer to the radiobiological and exponential growth characteristics of the tumor, and

(iii) the quantities D and τ which are basic to the treatment schedule.

The final surviving fraction Y is now regarded as being a function of the two continuous variables D and τ. Necessary conditions for an optimum of Y are that $\partial Y/\partial D$ and $\partial Y/\partial \tau$ simultaneously vanish, which requires that

$$D_o \ \ell n(1 - \theta^n) + aD n\theta^{n-1} e^{-D/D_o} / (1 - \theta^n) + \lambda\tau = 0 \qquad (6.4)$$

$$b \ \ell n(1 - \theta^n) + (a + b)\lambda\tau - \lambda a\tau/[(R_f/D)^{1/a} \tau^{b/a}] = 0, \qquad (6.5)$$

and, here, the quantity

$$\theta = 1 - \exp(-D/D_o).$$

If it is assumed that

$$\lambda a\tau/[(R_f/D)^{1/a} \tau^{b/a}] \approx 0, \qquad (6.6)$$

then

$$\tau = \tau^* = - \frac{b}{(a + b)\lambda} \ \ell n(1 - \theta^n). \qquad (6.7)$$

Thus, the result (6.6) has allowed for the mathematical simplification of being able to express τ directly as an explicit function of θ. It now follows that τ can be eliminated from (6.4) so that θ is the solution of the transcendental equation

$$(1 - \theta^n) \ \ell n(1 - \theta^n) - (a + b)n\theta^{n-1} (1 - \theta)\ell n(1 - \theta) = 0. \qquad (6.8)$$

This is Eq. (13) of Wheldon and Kirk (1976). (Note that there is a printing error in their Eq. (13); $n\ell\phi$ should be $\ell n\phi$.)

Define the function

$$\Theta(\theta) = [(1 - \theta^n)\ell n(1 - \theta^n)]/\theta^{n-1}(1 - \theta)\ell n(1 - \theta), \ 0 < \theta < 1.$$

$$= \frac{(1 + \theta + \ldots + \theta^{n-1})}{\theta^{n-1}} \left[1 + \frac{\ell n(1 + \theta + \ldots + \theta^{n-1})}{\ell n(1 - \theta)} \right], \ 0 < \theta < 1.$$

It is possible to show that $\Theta(\theta)$ is monotonic increasing in (0,1). Before demonstrating this conclusion a preliminary result is needed.

Introduce the function

$$\zeta(\theta) = \frac{\ell n(1 - \theta^n)}{\ell n(1 - \theta)}, \ 0 < \theta < 1, \ n > 1.$$

Assume that it is possible for $d\zeta/d\theta$ to be zero somewhere in (0,1). Now $d\zeta/d\theta = 0$ implies that

$$\frac{\ell n(1 + \theta + \ldots + \theta^{n-1})}{\ell n(1 - \theta)} = g(n,\theta),\ 0 < \theta < 1,$$

where the left-hand side is a positive quantity, and

$$g(n,\theta) = [-1 + (1 - n)\theta^n + n\theta^{n-1}]/(1 - \theta^n).$$

This expression for $g(n,\theta)$ can be factorized so that

$$g(n,\theta) = \frac{-(1 - \theta)^2}{1 - \theta^n}\,[(n - 1)\theta^{n-2} + (n - 2)\theta^{n-3} + \ldots + 4\theta^3 + 3\theta^2 + 2\theta + 1] < 0.$$

It follows that $d\zeta/d\theta$ cannot vanish and hence $\zeta(\theta)$ is a monotonic function of θ. For θ small,

$$\zeta(\theta) = (\theta^{n-1} + \tfrac{1}{2}\,\theta^{2n-1} + \ldots)/(1 + \tfrac{1}{2}\,\theta + \ldots)$$

$$\to 0, \text{ as } \theta \to 0 \text{ for } n > 1.$$

For θ near 1,

$$\zeta(\theta) = 1 + [\ell n(1 + \theta + \ldots + \theta^{n-1})]/\ell n(1 - \theta)$$

$$\to 1, \text{ as } \theta \to 1.$$

On collection of results it is now evident that $\zeta(\theta)$ is monotonic increasing in $0 < \theta < 1$ with $\zeta(\theta) = 0$ $(n > 1)$, $\zeta(1) = 1$; $n = 1$ does not appear to be of any interest.

Consider two values of θ in $(0,1)$ such that $\theta_1 < \theta_2$. Then, since $\zeta(\theta_1) < \zeta(\theta_2)$,

$$\Theta(\theta_1) - \Theta(\theta_2) = \frac{1 + \theta_1 + \ldots + \theta_1^{n-1}}{\theta_1^{n-1}}\,\zeta(\theta_1) - \frac{1 + \theta_2 + \ldots + \theta_2^{n-1}}{\theta_2^{n-1}}\,\zeta(\theta_2)$$

$$< \zeta(\theta_2)[(1 + \theta_1 + \ldots \theta_1^{n-1})\theta_1^{1-n} - (1 + \theta_2 + \ldots + \theta_2^{n-1})\theta_2^{1-n}$$

$$< A,$$

where A is some positive number. The difference $\Theta(\theta_1) - \Theta(\theta_2)$ is readily shown to be bounded below by a positive number by choosing $\theta_1 = 0$, $\theta_2 = \varepsilon$, where ε is a small positive number. Finally, by means of L'Hôpital's rule, $\Theta(0) = 1$ and $\Theta(1) = n(>1)$. Hence it follows that $\Theta(\theta)$ is monotonic increasing in $(0,1)$.

Equation (5.19) is of the form $\Theta(\theta) = (a + b)n$. This equation will have a unique solution Θ^* so long as

$$1 < (a + b)n < n.$$

Upon specification of the normal connective tissue parameters a and b and the extrapolation number n it is easy to check this condition.

At this stage in the mathematical solution only the necessary conditions for an optimum have been satisfied and it has been shown that the optimum is unique. Under the assumption that (6.6) applies then the following statements are true: - With τ fixed an increase in the value of D from zero results first in negative values of $\partial Y/\partial D$ and subsequently, after passage through zero, it increases through positive values. Now keep D fixed and vary $\partial Y/\partial \tau$. The result of doing this indicates that in fact the pair of values (D^*, τ^*) actually do provide a local minimum of the survival fraction Y. It is then straightforward to see that the minimum is also global.

Equation (6.8) is now solved numerically by a suitable root finding method to produce θ^* (and hence D^*) and the result can be used in (6.7) to determine τ^* for a specified value of λ.

For example, take the case of n = 2 and D_o = 400 rads. Define (compare (5.19)) the function

$$F(\theta) = (1 + \theta)\, \ell n(1 - \theta^2) - 1.52\, \theta\, \ell n(1 - \theta).$$

Now F(0.8966) = 0.00274 and F(0.8992) = -0.00347 which indicates that the value of θ^* is in the interval (0.8966, 0.8992). The bisection method gives F(0.8979) = 0.00033 and the method can be continued to give a more accurate estimate of the root. For $\theta^* \approx 0.89855$ the corresponding value of $D^* \approx 915$ rads (after rounding). Proceeding in this manner it is possible to generate graphs, which are rays of constant n entering the origin, of D^* versus D_o and τ^* versus tumor doubling time t_d, where

$$t_d = (\ell n\ 2)/\lambda;$$

see Wheldon and Kirk (1976). Here t_d is identical to the variable τ which they use.

For n = 2, D_o = 150 rads then the optimal dose $D^* \approx 350$ rads. If t_d = 10 days then (6.7) gives $\tau^* \approx 3.53$ or 4 days as the optimal time between fractions. The number of fractions

$$K = [R_f(\tau^*)^{0.11}/D^*]^{1.54} = 16$$

and the expression (6.2) can be used to calculate the fractional cell survival at the completion of the optimal schedule. Wheldon and Kirk (1976) give several tables of numerical results, for an extrapolation number of size 2 and a D_o of 150 rads, which include a range of tumor volume-doubling times from 10 to 130 days, the time interval between fractions and the total number of fractions. Their numerical results indicate that the optimal schedules are considerably more protracted than conventional schedules. Also, as the tumor volume-doubling time increases so does the superiority of the optimal schedules. However this is not significant for those tumors with doubling times of the order of a week or less.

Because of the constraint (6.6) the level of normal tissue damage, as given by R_f, does not enter into the determination of the optimal interval between fractions and the optimal dose. However it does enter into the determination of the number of fractions. The calculations of this Section are influenced by the use of the Kirk CRE formula. As with any mathematical model of the present type it is important to check the size of R_f to ensure that it comes within an acceptable clinical range. Overall, the main conclusion to be drawn from the minimization of the cumulative surviving fraction is that the optimal schedules are significantly better than those in conventional schedules in current use.

More recently, Hethcote et al. (1976) compared five radiation fractionation models by testing their ability to fit a varity of isoeffect data. They demonstrated that the power model, that forms the basis for the Ellis conventions, was inadequate. Furthermore, they noted that the exponential-quadratic survival function (3.1) was judged to be one of the better models.

It is therefore worthwhile considering the use of (3.1) with the Kirk CRE-formula in a preliminary investigation of the optimal radiotherapy of tumor cells, and this is examined in the next section.

6.3 Optimal Radiotherapy of Tumor Cells Based on Cumulative Radiation Effect and an Exponential-quadratic Survival Expression

The previous section considered the situation of Figure 5.1 with exponential regrowth of the tumor between fractions and is based on the Kirk CRE-formula (6.1) together with the cell survival function (2.1). In the present section the results for the survival function (3.1) from the molecular theory of single and double strand breaks in chromosomal DNA is used

$$S = \exp(-\alpha D - \beta D^2).$$

This survival expression was derived in Chapter 3. The Kirk CRE-formula is retained and it is assumed that there is an exponential regrowth of the tumor between fractions.

Define $y(D,\tau)$ to be the final surviving fraction when the treatment schedule is terminated, with, see (6.2) $y(D,\tau) \equiv L_f/L_i$. Then it follows that

$$y(D,\tau) = \exp[(\lambda\tau - \alpha D - \beta D^2)\left(\frac{R_f}{D}\right)^{1/a} \tau^{b/a} - \lambda\tau],$$

assuming that there is exponential regrowth of the tumor between fractions. If it is assumed that (6.6) holds then the solution of $\partial y/\partial D = \partial y/\partial\tau = 0$ produces

$$D^* = \frac{\alpha}{\beta} \cdot \frac{1 - (a + b)}{2(a + b) - 1}, \quad \tau^* = \frac{b[\alpha D^* + \beta(D^*)^2]}{\lambda(a + b)}, \tag{6.9}$$

with $1/2 < a + b < 1$. Introduce the symbols

$$A = \left(\frac{\partial^2 y}{\partial D^2}\right)_{D=D^*,\ \tau=\tau^*}, \quad B = \left(\frac{\partial^2 y}{\partial \tau \partial D}\right)_{D=D^*,\ \tau=\tau^*}, \quad C = \left(\frac{\partial^2 y}{\partial \tau^2}\right)_{D=D^*,\ \tau=\tau^*}.$$

It is straightforward to show that $B^2 = AC < 0$. This means, e.g. Gottfried and Weisman (1973, pp. 37, 38), that the function $y(D,\tau)$ has a saddle point at $D = D^*$, $\tau = \tau^*$. There are therefore no optimal uniform schedules. The fraction number K is calculated from the Kirk CRE-formula; see Table 6.1. It is convenient to refer to this non-optimal schedule as the W-schedule.

Tumor doubling time (t_d days)	Dose (D^* rad)	Interval (τ^* days)	Treatment number (K)	Surviving fraction	Conventional surviving fraction
1	230.8	0.14	17.28	5×10^{-5}	5.4×10^{-5}
10	230.8	1.41	25.51	4×10^{-7}	4×10^{-7}
30	230.8	4.23	30.72	3×10^{-8}	1×10^{-7}
70	230.8	9.86	35.46	1×10^{-9}	7×10^{-8}
100	230.8	14.09	37.66	4×10^{-10}	6×10^{-8}
150	230.8	21.13	40.34	8×10^{-11}	6×10^{-8}

Table 6.1 A comparison of the schedule calculated from (6.9) and a conventional schedule. The survival parameters $\alpha = 2.0 \times 10^{-3}$ rad^{-1}, $\beta = 4.0 \times 10^{-6}$ rad^{-2}. For the conventional schedule D = 200 rads, τ = 1 day and the fraction number K = 30. (Wheldon, et al. (1977), with permission.)

Inspection of the numerical values in Table 6.1 suggests that the W-schedule is of benefit for tumors which grow very slowly or very fast. For a 10 day doubling time there is no difference between the W-schedule and a conventional schedule.

Usher (1980) also examines the work of Wheldon and coworkers. His representation for tumor growth is the equation

$$\frac{dL(t)}{dt} = \frac{\lambda}{\alpha} L(t) \left\{1 - \left[\frac{L(t)}{\theta}\right]^{\alpha}\right\}, \quad \alpha > 0,\ \lambda > 0,\ \theta > 0.$$

Gompertz growth occurs when $\alpha \to 0$; logistic growth occurs when $\alpha \to 1$; exponential growth occurs when $\alpha \to 1$, $\theta \to \infty$; see Swan (1977, Chapter 1), or Chapter 1 of the present book. The survival expressions (2.1), (2.3) and (3.1) are considered, as well as the Kirk CRE-formula (6.1). Usher produces a number of tables of numerical results for optimal schedules.

Recently Wheldon (1979) presents his findings on the fractionation of tumors such as melanoma, osteosarcoma, and rhabdomyosarcoma which have wide-shouldered survival curves. His results include use of the exponential quadratic survival expression.

6.4 Fractionation Scheme with a Four Level Population Tumor Model

Section 1.3 presents some mathematical models of tumors. For the most part these models consist of a description in terms of some measure of the size of the tumor. More realistic tumor models are expected to incorporate several distinct populations comprised of hypoxic and well oxygenated cells. In the present section a tumor model due to Fischer (1971a) is introduced and used in a fractionation scheme. His model involves live- and dead-oxygenated as well as anoxic cells and so involves four subpopulations.

Prior to irradiation the tumor cell population is assumed to consist of live well oxygenated cells at the level L_1 as well as live anoxic cells at the level L_3. After this population of clonogenic cells is irradiated certain fractions of them will suffer radiation damage. These damaged cells will exist in some intact form and will contribute to the bulk of the tumor even though they are unable to propagate. Fischer (1971a) considers death of a cell to be defined when it cannot reproduce indefinitely to perpetuate the cell line. "Death specifically does not imply that the cell has ceased to exist as a grossly intact, metabolizing entity." Experimental evidence suggests that most cells, with the possible exception of lymphocytes do not undergo intermitotic metabolic death after exposure to radiation at the dose levels used in therapy. It is assumed that each "dead" cell disintegrates at its first attempted division. For bookkeeping purposes it is helpful to identify L_2 as the level of "dead" oxygenated cells and L_4 as the level of "dead" anoxic cells. During a fractionation scheme it is therefore necessary to keep track of the four populations (L_1, L_2, L_3 and L_4).

From the discussion in Elkind and Whitmore (1967) it is appropriate to introduce the effect of radiation-induced mitotic delay. The delay time Δt is assumed to be linearly related to the radiation dose D in the manner

$$\Delta t = \gamma D.$$

In a model of fractionated treatment the reproduction of oxygenated living cells and the disintegration of oxygenated dead cells begins only after an elapse of this delay period.

The sequence of calculations in the fractionation scheme proceeds through the three phases of radiation kill, reproduction, and then reoxygenation.

Phase 1: radiation kill

At time $t = 0$ the first radiation fraction is delivered to the tumor consisting of live oxygenated and live anoxic cells. Let F(L) denote the fraction of well oxygenated cells with L denoting the size of the tumor (e.g., total number of cells). Then L can be decomposed into the two levels

$$L_1 = F(L)L, \quad L_3 = [1 - F(L)]L.$$

Assume that the radiation reduces the level L_1 by a fraction S_1 and L_3 by a fraction S_3 so that just immediately after irradiation (compare Fig. 5.1)

$$\begin{aligned}
&\text{the level of oxygenated cells} = L_1^I = S_1L_1,\\
&\text{the level of "dead" oxygenated cells} = L_2^I = L_1 - L_1^I,\\
&\text{the level of live anoxic cells} = L_3^I = S_3L_3,\\
&\text{the level of "dead" anoxic cells} = L_4^I = L_3 - L_3^I .
\end{aligned}$$

The form of the survival expression S is at one's disposal and it is assumed that S_1 and S_3 will, in general, have different parameter values. Note: If prior to irradiation the tumor cell population is assumed to consist of live, as well as dead, oxygenated and hypoxic cells then

$$\begin{aligned}
&\text{the level of "dead" oxygenated cells} = L_2^I = L_1 + L_2 - L_1^I,\\
&\text{the level of "dead" anoxic cells} = L_4^I = L_3 + L_4 - L_3^I.
\end{aligned}$$

Phase 2: reproduction

Assume that the irradiated level of well oxygenated cells has a specific growth rate λ and that the level grows exponentially according to the equation

$$L_1^{II} = L_1^I e^{\lambda\tau}.$$

Here τ is the value of the actual time period between treatments, t, less the amount due to the mitotic delay so that $\tau = t - \Delta t$.

Assume that there is exponential decay of the "dead" oxygenated cells with the same magnitude λ as before. Mathematically, this means that

$$L_2^{II} = L_2^I e^{-\lambda\tau}.$$

There is no division of the hypoxic cells and (using the superscript notation II to indicate phase 2) so

$$L_3^{II} = L_3^I , \quad L_4^{II} = L_4^I.$$

Also, the ratio of oxygenated to anoxic cells is given by

$$R^{II} = (L_1^{II} + L_2^{II}) \;/\; (L_3^{II} + L_4^{II}).$$

Phase 3: reoxygenation phase

Quantities with a superscript III represent cellular population levels associated with the reoxygenated phase. The new total cell population is given by

$$L^{III} = L_1^{II} + L_2^{II} + L_3^{II} + L_4^{II}$$

and, at this point in the development, the right-hand side is a known number. Represent the total cell population as the sum of component populations from phase 3 in the manner

$$L_1^{III} + L_2^{III} + L_3^{III} + L_4^{III} = L^{III}. \qquad (6.10)$$

If the fraction of well oxygenated cells has the same mathematical form as F(L) then the ratio

$$R^{III} = \frac{\text{oxygenated cells}}{\text{anoxic cells}} = \frac{F(L^{III})}{1 - F(L^{III})}$$

can be computed, and R^{III} is thus a known number. Since, by definition

$$R^{III} = (L_1^{III} + L_2^{III})/(L_3^{III} + L_4^{III}) \qquad (6.11)$$

this equation can be rearranged to give a second (independent of (6.10)) equation connecting the four populations.

It is reasonable to expect that the number of living cells at the end of the reproductive phase is the same as the number of cells which are living during reoxygenation; thus

$$L_1^{III} + L_3^{III} = L_1^{II} + L_3^{II}. \qquad (6.12)$$

Assume that the oxygenation procedure is unable to distinguish between living and "dead" hypoxic cells in selecting which ones are to change their state of oxygenation. The consequences which follow from this assumption are now examined. Consider, first, the situation when the proportion of anoxic cells after reoxygenation is the same as the proportion of anoxic cells prior to reoxygenation. That is,

$$L_3^{III}/L_4^{III} = L_3^{II}/L_4^{II} .$$

This equation can be solved for L_3^{III} and this quantity can then be eliminated from the defining expression for R^{III}. Now use (6.10) in the result and again eliminate L_3^{III} to produce

$$\frac{R^{III}}{R^{II}} = \frac{L_4^{II}\, L^{III} - L_4^{III}(L_3^{II} + L_4^{II})}{L_4^{III}\, L^{III} - L_4^{III}(L_3^{II} + L_4^{II})}.$$

There is the possibility of a decrease in the level of "dead" anoxic cells which implies that $L_4^{II} > L_4^{III}$ and hence $R^{III} > R^{II}$. A high value of R^{III}, in comparison with R^{II}, indicates that more cells are being reoxygenated; that is, a move from the anoxic group to the oxygenated group.

However, if the proportion of alive oxygenated cells is conserved, there is the alternative equation

$$L_1^{III}/L_2^{III} = L_1^{II}/L_2^{II}.$$

On proceeding as before, but this time eliminating L_1^{III} and using (6.10), then

$$\frac{R^{III}}{R^{II}} = \frac{L_2^{III}\, L^{III} - L_2^{III}(L_1^{II} + L_2^{II})}{L_2^{II}\, L^{III} - L_2^{III}(L_1^{II} + L_2^{II})}.$$

The possibility of a decrease in the level of "dead" oxygenated cells means that $L_2^{III} < L_2^{II}$ and it therefore follows that $R^{III} < R^{II}$.

In summary:

$$L_3^{III}/L_4^{III} = L_3^{II}/L_4^{II}, \quad R^{III} > R^{II}; \tag{6.13a}$$

$$L_1^{III}/L_2^{III} = L_1^{II}/L_2^{II}, \quad R^{III} < R^{II}. \tag{6.13b}$$

Equations (6.10) - (6.13 a or b) provide a set of four linearly independent equations for the determination of L_1^{III}, L_2^{III}, L_3^{III} and L_4^{III}. Thus:

If $R^{III} > R^{II}$, then

$$L_1^{III} = L_1^{II} + L_3^{II} - L_3^{II}A/L_4^{II}, \quad L_2^{III} = L_2^{II} + L_4^{II} - A, \tag{6.14}$$

$$L_3^{III} = L_3^{II}A/L_4^{II}, \quad L_4^{III} = A,$$

where the symbol A is defined by

$$A = L^{III}/[(1 + R^{III})(1 + L_3^{II}/L_4^{II})].$$

If $R^{III} < R^{II}$, then

$$\left.\begin{array}{l} L_1^{III} = L_1^{II}\ B/L_2^{II},\ L_2^{III} = B, \\ L_3^{III} = L_1^{II} + L_3^{II} - L_1^{II}\ B/L_2^{II},\quad L_4^{III} = L_2^{II} + L_4^{II} - B, \end{array}\right\} \tag{6.15}$$

where the symbol B is defined by

$$B = R^{III}\ L^{III}/[(1 + R^{III})\ (1 + L_1^{II}/L_2^{II})].$$

The manner in which the cell populations from these three phases are utilized is as follows: After a single dose of irradiation determine the four levels L_1^I, L_2^I, L_3^I and L_4^I by means of appropriately chosen survival expressions. Those newly killed cells are then added to the populations of dead cells, as described earlier, without changing the oxygenation of the individual cells. The fraction of cells which are oxygenated can also be determined. This completes phase 1 dealing with radiation kill.

Phase 2 consists of the cell populations after reproduction has taken place through the period of time between treatments, suitably reduced by the mitotic delay time Δt.

Phase 3 now deals with reoxygenation. A new total cell population L^{III} is determined and is used to realign the cell count in order to obtain the proper oxygenated-to-anoxic ratio. The appropriate equations are either (6.14) or (6.15) and provide the initial values of the four cell populations immediately prior to the next dosage of irradiation.

As a numerical example the following expression and values are taken from Fischer (1971a). The fraction of well oxygenated cells is assumed to be of the form $F(L) = \exp(-\mu L)$ with $\mu = 10^{-10}$ and the initial size of the tumor is comprised of 10^{10} cells. Hence $L_1 = 3.68 \times 10^9$ well oxygenated cells and $L_3 = 6.32 \times 10^9$ hypoxic cells. (This particular example indicates that about 63 percent of the total tumor cell population is hypoxic.) Fischer considers the survival expression (2.1) with $n = 4$ and $k = (100\ \text{rads})^{-1}$ for the well oxygenated cells; also $n = 1$ and $k = (250\ \text{rads})^{-1}$ for the hypoxic cells. For the five day treatment week the radiation dose D is 200 rads. Thus $S_1 = 0.441$ and $S_2 = 0.449$ and after a single fraction

$$L_1^I = 1.62 \times 10^9,\ L_2^I = 2.06 \times 10^9,\ L_3^I = 2.84 \times 10^9,\ L_4^I = 3.48 \times 10^9.$$

The parameter $\gamma = 0.005$ hr/rad, the specific growth (and death) rate $\gamma = 0.004$/hr and radiation is delivered at daily intervals ($t = 1$ day). Thus the mitotic delay time $\Delta t = 1$ hr and $\tau = 23$ hrs. Note that if $V(\tau) = V_o e^{\lambda\tau}$ with

$$V(\tau_1) = V_o\ \exp(\lambda\tau_1),\ V(\tau_2) = V_o\ \exp(\lambda\tau_2) = 2V(\tau_1)$$

then $(\tau_2 - \tau_1)\lambda = \ln 2$. If $\tau_2 - \tau_1 = 1$ week then $\lambda \approx 0.004126$/hr. Hence the inherent doubling time of the tumor is about a week. For the reproduction phase

$$L_1^{II} = 1.62 \times 10^9 \exp[(0.004)(23)] = 1.78 \times 10^9,\ L_2^{II} = 1.88 \times 10^9,$$

$$L_3^{II} = 2.84 \times 10^9,\quad L_4^{II} = 3.48 \times 10^9,\quad R^{II} = 0.578.$$

The sum of these four cell populations gives $L^{III} = 9.98 \times 10^9$ and the sizes of each of the component cell populations in the reoxygenation phase can be found as follows. In this example the fraction of well oxygenated cells is given by $F(L) = \exp(-\mu L)$. Hence the ratio

$$R^{III} = \frac{\text{level of oxygenated cells}}{\text{level of anoxic cells}} = \frac{\exp(-\mu L^{III})}{1 - \exp(-\mu L^{III})} = 0.584.$$

It is evident upon inspection that $R^{III} > R^{II}$ and consequently the formulae (6.14) are now used. This results in

$$L_1^{III} = 1.79 \times 10^9,\ L_2^{III} = 1.89 \times 10^9,\ L_3^{III} = 2.83 \times 10^9,$$

$$L_4^{III} = 3.47 \times 10^9,$$

and the sum of these four populations gives the value for L^{III} (and provides a numerical check). The values given in the last display are the cellular population sizes just prior to the next irradiation.

Continuation of the calculations is straightforward and is best done on a computer. It is useful to compute the probability of cure of the tumor, P_c, which is the probability that no cells remain alive after treatment and is obtained from the Poisson distribution $P_c = \exp(-s)$ where s is the expected number of cells surviving.

The present mathematical model has utilized the (inherent) assumption that the level of hypoxic cells is linearly related to the total number of cells present in the tumor. Such a situation may possibly arise if the tumor cells multiply at such a fast rate than an adequate vasculature cannot develop. It is natural to assume, compare Swan (1977, pp. 9-47), that the state of oxygenation of a given cell would depend on its location in a specific part of the tumor. When the tumor size is diminished then reoxygenation of the hypoxic cells would occur. One way in which this is achieved has been described in the present section. Fischer (1978) makes a number of comments in connection with his model.

6.5 A Dynamic Programming Solution to the Problem of the Determination of Optimal Treatment Schedules

The previous section described some of the interactions between the different levels of a tumor model in which there are four subpopulations of cells. In this section a similar, but simpler, tumor model is discussed, and its use in the determination of optimal treatment schedules for radiation therapy is examined. The material of this section is based on Hethcote and Waltman (1973).

In order to simplify the Fischer (1971a) tumor model Hethcote and Waltman (1973) introduce the additional assumption--that cells disappear from the tumor volume when "killed" rather than at the time of the first attempted division. This means, in terms of the notation of the previous section, that the population levels L_2 (the "dead" oxygenated cells) and L_4 (the "dead" anoxic cells) are excluded from the simpler tumor model. As before L_1 is the level of live well oxygenated cells and L_3 is the level of live anoxic cells. Throughout the present section the multitarget single-hit expression (2.1) is used. For the tumor introduce the following notation--

NO = extrapolation number for oxygenated cells,
DO = characteristic dose for oxygenated cells,
NA = extrapolation number for anoxic cells,
DA = characteristic dose for anoxic cells.

The oxygenated fraction of the tumor is assumed to be described by $\exp(-\mu L)$, where L is the total number of cells in the tumor and μ is a prescribed constant; see the discussion on mathematical models for tumors in Section 1.3. This expression approximates to the behavior of the oxygenated cells at small and large values of L. Any other mathematical expression which gives the same qualitative behavior could also be used.

The radiation-induced mitotic delay $\Delta t = \gamma D$ (c.f. Section 6.4) is provided for. Introduce the quantity

$$R = \exp(-\mu L), \tag{6.16}$$

where L is the current level of cells in the tumor divided into RL oxygenated cells and (1 - R)L anoxic cells. The total number of live cells after irradiation by a dose D followed by a recovery time t with exponential growth is given by the expression

$$RL\{1 - [1 - \exp(-D/DO)]^{NO}\}\exp[\lambda(t - \gamma D)] + (1 - R)L\{1 - [1 - \exp(-D/DA)]^{NA}\}. \tag{6.17}$$

During the irradiation of the tumor normal tissue will be affected. Assume that all of the normal cells are well oxygenated. Live normal cells are assumed to be killed according to the multitarget single-hit expression (2.1). The surviving fraction of these cells is therefore of the form

$$S = 1 - [1 - \exp(-D/DB)]^{NB}, \tag{6.18}$$

where DB and NB are the characteristic dose and extrapolation number for the normal cells. As discussed in the last paragraph of Section 5.3 this expression is assumed to account for the rapid sublethal recovery which occurs during the first day after irradiation. After one day then it is more appropriate to use a recovery expression of the logistic type (5.10).

Assume that there are K treatments $i = 1,2,\ldots,K$ with corresponding dose levels D(1), D(2), ..., D(K). Define

$L(i + 1) \equiv$ total number of cells in the tumor after irradiation by a dose D(i) followed by a recovery time t with exponential growth; $i = 1,\ldots,K$.

Hence, on rewriting (6.16) and (6.17),

$$L(i + 1) = L(i)\exp[-\mu L(i)]\{1 - [1 - \exp(-D(i)/DO)]^{NO}\} \exp\{\lambda[t - \gamma D(i)]\}$$
$$+ L(i)\{1 - \exp[-\mu L(i)]\}\{1 - [1 - \exp(-D(i)/DA)]^{NA}\},$$
$$i = 1,\ldots,K. \tag{6.19}$$

Equation (6.18) can be rewritten as

$$S(D(i)) = 1 - [1 - \exp(-D(i)/DB)]^{NB}. \tag{6.20}$$

The basic problem can now be formulated: Assume that the initial size of the tumor is prescribed

$$L(1) = m \text{ cells}, \tag{6.21}$$

with m being the sum of well oxygenated and anoxic cells. Determine the irradiation dose levels D(i), $i = 1,\ldots,K$, such that the surviving fraction of normal cells, see (5.18),

$$\prod_{i=1}^{K} S(D(i)) \tag{6.22}$$

is maximized, and the final size of the tumor is less than one cell, that is,

$$L(K + 1) = \rho < 1. \tag{6.23}$$

with the constraint that L(i) satisfies the nonlinear difference equation (6.19). The expression given by (6.20) is used in the product (6.22).

The mathematical description (6.19) can be referred to as being a system with <u>states</u> L(1), L(2),...,L(K + 1) and <u>controls</u> D(1), D(2),...,D(K). In the language of control theory the present problem involves a system of nonlinear difference equations for the determination of the states. The controls appear in these equations in a nonlinear manner, and when their values are specified then (6.19), with initial condition (6.21) prescribed, can be used to compute the number of tumor cells; the cumulative surviving fraction (6.22) for the normal cells can also be computed. With each dose of irradiation there is assumed to be instantaneous cell kill. While, in principle, it appears that allowable values of $D(i)$, $i = 1,\ldots,K$ may exist, there is no *a priori* guarantee that in fact this is the case. In the present situation it is assumed that a control sequence $D(1)$, $D(2)$,... does exist, which, when implemented in a fractionation scheme, will reduce the tumor of given size to less than one cell. It is convenient to refer to each specific value of i as denoting particular *stage* in the treatment schedule.

Decide on values for the number of treatments K, the initial size of the tumor m, and the final state $L(K + 1) = \rho$, where $\rho < 1$. Since (6.20) is being used it is appropriate to select the recovery time t in (6.19) to be unity, this is done in Problem 1 below.

It is apparent that the applied doses must be selected from a preassigned set $\{D\}$.

<u>Problem 1</u>: The following tumor data are taken from Fischer (1971a, b): $\lambda = (0.004)(24)/\text{day}$, $\mu = 10^{-10}$, $\gamma = (0.005/24)\text{day}/\text{rad}$, $NO = 4$, $DO = 100$ rads, $NA = 1$, $DA = 250$ rads. The initial size of the tumor is assumed to consist of 10^{10} cells.

For the normal tissue the parameter values $DB = 120$ rads and $NB = 4$ are used.

Assume that there are 40 treatments, then $K = 40$. Also assume that the final size of the tumor is 0.9928. Then the state equation (6.19) has the initial condition $L(1) = 10^{10}$ and the final condition $L(41) = 0.9928$. The performance criterion to be used is given by (6.22). To determine the values $D(1),\ldots,D(40)$ the dynamic programming technique of Section 7.8 can be used. The basic iterative functional equation, which is a mathematical statement of Bellman's principle of optimality, for a maximization problem, can be written in the form

$$V(\underset{\sim}{x},k) = \max_{\underset{\sim}{u}} \{p(\underset{\sim}{x},\underset{\sim}{u},k) + V(f(\underset{\sim}{x},\underset{\sim}{u},k), k+1)\}.$$

This equation can be manipulated in order to deal with the product form in (6.22). Define

$$V(\underset{\sim}{x},k) = \ln v(\underset{\sim}{x},k), \quad p(\underset{\sim}{x},\underset{\sim}{u},k) = \ln S(D(k))$$

where

$$v(\underset{\sim}{x},k) = \max_{\substack{D(j) \\ j=k,k+1,\ldots,K}} \sum_{j=k}^{K} S(D(j)), \quad k = 1,2,\ldots,K.$$

Since the control variable $\underset{\sim}{u}$ has elements D(1),...,D(K) the maximization of the product (6.22) can now be expressed in the dynamic programming format:

$$v(\underset{\sim}{x},k) = \max_{D(j)} S(D(j))\, v(\underset{\sim}{f},(\underset{\sim}{x},\underset{\sim}{u},k),\ k + 1).$$

Note that $\underset{\sim}{x}$ is the state vector and has elements L(1),L(2),...,L(K + 1) and that $\underset{\sim}{f}(\underset{\sim}{x},\underset{\sim}{u},k)$ is just the right-hand side of (6.19).

In the present problem, as well as in Section 7.8, it is required to solve the optimal control problem, when boundary constraints are placed at the initial (i = 1) and final (i = 40) stages. Guess ranges of values for each of D(1),...,D(40) and compute (6.22) by means of (6.20) as well as L(41) from the state equation (6.19). With greater refinement (see Table 7.3 for the procedure followed in a non-radiotherapy problem) the dynamic programming method eventually produces the results in Table 6.2. Hethcote and Waltman (1973) used the term tumor bed to describe all normal tissue affected by irradiation of the tumor. Note, also, that the elements in the last column of the table are produced from (6.22).

It is interesting to note from Table 6.2 that, when there are less than four tumor cells left, one needs 256.50 rads to reduce their number.

The results in Table 6.2 indicate that the dose size increases as the oxygenated fraction of the tumor increases and that the dose size is approximately constant when the tumor is fully oxygenated. Initially it is mainly the oxygenated tumor cells that sustain damage and die, since the anoxic cells are more resistant to radiation damage. One might argue that, as a result, there is a reduction in tumor size and a consequent phase of reoxygenation of the tumor. The increasingly larger doses of radiation kill the oxygenated cells as the percentage of the tumor which is oxygenated increases during a treatment course. An alternative explanation of this increase in doses may be that the type of control problem leads to solutions for the controls (doses) which increase as time increases. In the context of a different problem involving the chemotherapy of human multiple myeloma Swan and Vincent (1977) found an increasing pattern in the control variable. The problems considered in the next section also give values of the control which increase.

Problem 2: In Section 5.3 a formula for the normal cell surviving fraction was derived on the basis of the logistic equation (5.9). Hethcote and Waltman (1973) use this equation to write, for $t \geq 1$,

$$\dot{S}(t) = \delta S(t)[H - S(t)],\quad S(t) \equiv S(D,t)$$

with solution

$$S(D,t) = \frac{HS(1)}{S(1) + [H - S(1)]\exp[-H\delta(t - 1)]},$$

Dose in rads	Recovery time in days	Tumor cell population	Oxygenated fraction of tumor, R	Tumor bed surviving fraction
		0.1000E 11	0.3678	0.1000E 01
33.00	1.0	0.9561E 10	0.3844	0.9967E 00
34.17	1.0	0.9148E 10	0.4006	0.9929E 00
36.00	1.0	0.8746E 10	0.4170	0.9884E 00
36.00	1.0	0.8398E 10	0.4320	0.9840E 00
37.57	1.0	0.8052E 10	0.4470	0.9788E 00
39.00	1.0	0.7725E 10	0.4618	0.9730E 00
39.73	1.0	0.7425E 10	0.4759	0.9669E 00
42.00	1.0	0.7123E 10	0.4905	0.9595E 00
44.84	1.0	0.6810E 10	0.5061	0.9505E 00
46.10	1.0	0.6518E 10	0.5211	0.9407E 00
48.00	1.0	0.6233E 10	0.5362	0.9296E 00
51.32	1.0	0.5934E 10	0.5525	0.9159E 00
52.60	1.0	0.5655E 10	0.5681	0.9014E 00
56.85	1.0	0.5353E 10	0.5855	0.8831E 00
61.28	1.0	0.5031E 10	0.6047	0.8605E 00
65.90	1.0	0.4690E 10	0.6256	0.8331E 00
70.73	1.0	0.4336E 10	0.6482	0.8003E 00
79.66	1.0	0.3917E 10	0.6759	0.7560E 00
96.85	1.0	0.3339E 10	0.7161	0.6849E 00
114.47	1.0	0.2659E 10	0.7665	0.5870E 00
138.10	1.0	0.1892E 10	0.8276	0.4588E 00
166.39	1.0	0.1144E 10	0.8919	0.3136E 00
186.00	1.0	0.6089E 09	0.9409	0.1928E 00
216.00	1.0	0.2585E 09	0.9745	0.9922E -01
240.03	1.0	0.8989E 08	0.9911	0.4375E -01
257.24	1.0	0.2688E 08	0.9973	0.1719E -01
258.00	1.0	0.7945E 07	0.9992	0.6714E -02
258.00	1.0	0.2353E 07	0.9998	0.2623E -02
258.00	1.0	0.6966E 06	0.9999	0.1025E -02
258.00	1.0	0.2062E 06	1.0000	0.4003E -03
258.00	1.0	0.6106E 05	1.0000	0.1564E -03
258.00	1.0	0.1808E 05	1.0000	0.6109E -04
258.00	1.0	0.5352E 04	1.0000	0.2387E -04
258.00	1.0	0.1585E 04	1.0000	0.9323E -05
258.00	1.0	0.4691E 03	1.0000	0.3642E -05
258.00	1.0	0.1389E 03	1.0000	0.1423E -05
257.20	1.0	0.4141E 02	1.0000	0.5589E -06
250.11	1.0	0.1314E 02	1.0000	0.2304E -06
256.50	1.0	0.3944E 01	1.0000	0.9094E -07
266.02	0.0	0.9928E 00	1.0000	0.3361E -07

Table 6.2 An optimal schedule with K = 40 treatments. The term tumor bed refers to all normal tissue affected by irradiation. All numbers are given in a computer format with E 09 meaning a factor of 10^9. (Hethcote and Waltman (1973), with permission.)

where S(D,t) is the surviving fraction as a function of the dose D in rads, t is the time in days and S(1) is the surviving fraction 1 day after irradiation. They consider the case when H = 1, which corresponds to normal tissue regeneration up to a maximum level equal to the tumor bed cell population just before irradiation. Since data on repopulation rates between doses does not appear to be available Hethcote and Waltman selected $\delta = 0.1$ in the logistic equation in order that the mean regeneration time (the time required for a cell population increase by a factor of e) during the early rapid regeneration period is approximately 10 days. They investigate the maximization of (6.22), as in Problem 1, but using the multitarget expression with the logistic expression to compute the tumor bed surviving fraction. The solution is produced by means of dynamic programming.

Other results for equal dose-equal recovery time treatment schedules are presented by Hethcote and Waltman and compared with those from Problems 1 and 2.

The overall most important conclusion from the sample computations is that there is a pattern of monotonic increasing doses as the treatment progresses and the tumor becomes more oxygenated. The results of Problem 2 suggest that larger doses with longer recovery times may be the best dose-recovery time combination after the tumor has become well oxygenated. It is interesting that these results vary from the more accepted treatment patterns involving uniform equal dose schedules.

The special nature of the dynamic programming technique is such that the global maximization of (6.22) is obtained. Other techniques which involve the vanishing of $\partial H/\partial u$, where the H function (see Section 7.2) may possibly give just a local maximum.

6.6 Optimal Treatment Schedules in Fractionated Radiation Therapy for Fischer's Tumor Model

The dynamic programming method used to solve the optimal radiation therapy problem of the last section encounters computer storage difficulties when the size of the problem is increased to include the four classes of cell populations in the Fischer tumor model of Section 6.4. Almquist and Banks (1976) pointed out that the conjugate gradient method could be used for the larger problem and proceeded to show results of its implementation. In addition they considered a number of different performance criteria. Their work is examined in this section.

The Fischer four cell population tumor model, as introduced in Section 6.4, is used in the present section. In order to simplify the discussion of the mathematical details and description of the application of the conjugate gradient method to the derivation of treatment schedules it is necessary to introduce some notation. Introduce

$x_1(i)$ = the level of live-oxygenated cells,

$x_2(i)$ = the level of dead-oxygenated cells,

$x_3(i)$ = the level of live-anoxic cells,

$x_4(i)$ = the level of dead anoxic cells,

$x_5(i)$ = the level of normal tissue cells (sometimes referred to as the "tumor-bed").

As in Phase 1 (the radiation kill), Section 6.4, there is the assumption of an instantaneous effect as a consequence of the applied irradiation. Strictly, therefore, the symbols $x_1(i)$, $x_2(i)$,... represent the levels of the cell populations (remaining)

immediately before the next treatment. It is convenient to think of i as indicating the appropriate treatment stage number. These five cellular populations can be collected into a vector $\underset{\sim}{x}(i)$:

$$\underset{\sim}{x}(i) = (x_1(i), x_2(i), x_3(i), x_4(i), x_5(i)).$$

Assume that there are K radiation treatments, $i = 1,2,\ldots,K$, with corresponding dose levels $u(i)$. (The quantity $u(i)$ has the same interpretation as $D(i)$ in the previous section. It is common usage to regard the symbol u as the control variable in optimal control theory. To facilitate the description of the fractionated therapy problem in optimal control theory it helps if the notation of the theory is used.)

Introduce

$\underset{\sim}{x}(i+1)$ = vector consisting of the four cell populations in the tumor, and the normal cell population, after irradiation by a dose $u(i)$, reproduction and reoxygenation followed by a recovery time t

$= (x_1(i+1), x_2(i+1), x_3(i+1), x_4(i+1), x_5(i+1))$.

It is also useful to have the vector of cell populations available at the beginning of the treatment. Designate this as the vector $\underset{\sim}{x}(0)$. For example

$$\underset{\sim}{x}(0) = (L_1, L_2, L_3, L_4, 10^a),$$

where 10^a (a some positive integer) is the number of normal cells present initially (prior to the first irradiation), and $L_1,\ldots,L_4$ are four tumor cell populations as used in Section 6.4. From the discussion in that section it follows that

$$\underset{\sim}{x}(1) = (L_1^{III}, L_2^{III}, L_3^{III}, L_4^{III}, 10^a S),$$

where S is defined either by (6.18) or by (5.10a). The quantities L_1^{III} etc. are computed either from (6.14) or from (6.15), these equations forming the basis for the calculation of $x_1(i+1),\ldots,x_4(i+1)$, $i = 0,\ldots,K-1$.

Assume that some mathematical expression is available which gives a usable approximation to the fraction of oxygenated cells in the tumor. One possible form has been used in the illustrative numerical example of Section 6.4 and is $F(L) = \exp(-\mu L)$, where L is the total number of cells in the tumor; see also Section 1.3. The following description parallels that of Section 6.4.

Phase 1: radiation kill

It is convenient to write

L_1^I = level of oxygenated cells after a single radiation of dose $u(i)$ has reduced the level L_1 of $x_1(i)$ by a fraction $S_1(u(i))$

$= S_1(u(i))x_1(i)$,

where, for the moment, the survival expression $S_1(u(i))$ is at our disposal. In the same way,

$$L_3^I = S_3(u(i))x_3(i).$$

Also the other tumor cell populations

$$L_2^I = L_1 + L_2 - L_1^I = x_1(i) + x_2(i) - S_1(u(i))x_1(i),$$

$$L_4^I = L_3 + L_4 - L_3^I = x_3(i) + x_4(i) - S_3(u(i))x_3(i).$$

Given the values of $x_1(i),\ldots,x_4(i)$ the dose u(i) and the mathematical forms for S_1 and S_3 then $L_1^I,\ldots,L_4^I$ can be computed.

Phase 2: reproduction

$$L_1^{II} = L_1^{II}\, e^{\lambda\tau},\; L_2^{II} = L_2^I\, e^{-\lambda\tau},\; L_3^{II} = L_3^I,\; L_4^{II} = L_4^I,$$

and these quantities are known whenever the tumor growth rate λ is specified. As before, $\tau = t - \Delta t$ where t is the time interval between radiation treatments and Δt is the mitotic delay time.

Phase 3: reoxygenation

The quantity L^{III} is known and computed from

$$L^{III} = L_1^{II} + L_2^{II} + L_3^{II} + L_4^{II}$$

Then

$$R^{III} = \frac{F(L^{III})}{1-F(L^{III})}$$

is known; F(L) being the oxygenated fraction of the tumor. Hence L_1^{III} is a known function of $x_1(i),\ldots,x_4(i)$ and u(i), which, for convenience is written, since $x_1(i + 1) \equiv L_1^{III}$,

$$x_1(i + 1) = f_1(x_1(i),x_2(i),x_3(i),x_4(i),u(i)).$$

Since $x_2(i + 1) \equiv L_2^{III}$, $x_3(i + 1) \equiv L_3^{III}$, $x_4(i + 1) \equiv L_4^{III}$ then the right-hand sides of these last three equations are known functions. Hence it is possible to write in the concise form

$$x_j(i + 1) = f_j(x_1(i),x_2(i),x_3(i),x_4(i),u(i)),\; j = 1,\ldots,4,$$

where each of the functions f_1, f_2, f_3 and f_4 are constructed either from (6.14) or from (6.15). Finally, for the normal cells,

$$x_5(i + 1) = f_5(x_5(i),u(i)),$$

with the particular form of the function f_5 remaining at our disposal. The particular form for F(L) introduced by Fischer (1971a) is $F(L) = \exp(-\mu L)$ and this is also used by Almquist and Banks (1976).

In many control theory applications the performance criterion is often better designated as a cost. Almquist and Banks (1976) consider the full equations for the Fischer tumor model. They include terms in the performance criterion which respectively apportion the "costs" associated with (i) remaining live tumor cells, (ii) damage to tumor bed, (iii) "real" cost of treatment, and (iv) violation of constraints on dosage levels. Mathematical expressions for simulating these costs are as follows:

(i) $J_1 = w_1[x_1(K) + x_3(K)]$. Here w_1 is a scalar weight factor. The sum $x_1(K) + x_3(K)$ denotes the total number of live tumor cells (oxygenated plus anoxic) which remain at the Kth treatment stage. In general K is the last stage at which treatment is given.

(ii) $J_2 = w_2\phi_2[x_5(K)]$, where $\phi_2(y) = [\ell n\ y]^2$, if $y < 1$ and $\phi_2(y) = -[\ell n\ y]^2$, if $y \geq 1$. The quantity w_2 is a scalar weighting factor. The quantity $x_5(K)$ signifies the amount of undamaged normal tissue left after treatment. The smaller the value of $x_5(K)$ then the larger the function ϕ_2 becomes.

(iii) $J_3 = w_3 \sum_{i=0}^{K-1} \{0.5 + (1/\pi) \arctan [0.12\ u(i) - 1.8]\}$. This term represents a cumulative "cost of treatments". With the numerical parameters as shown the arctan function approximates a function which is zero if there is no treatment at stage i and is unity when there is a treatment at i. The idea behind this expression is to drive to zero any insignificant doses, say 10 rads, which clinically are so small that in practice one would not administer them. One is charged an approximate "cost" of 1 (scaled by the weight factor w_3) for the treatment when $u(i) \geq 30$ rads, for the chosen parameter values.

(iv) $J_4 = \sum_{i=0}^{K-1} \phi_4[u(i)]$, where $\phi_4(z) = 0$, if $z \leq 500$ and $\phi_4(z) = (z - 500)^2$, if $z > 500$. This is a "penalty" term, which is introduced to keep all doses within some acceptable range. The maximum desirable dose is assumed to be 500 rads.

A cumulative cost (or payoff) is written as

$$J = J_1 + J_2 + J_3 + J_4. \tag{6.24}$$

To solve for the controls u(i) in the multistage optimal control problem where the cost (6.24) is to be minimized subject tothe state equation in its component form (6.23) Almquist and Banks propose the usage of the second algorithm in Section 7.7, which uses the conjugate gradient approach. Tumor model parameter values are the same as in Problem 1 in Section 6.5. Initial values for the cell populations were

$$x_1(0) = 3.679 \times 10^9,\ x_2(0) = 0.0,\ x_3(0) = 6.321 \times 10^9,\ x_4 = 0.0,$$

$$x_5(0) = 10^8.$$

Eventually, after many runs on the computer in which the weight factors in (6.24) varied it was decided to select the values $w_1 = 100$, $w_2 = 100$, and $w_3 = 50$. These values were used in calculating the schedules shown in Tables 6.3 and 6.4.

Table 6.3 shows a representative collection of results. When the number of treatments K and the period of time δt between treatments is given then the first block of results show the optimal variable-dose treatment programs. The second block represents the final results if one uses the same treatment calendar and the same total dose as in the corresponding program in the "optimal variable-dose program" but, instead of optimizing, gives the dose in K equal treatments. The third block shows results designated "optimal equal-dose programs" and were derived as follows. The same treatment calendar as in the corresponding program block one is used. One then asks to discover the treatment program that minimizes J among the class of all programs (with the given calendar) with equal doses.

Table 6.4 presents the optimal variable-dose schedules for the programs given in the first block of Table 6.3.

	Treatment code number	k46	k53	k54	k59	k72	k71	k82
	K (number of treatments)	10	15	20	25	30	35	40
	δt (time between treatments, in days)	7	3.5[a]	2	1	1	1.4[a]	1.4[a]
Optimal variable dose program	Total dose (in rads)	4167	4635	5135	5669	5687	5968	6150
	Live tumor cells left	7.0	2.8	1.24	0.41	0.68	0.56	0.53
	Undamaged tumor bed	0.05	0.21	0.52	0.82	0.70	0.71	0.73
	Payoff (adjusted)	1638	516	157	29	106	104	120
Equal dose program	Total dose	4167	4635	5135	5669	5687	5968	6150
	Live tumor cells left	21.0	10.6	3.9	0.89	66.9	410.2	3995.9
	Undamaged tumor bed	0.06	0.32	0.82	0.11	25.2	77.4	302.4
	Payoff (adjusted)	2942	1180	381	72	5630	39,102	396,285
Optimal equal dose program	Total dose	4289	4758	5238	5727	6301	6836	7355
	Live tumor cells left	8.6	4.43	1.90	0.55	0.67	0.72	0.84
	Undamaged tumor bed	0.02	0.13	0.40	0.77	0.66	0.63	0.57
	Payoff (adjusted)	2369	860	274	62	83	93	115

[a]The programs with $\delta t = 3.5$ and $\delta t = 1.4$ refer to treatment calendars with 2 and 5 treatments per week respectively. The time intervals between treatments for these cases were {4,3,4,3,4,3,...} for the twice-weekly treatments and {1,1,1,1,3,1,1,...} for the calendars specifying 5 treatments per week (corresponding to daily treatments, Monday through Friday).

Table 6.3 Comparison of optimal variable-dose, equal-dose, and optimal equal-dose treatment schedules. (Almquist and Banks (1976), with permission.)

The following specific conclusions can be drawn from these results (and from unpublished related results):

1. A comparison of the optimal variable-dose program results (first block of Table 6.3) with those for the equal-dose program (second block) with the same dose

Treatment code no.	k46 (K=10)	k53 (K=15)	k64 (K=20)	k69 (K=25)	k72 (K=30)	k71 (K=35)	k82 (K=40)
	364.2	243.9	213.1	202.2	0.0	0.0	0.0
	287.9	223.3	197.3	188.2	0.0	0.0	0.0
	279.8	226.8	192.8	184.0	0.0	0.0	0.0
	351.4	228.6	192.8	183.7	0.0	0.0	0.0
	424.2	232.6	195.8	185.3	0.0	0.0	0.0
	468.7	240.3	201.2	188.0	165.7	0.0	0.0
	489.7	252.1	208.3	191.4	173.9	0.0	0.0
	501.3	272.1	216.4	195.2	178.8	85.0	0.0
	500.9	292.9	224.9	199.1	181.6	114.1	0.0
	499.3	322.3	233.6	203.1	182.7	133.0	0.0
		348.2	242.3	207.0	185.7	163.7	62.9
		382.7	251.1	211.0	187.9	170.4	98.5
		412.5	260.0	215.0	191.6	176.2	130.4
		456.1	269.6	219.1	196.3	182.1	146.4
		501.4	280.3	223.3	201.6	188.0	154.8
			293.2	227.8	214.2	200.8	169.6
			309.8	232.7	218.7	205.1	174.5
			333.7	238.1	223.3	209.1	179.0
			372.3	244.3	227.9	213.0	183.4
			446.3	251.7	232.6	216.7	187.6
				260.8	243.6	224.6	197.3
				272.5	247.6	227.2	200.9
				288.3	251.9	229.8	204.4
				310.9	256.7	232.5	207.8
				346.0	262.2	235.1	211.2
					276.9	241.5	219.2
					282.9	243.9	222.0
					290.4	246.4	224.9
					300.0	249.1	227.8
					312.4	252.0	230.7
						259.5	237.6
						262.3	240.1
						265.5	242.7
						269.0	245.4
						272.9	248.3
							255.2
							257.7
							260.3
							263.2
							266.4

Table 6.4 Optimal variable-dose treatment schedules.
(Almquist and Banks(1976), with permission.)

indicates that the payoff is substantially smaller for the variable-dose treatments. In addition the resulting final values for normal tissue are improved for the variable-dose programs.

2. In comparing the optimal variable-dose programs with the optimal equal-dose programs it is noted that the optimal equal-dose program required a larger dose to produce either approximately the same final results with regard to the surviving normal tissue and tumor (see, e.g., k71, k72), or, as in most cases (see k53), less desirable final values for these quantities.

3. Either the doses u(i) are increasing as i increases (e.g. k71) or in the case of a small number of treatments (see k46) there was an initial drop in the size of u(i) for early values of i after which u(i) increased with i.

An increasing pattern for u(i) was found in the work of Hethcote and Waltman (1973). See the discussion at the end of Section 6.5.

4. Perhaps the most surprising feature in Table 6.4 is the presence of so many zeroes. For example k82 would appear to suggest that one should not treat the patient until the eleventh treatment and then only give 63 rads.

5. The mathematical model, as used by Almquist and Banks (1976) does not include terms which could account for growth of undamaged normal tissue.

6.7 Optimal Radiation Schedules with Cell Cycle Analysis

Section 6.5 presented a simplification of the Fischer tumor model to include two main subpopulations of cells. An extension of this simplified model to account for the effects of radiation on the individual populations distributed through the cell cycle is presented by Ivanov (1978). This work is examined in the present Section. When the total experimental time is an appreciable portion of the cell cycle time then it appears reasonable to try to incorporate the effects of irradiation on the cell cycle.

Fischer (1971a) assumed that the fraction of the total number of cells present in the tumor which are well oxygenated can be represented by the mathematical quantity $\exp(-\mu L)$; see Section 1.3. Define

$$L_{0x} = \text{number of well oxygenated cells in tumor;}$$

then it follows that

$$L_{0x}/L = \exp(-\mu L).$$

Earlier in Section 1.3 the cell cycle model due to Baserga was introduced. The main phases are G_0, G_1, S, G_2 and M. Frequently the last two are lumped together and written as $G_2 + M$. In the Ivanov (1978) work they are kept distinct. Hypoxic cells are assumed to be in the rest phase G_0, from which they can enter the cell cycle and become potentially proliferative. Let ℓ_{10x}, ℓ_{20x}, ℓ_{30x} and ℓ_{40x} respectively denote the populations of well oxygenated cells in the G_1, S, G_2 and M phases so that

$$\ell_{10x} = \alpha_1 L_{0x}, \ \ell_{20x} = \alpha_2 L_{0x}, \ \ell_{30x} = \alpha_3 L_{0x}, \ \ell_{40x} = \alpha_4 L_{0x},$$

$$\alpha_1 + \alpha_2 + \alpha_3 + \alpha_4 = 1.$$

In the interests of clarity the following assumptions are introduced:

(a) The effect of irradiation on the populations of tumor cells in the phases G_1, S, G_2, M, G_0 and on healthy normal tissue cells can be described by survival expressions of the form (2.1)

$$S_j(D) = 1 - [1 - \exp(-D/D_{0j})]^{n_j}, \quad j = 1,\ldots,6. \tag{6.25}$$

(b) There is a mitotic delay of length $\Delta t = \gamma D$ after application of a certain dose D.

(c) There are only K treatments.

(d) Decrease in the population sizes of both normal and tumor cells is instantaneous after a single discrete irradiation.

These four assumptions are precisely the same as those already considered in this Chapter. In addition Ivanov makes one further assumption:

(e) The effect of irradiation on normal tissue consists of two components--reversible and irreversible injury.

The notation R, given in (6.16), for the fractionated portion of the tumor is used here. In using the definitions (6.25), the total number of live cells in the tumor after irradiation by a dose D followed by a recovery time t with exponential growth is given by the expression

$$\begin{aligned} &\text{number of well oxygenated cells + number of anoxic cells} \\ &= R[\ell_{10x}S_1(D) + \ell_{20x}S_2(D) + \ell_{30x}S_3(D) + \ell_{40x}S_4(D)] \exp \lambda(t - \gamma D) \\ &\quad + (1 - R)\, L\, S_5(D) \\ &= RL \exp \lambda(t - \gamma D) \sum_{j=1}^{4} \alpha_j S_j(D) + (1 - R)L\, S_5(D). \end{aligned} \tag{6.26}$$

The first expression in (6.26) reflects the effect of radiation on oxygenated cancerous cells in the cell cycle phases G_1 through M and their post irradiation proliferation after the time delay γD. The second term gives the contribution from the effect of irradiation on hypoxic cells. The complete expression given by (6.26) is just the extension of (6.17) to include radiation effects on tumor cell cycle phases.

In connection with the irradiation of normal tissue a mathematical model introduced by Sacher and Trucco was considered in Section 5.3. This led to the formulae (5.11) and (5.13). After an irradiation the normal cells are assumed to recover to a certain level $H(\leq 1)$, which has been expressed in terms of a number of theoretical equations by Cohen and coworkers; see Section 5.4. An alternative representation is given by Ivanov (1978): Assume that η is the minimum allowable regeneration interval. If, as in Sections 5.3, 5.4, τ is the time interval between fractions then $\tau \geq \eta$. The logistic equation for the surviving fraction S(D,t) of normal cells is

$$\frac{dS(D,t)}{dt} = \frac{S(D,t)}{\rho}[H(D) - S(D,t)], \; S(D,\eta) = S_6(D),$$

where the recovery level H is assumed to depend on the dose D so that $H \equiv H(D)$. The solution is given by the expression

$$S(D,t) = \frac{H(D)S_6(D)}{S_6(D) + [H(D) - S_6(D)]\exp[-H(D)(t - \eta)/\rho]} . \tag{6.27}$$

Ivanov assumed that

$$H(D) = 1 - \psi D/D_{max}, \tag{6.28}$$

where

$\psi \equiv$ fraction of irreversible irradiation damage,

D_{max} = maximum permissible radiation dose.

Davidson (1957) considered the structure of a radiation lesion and its post-irradiation biological restoration. This led him to consider that the influence of radiation on normal tissue consisted of two parts--reversible and irreversible damage. Define

r = constant of normal tissue restoration; dimensions of $(\text{time})^{-1}$.

Then Davidson wrote the residual damage due to a radiation dose D in the form

$$[\psi + (1 - \psi)e^{-rt}]D. \tag{6.29}$$

It appears reasonable in (6.27) to make the identification $\rho = 1/r$. If $N(\tau_-)$, $N(\tau_+)$ respectively denote the normal cell populations immediately prior to and immediately after irradiation by a dose D at time $t = \tau$, then

$$N(\tau_+) = S(D,\tau)N(\tau_-). \tag{6.30}$$

With the assumption that there are K treatments $i = 1,2,\ldots,K$ with corresponding dose levels $D(1),D(2),\ldots,D(K)$ then, on using the same notation for $L(i)$, $L(i + 1)$ as in (6.19),

$$L(i + 1) = L(i)\exp[-\mu L(i)]\exp\{\lambda[t - \gamma D(i)]\} \sum_{j=1}^{4} \alpha_j S_j(D(i)) + L(i)\{1 - \exp[-\mu L(i)]\}S_5(D(i)), \; i = 1,\ldots,K, \tag{6.31}$$

which is a difference equation for $L(i)$. Introduce

$N(i + 1) \equiv$ population level of normal cells after irradiation by a dose $D(i)$.

Hence (6.30) may be rewritten in the difference equation form

$$N(i + 1) = S(D(i),\tau)N(i). \tag{6.32}$$

Equations (6.31) and (6.32) form the basic system. To them one needs to add conditions on the initial sizes of the tumor and normal cell populations.

Ivanov is interested in maximizing the survival fraction of normal cells (6.22). In the absence of any other constraint Ivanov presents a proof (dependent on the special form (2.1) or (6.25)) that the maximum is obtained when $D(1) = D(2) = \ldots = D(K) = C/N$, where C is the total dose given. However a much better proof of this result is in Dienes (1971) who does not need to include any particular mathematical form for the survival fraction.

Table 6.5 shows an example of an optimal radiation treatment schedule and is based on the following parameter values:

$L(1) = 0.819 \times 10^7$ tumor cells (see (6.21)), $\mu = 0.819 \times 10^{-7}$;

$\alpha_1 = 0.53$, $\alpha_2 = 0.41$, $\alpha_3 = 0.04$, $\alpha_4 = 0.02$;

$D_{01} = 160$ rads, $D_{02} = 160$ rads, $D_{03} = 140$ rads, $D_{04} = 120$ rads,

$D_{05} = 400$ rads, $D_{06} = 250$ rads; $\psi = 0.1$, $r = 0.693/3$ (day)$^{-1}$;

$n_1 = 2$, $n_2 = 2$, $n_3 = 1$, $n_4 = 1$, $n_5 = 1$, $n_6 = 5$; $\gamma = 0.01/24$ (days/rad).

Inspection of Table 6.5 indicates that K = 30 treatments and that the terminal condition for the state equation (6.31) is selected to be $L(31) = 0.9812$. The results appear to have been produced by means of the method of dynamic programming.

An experiment involving irradiated extremities of mice gives results which indicate that a uniform dose fractionation reduces the degree of radiation injury to the skin.

Earlier work by Ivanov and coworkers has appeared in the Russian journal Meditsinskaia Radiologiya in 1975 and 1976 but unfortunately the present author has not been able to see these papers.

A subsequent paper, which purports to deal with optimization in radiation therapy, is by Ivanov et al. (1977). They consider a fractionation scheme with assumptions of the same type as introduced in this Chapter. The macroscopic growth of the tumor under such a fractionation treatment is assumed to follow the equation

$$\frac{dL}{dt} = \Phi(L) \sum_{i=1}^{K} [1 - \phi_i(t)] - \sum_{i=1}^{K} L(\tau_{i-})[1 - S(D_i)]\delta(t - \tau^i),$$

Dose	Regeneration Interval	Fraction of dividing tumor cells	Number of tumor cells	Fraction of surviving healthy tissue
120.00	1.0000	0.36788	0.62528E07	0.99196
120.00	1.0000	0.55531	0.37329E07	0.98395
120.00	1.0000	0.70750	0.22220E07	0.97604
120.00	1.0000	0.81584	0.13181E07	0.96818
140.00	1.0000	0.83716	0.71394E06	0.95415
140.00	1.0000	0.91399	0.42064E06	0.94032
140.00	1.0000	0.95942	0.24768E06	0.92669
140.00	1.0000	0.97592	0.14578E06	0.91325
140.00	1.0000	0.98577	85781	0.90002
140.00	1.0000	0.99160	50470	0.88697
140.00	1.0000	0.99505	29692	0.87411
140.00	1.0000	0.99709	17467	0.86144
140.00	1.0000	0.99829	10275	0.84896
140.00	1.0000	0.99899	6044.4	0.83665
140.00	1.0000	0.99941	3555.6	0.82452
140.00	1.0000	0.99965	2091.5	0.81257
140.00	1.0000	0.99979	1230.3	0.80079
140.00	1.0000	0.99988	723.72	0.78918
140.00	1.0000	0.99993	425.72	0.77774
140.00	1.0000	0.99996	250.42	0.76647
140.00	1.0000	0.99998	147.31	0.75536
140.00	1.0000	0.99999	86.652	0.74441
140.00	1.0000	0.99999	50.972	0.73362
140.00	1.0000	0.99999	29.983	0.72299
140.00	1.0000	1.0000	17.637	0.71251
140.00	1.0000	1.0000	10.375	0.70218
140.00	1.0000	1.0000	6.1029	0.69200
140.00	1.0000	1.0000	3.5899	0.68197
140.00	1.0000	1.0000	2.1117	0.67208
160.00	1.0000	1.0000	0.98102	0.65765

Table 6.5 Example of optimal treatment schedule taking into account effects on the cell cycle; Ivanov (1978).

where $\phi_i(t) = 1$ in the interval $(\tau_i, \tau_i + \alpha D_i)$ and is zero outside the same interval. This equation is a generalization of (5.6) which dealt with exponential growth and $\Phi(L) = \lambda L$.

They introduce the degree of restoration of normal tissue, designated by y(t), which takes into account the proliferation delay after application of the dose. Also, a quantity v(t) is introduced, but not defined. The following equations for y(t) and v(t) are presented:

$$\dot{y}(t) = -r[y(t) - v(t)] \sum_{i=1}^{K} [1 - \phi_i(t)] + \frac{1}{D_k} \sum_{i=1}^{K} D_i \delta(t - \tau_i) ,$$

$$\dot{v}(t) = \frac{\psi}{D_k} \sum_{i=1}^{K} D_i \delta(t - \tau_i),$$

where D_i is some critical value for the value of the utilized effective dose and is determined by the stromal elements of normal tissue; ψ and r are the same quantities introduced earlier in this Section.

The paper by Ivanov et al. (1977) then presents a variety of mathematical results in which (2.1) plays a part. Finally, they present a table of numerical values in decimals of the observed effects (such as appearance of weak erythema, beginning of dry peeling, formation of ulcer, etc.)

Chapter 7
NUMERICAL SOLUTION OF MULTISTAGE OPTIMAL CONTROL PROBLEMS

7.1 Introduction

In many engineering problems one is given a known system which has a description in terms of one or more states. Relations, such as differential equations, provide the connections between these states and the input to the system. Often it is desired to determine the control which changes the state in order that some desirable objective be reached. This is a general statement of one kind of control problem.

Prior to the second world war control system design was mainly an art. From the end of the war up to the fifties the theory of servomechanisms developed rapidly. Then began an era of rapid technological change and aerospace exploration. One of the early engineering applications of control theory was to the problem of achieving a satellite rendezvous with another object in space. This problem embodied the classical ideas of optimal control--dynamical system equations governed the motions of the objects in space and an optimal trajectory (the trajectory which accomplished rendezvous consistent with the requirements on allowable fuel and/or time) had to be found. Lawden (1963) describes space navigation topics of this kind.

In the period from 1953 to 1957 Bellman and LaSalle in the United States and Gamkrelidze and Krasovskii in the Soviet Union developed the basic theory of minimum-time problems, and presented results concerning the existence, uniqueness, and general properties of the time-optimal control problem. Bellman (1957) produced his fundamental work on dynamic programming. The correspondence between control problems and the calculus of variations was examined in greater detail. However variational theory could not readily handle many of the constraints commonly imposed in a control problem. This difficulty led Pontryagin in the Soviet Union to conjecture his maximum principle; see Pontryagin et al. (1961).

Modern control theory and practice can be viewed as the coming together of three areas: servomechanism theory, the calculus of variations and computer development.

Within a short time after the initial applications of optimal control theory numerous research papers and a small number of books on the theory and application of optimal control appeared. Unhappily, there is no easy straightforward introduction to the area but the interested reader may care to vent some energy on looking at the books by Athans and Falb (1966), Lee and Markus (1966), Leitmann (1966), and Bryson and Ho (1969). Some engineering students in an introductory course use Brogan (1974).

In addition to the traditional engineering applications, optimal control theory has been applied to a myriad of problems in various disciplines. In fact, the concepts of optimal control theory can be applied to any problem for which the system considered can be described by differential or difference equations, there is some quantity which can be used to influence (control) the system, and some quantity, that is a function of the variables used to describe the system, is to be maximized or minimized. Within this framework there can occur many variants, for example there may be constraints on the control function or on some of the variables which describe the system. (For a brief description of the mathematical formulation of the optimal control problem see Sections 7.2 and 7.3.) This does not imply that optimal control theory provides a simple and routine solution to all problems. There are in fact many difficulties in applying the theory to specific problems. Each problem usually has aspects which require special treatment; however, there are many instances where the approach of optimal control theory has led to significant improvement. Banks (1974) gives a number of control problems in biology and biochemistry. Optimal control theory has been successfully applied in solving problems in the following areas:

1. Epidemic control, Wickwire (1977);
2. Harvesting and control of biologically renewable resources, Clark (1976);
3. Pest control, Wickwire (1977);
4. Endocrine regulation, Stear (1973, 1975);
5. The immune system, Perelson et al. (1976, 1978), and Perelson (1978);
6. Biochemical (enzyme) systems, Rapp (1978a, b);
7. Biomedical engineering, Swan (1981a, b).

The idea of applying optimal control theory to problems in cancer research occurred to the author during the spring of 1975 when he was in the Theoretical Biology Group at the University of Utrecht in The Netherlands. One outcome of this was the joint work, Swan and Vincent (1977) concerned with the chemotherapy of multiple myeloma. This paper appears to be the first application of optimal control to a human tumor problem. Also in Chapter 7 of Swan (1977) I presented the first published survey of the use of modern optimal control theory in cancer research. Problems in theoretical immunology involving antibody production due to stimulating antigen, which have a natural interpretation in terms of optimal control are also discussed in that Chapter. A more recent paper, Swan (1980), examines a number of different performance criteria and the nature of the solution when the control (related to the concentration of anticancer drug) must satisfy bounded constraints.

In human cancer radiotherapy some of the current problems appear to be able to be interpreted in terms of control problems. For example: An externally applied dosage of radiation may be required to reduce a tumor from a certain undesirable level to some other lower (desirable) level. The radiation dosage can be interpreted as the control to be applied at some initial stage in the therapy and the volume of the tumor can be taken as a state variable of the tumor system. Another possibility might be to take some sub-population of cells within the tumor model as the representative state variable.

Earlier in Chapters 5 and 6 a theory was developed for dealing with fractionated therapy. At each new time point a decision has to be made on what the radiation dose level should be. These radiation dose levels are the controls and a control problem can be formulated when something is said about the mathematical model which approximates the tumor model. The control problem also requires that some objective criterion (or performance criterion or cost function) be specified. Many clinicians believe that the surviving fraction gives some measure of tissue response to irradiation. Consequently, as in Chapter 6 (see Section 6.5) one type of control problem is to determine the controls so that the surviving fraction of normal cells

$$\prod_{i=1}^{K} S(D(i))$$

is maximized and the tumor size is below a single cell. A problem of this type comes in the class of difficult multistage multi-variable two-point boundary condition optimal control problems. In the present Chapter is presented a synopsis of some of the techniques which are possible candidates for use in the numerical solution of such problems.

Polak (1973) presents a primarily mathematical review of computational procedures in optimal control theory. A more applications-oriented presentation is given in Sage and White (1977), Chapter 10. Current analytical techniques for solving optimal control problems depend on the costate variable (see Section 7.2). Determination of the value of the costate variable plays a fundamental role in the numerical solution of multistage multi-variable optimal control problems. The technique of quasilinearization is not discussed and the reader is referred to the last section of Chapter 10 in the book by Sage and White (1977). Also space does not permit the inclusion of a satisfactory discussion of nonlinear programming methods for multistage multi-variable optimal control problems; see Canon et al. (1970) and Tabak and Kuo (1971). Some computational procedures in the area of dynamic programming are given in the review article by Larson (1967). A number of applications and survey of numerical methods for their solution are presented in the extensive report by Garg (1977). Gradient methods are of interest and the book by Hasdorff (1976) provides a useful discussion of them. A number of useful features for consideration of the numerical solution of optimal control problems are presented in the recent report by Mehra et al. (1979). Although this report is concerned with applications to aircraft trajectory optimization many of the sections are presented in a framework which can allow for interpretation in other disciplines. Some of the techniques are however based on singular perturbation theory, and as yet that has not found an application in any area of cancer research that the author is aware of.

As more mathematical techniques become utilized in various optimization problems in radiation therapy it is certain that an understanding of the details of the numerical solution of multistage optimal control problems will become of considerable importance. For that reason the author felt that it would be worthwhile to collect in one place details of some of these numerical approaches. Accordingly, it follows that most of the examples in this chapter are of an expository nature, and are of no direct application to the optimization of human cancer radiotherapy. The material in this chapter does not appear to be generally available in other publications. A reading of the majority of recent papers dealing with quantitative aspects of human cancer radiotherapy indicates that they utilize results and the approaches of various portions of this chapter.

7.2 Continuous Time Optimal Control

The optimal control problem typically involves some system whose behavior can be described by differential equations. The first step in attacking an optimal control problem is to convert these equations to a set of first order differential equations. Thus the system equations become

$$\dot{\tilde{x}} = f(\tilde{x},\tilde{u},\tilde{t}),$$

where $\tilde{x}$ is an n dimensional vector referred to as the state vector, $\tilde{u}$ is an m dimensional vector called the control vector, t is time, and $\tilde{f}$ is an n dimensional vector whose components are the functions relating $\tilde{x}$, $\tilde{u}$ and t to the derivative of the state vector. The components of the state vector are called the state variables. A cost functional J(u) is defined as

$$J(u) = \theta[x(t_f)] + \int_{t_o}^{t_f} f_o(\tilde{x},\tilde{u},t)dt, \tag{7.1}$$

where t_o and t_f are the initial and final times respectively. The final time t_f need not necessarily be fixed a priori. It is assumed that the control vector $\tilde{u}(t)$ can be varied subject to the constraint that $M_i \le U_i \le N_i$, $i = 1,2,\ldots,m$. The optimal control $\tilde{u}(t)$ is the control vector which maximizes (or minimizes depending on how the problem is formulated) the cost functional J as the state vector changes from $\tilde{x}(t_o)$ to $\tilde{x}(t_f)$. All the components of the initial state $\tilde{x}(t_o)$ and the final state $\tilde{x}(t_f)$ need not necessarily be specified. There may be additional constraints on the state variables. For example, some of the state variables may be constrained such that

$$P_i \le x_i(t) \le Q_i,$$

where P_i and Q_i are respectively the minimum and maximum allowable values of the ith component of the state vector.

When the optimal control $\hat{\tilde{u}}(t)$ is obtained as a function of time, this solution is referred to as an optimal open loop solution. If the optimal control is found as a function of the state vector, i.e. $\hat{\tilde{u}} = \tilde{f}_c(\tilde{x})$, the solution is referred to as the optimal closed loop or optimal feedback control solution. Generally the closed loop solution is preferred--and it is more difficult to obtain.

For continuous time optimal control problems Athans and Falb (1966) in their Section 5.7, discuss necessary conditions for the minimization of the performance functional J(u). By heuristic arguments they demonstrate, for free end-point problems and fixed terminal time, that it is plausible to consider the introduction of the auxiliary scalar called the H function (often loosely referred to an the Hamiltonian):

$$H(\underset{\sim}{x},\underset{\sim}{\lambda},\underset{\sim}{u},t) = f_o(\underset{\sim}{x},\underset{\sim}{u},t) + \underset{\sim}{\lambda}^T\underset{\sim}{f}(\underset{\sim}{x},\underset{\sim}{u},t).$$

The costate vector $\underset{\sim}{\lambda}(t)$ satisfies the equations

$$\frac{d\underset{\sim}{\lambda}}{dt} = -\frac{\partial H}{\partial \underset{\sim}{x}}, \quad \underset{\sim}{\lambda}(t_f) = \frac{\partial \theta}{\partial \underset{\sim}{x}(t_f)}.$$

Athans and Falb present a discussion which suggests that the minimization of the functional J(u) corresponds to the minimum of the H function so that one can adjoin the additional necessary condition for a local extremum

$$\partial H/\partial \underset{\sim}{u} = \underset{\sim}{0}.$$

The equations of the previous paragraph lead to a basic theorem in optimal control theory--the Pontryagin minimum principle. This theorem has a rather complicated proof and so is usually omitted from elementary discussions such as the present one.

The reader should keep in mind, however, that the automatic solution of the basic equations of optimal control theory does not by itself guarantee that a globally optimal solution has been found. Recourse often has to be made to the use of sufficiency or the use of other procedures to establish the globally optimal solution.

For illustrative examples of many types of optimal control problems, see, e.g., Athans and Falb (1966), Leitmann (1966), Lee and Markus (1966), Bryson and Ho (1969), Intriligator (1971), Sage and White (1977).

Many applications require knowledge of the controls and state variables only at discrete points in time. A brief introduction to these discrete time optimal control problems, or multistage optimization problems, is presented in the section following.

7.3 Optimization of Multistage Systems.

Let $x_i(t_m)$ denote the ith component of the state vector $\underset{\sim}{x}$ at the time t_m. It is convenient to write $x_i(m)$ instead of $x_i(t_m)$, where m is now regarded as being a time counter and takes on discrete values. Assume that the column vector $\underset{\sim}{x}$ has n components. The state vector at m + 1 may be given as some function of $\underset{\sim}{x}$ at m as in the equation

$$\underset{\sim}{x}(m + 1) = \underset{\sim}{f}[\underset{\sim}{x}(m),m],$$

or in component form,

$$x_i(m+1) = f_i[x_j(m), m], \quad i,j = 1,2,\ldots,m,$$

with $m = 0,1,\ldots,N-1$. The last displayed equation indicates that the values of the components x_i, $i = 1,\ldots,n$ are produced at the end of each equal interval of time, that is, at the end of each stage. As the subscript i changes then the functions on the right-hand side (in general) also change, which is the reason for the subscript on f. Since numerical values of the right-hand side will (in general) also change from stage to stage, it is important to include the counter m in the symbolic representation of f. The above illustration indicates that it is an example of an N-stage system. When $\underset{\sim}{x}(0)$ and the form of the functions f_i are prescribed then the equation can be used in a recursive manner and this is a useful consideration in numerical work.

An alternative mathematical representation would be to write

$$x_i^{m+1} = f_i^m(x_j^m)$$

with the superscript notation denoting stage.

Now consider the situation when certain external bounded influences (or controls) are impressed on the system at the end of each stage. Symbolically, a representation of this situation is given by

$$\underset{\sim}{x}(m+1) = \underset{\sim}{f}[\underset{\sim}{x}(m), \underset{\sim}{u}(m), m], \qquad (7.2)$$

or, in component form,

$$x_i(m+1) = f_i[x_j(m), u_k(m), m], \quad m = 0,1,\ldots,N-1,$$

where $i, j = 1,2,\ldots,n$ and $k = 1,2,\ldots,r$. Here $u_k(m)$ denotes the value of the kth element in the control vector $\underset{\sim}{u}$ at the time t_m. Also the dimension of $\underset{\sim}{u}$, in general, is not the same as the dimension of the state vector $\underset{\sim}{x}$. When the initial state $\underset{\sim}{x}(0)$ and the control variables are specified at each stage then the components of the stage vector can be computed for the next stage, if the form of the functions f_i are prescribed.

Frequently, it is desired to maximize or minimize a certain scalar performance criterion of the form

$$J = \theta[\underset{\sim}{x}(N)] + \sum_{m=0}^{N-1} L[\underset{\sim}{x}(m), \underset{\sim}{u}(m), m]$$

subject to the equality constraints given by (7.2). Here $\theta[\ ]$ is some function of the stage vector at the stage N. Assume that $\underset{\sim}{x}(0)$ is given and that there is a fixed number of stages. It is now required to determine the sequence of control vectors $\underset{\sim}{u}(m)$. One way to solve this problem is now presented.

By means of the Lagrange multiplier sequence $\underset{\sim}{\lambda}^T(m + 1)$, where $\underset{\sim}{\lambda}(m)$ is a column vector and T denotes its transpose, adjoin the equality constraints (7.2) to the performance criterion to produce

$$J = \theta[\underset{\sim}{x}(N)] + \sum_{m=0}^{N-1} [L[\underset{\sim}{x}(m),\underset{\sim}{u}(m),m] + \underset{\sim}{\lambda}^T(m + 1)\{f[\underset{\sim}{x}(m),\underset{\sim}{u}(m),m] - \underset{\sim}{x}(m + 1)\}],$$

$$m = 0,\ldots,N-1.$$

Introduce the Hamiltonian function (a scalar function of m)

$$H(m) \equiv H[\underset{\sim}{x}(m),\underset{\sim}{u}(m),\underset{\sim}{\lambda}(m + 1),m]$$

$$= L[\underset{\sim}{x}(m),\underset{\sim}{u}(m),m] + \underset{\sim}{\lambda}^T(m + 1)\underset{\sim}{f}[\underset{\sim}{x}(m),\underset{\sim}{u}(m),m], \quad m = 0,\ldots,N-1. \quad (7.3)$$

Upon rearrangement of some terms,

$$J = \theta[\underset{\sim}{x}(N)] - \underset{\sim}{\lambda}^T(N)\underset{\sim}{x}(N) + \underset{\sim}{\lambda}^T(0)\underset{\sim}{x}(0) + \sum_{m=0}^{N-1} [H(m) - \underset{\sim}{\lambda}^T(m)\underset{\sim}{x}(m)].$$

Arbitrary variations $\delta\underset{\sim}{u}$ in the control vector lead to corresponding variations $\delta\underset{\sim}{x}$ in the state vector which in turn lead to a variation in the performance criterion δJ. Since $\underset{\sim}{x}(0)$ is fixed $\delta\underset{\sim}{x}(0)$ is zero and

$$\delta J = [\frac{\partial\theta}{\partial\underset{\sim}{x}(N)} - \underset{\sim}{\lambda}^T(N)]\ \delta\underset{\sim}{x}(N) + \sum_{m=0}^{N-1}\{[\frac{\partial H(m)}{\partial\underset{\sim}{x}(m)} - \underset{\sim}{\lambda}^T(m)]\ \delta\underset{\sim}{x}(m) + \frac{\partial H(m)}{\partial\underset{\sim}{u}(m)}\ \delta\underset{\sim}{u}(m)\}.$$

A necessary condition for an extremum is that this first variation in J vanish and, since the variations in $\delta\underset{\sim}{x}$ and $\delta\underset{\sim}{u}$ are arbitrary, hence

$$\underset{\sim}{\lambda}^T(N) = \frac{\partial\theta}{\delta\underset{\sim}{x}(N)}, \quad (7.4)$$

$$\underset{\sim}{\lambda}^T(m) = \frac{\partial H(m)}{\partial\underset{\sim}{x}(m)}, \quad m = 0,1,\ldots,N-1, \quad (7.5)$$

$$\frac{\partial H(m)}{\partial\underset{\sim}{u}(m)} = 0, \quad m = 0,1,\ldots,N-1. \quad (7.6)$$

It is important to realize that these are only necessary conditions for a maximum or minimum of the performance criterion. (If H(m) is linear in the control variable then the last equation is not appropriate. In this event a search is made through all the viable controls to determine when the H function is maximized or minimized.) The expanded forms of the above conditions are:

$$\underset{\sim}{\lambda}^T(N) = \left[\frac{\partial\theta}{\partial x_1(N)} \; \frac{\partial\theta}{\partial x_2(N)} \cdots \frac{\partial\theta}{\partial x_n(N)}\right],$$

$$\underset{\sim}{\lambda}^T(m) = \left[\frac{\partial H(m)}{\partial x_1(m)} \; \frac{\partial H(m)}{\partial x_2(m)} \cdots \frac{\partial H(m)}{\partial x_n(m)}\right], \quad m = 0,\ldots,N-1,$$

$$\frac{\partial H(m)}{\partial u_1(m)} = \frac{\partial H(m)}{\partial u_2(m)} = \ldots = \frac{\partial H(m)}{\partial u_r(m)} = 0, \quad m = 0,\ldots,N-1.$$

In Section 7.2 on continuous time optimal control problems the minimization of the performance functional (7.1) is cast in terms of the minimization of the H function. It is natural to think that the same procedure is valid when dealing with discrete time optimal control problems. First form the H function (7.3). A necessary condition for the minimization of J(u) would then imply that $\partial H/\partial u(m) = 0$ provides the necessary condition for the minimization of H(m). However, the following example illustrates that the previous remark is <u>not</u> entirely correct.

Consider the following discrete-time two-stage process:

$$x(1) = x(0) - 2u(1) - \frac{1}{2}u^2(1), \quad x(0) = 1,$$

$$y(1) = y(0) + u(1), \quad y(0) = 1,$$

$$x(2) = x(1) + y^2(1) + u^2(2), \quad y(2) = f(x(1),y(1),u(2)),$$

where f(x(1),y(1),u(2)) is some arbitrary function. The objective is to minimize x(2).

At stage 1 the H function is given by

$$H(1) = \lambda(1)\, x(1) + \mu(2)\, y(1)$$

$$= \lambda(1)[1 - 2u(1) - \frac{1}{2}u^2(1)] + \mu(1)[1 + u(1)],$$

where $\lambda(1)$ and $\mu(1)$ are costate variables. Now

$$\frac{\partial H(1)}{\partial u(1)} = -\lambda(1)[2 + u(1)] + \mu(1), \quad \frac{\partial^2 H(1)}{\partial u^2(1)} = -\lambda(1),$$

since $\lambda(1)$ and $\mu(1)$ are held as constants during the differentiations. For stage 2, the appropriate H function is

$$H(2) = \lambda(2)[x(1) + y^2(1) + u^2(2)] + \mu(2)f(x(1),y(1),u(2)).$$

By virtue of (7.4) the terminal conditions on the costate variables are given by

$$\begin{bmatrix} \lambda(2) \\ \mu(2) \end{bmatrix} = \begin{bmatrix} \partial\theta/\partial x(2) \\ \partial\theta/\partial y(2) \end{bmatrix} = \begin{bmatrix} 1 \\ 0 \end{bmatrix} .$$

Also,

$$\lambda(1) = \partial H(2)/\partial x(1) = \lambda(2) + \mu(2)\partial f/\partial x(1),$$

$$\mu(1) = \partial H(2)/\partial y(1) = 2\lambda(2)y(1) + \mu(2)\partial f/\partial y(1).$$

These equations simplify to $\lambda(1) = 1$ and $\mu(1) = 2y(1) = 2 + 2u(1)$. It follows that $\partial^2 H/\partial u_2(1) < 0$ and $H(1)$ is being maximized. However $H(2)$ is being minimized. The controls $u(1)$ and $u(2)$ are found from the necessary conditions to be zero.

The main point about this example is that the H function is not minimized at each stage. It appears that Horn and Jackson (1965) were the first to point out that if one only uses the necessary conditions for a local optimum then one cannot assume, without checking the sufficiency conditions, that the H function is being minimized at every stage.

Example 7.1:

Minimize

$$J = \prod_{m=0}^{1} S(m), \quad S(m) = \exp[-u(m)],$$

subject to $x(m + 1) = x(m) - \alpha u^2(m)$, $x(0) = 10$ and $x(2) = 4$. This problem involves the minimization of a product in contrast to a sum, which appears in the earlier discussions. Define $j = \ln J$ then

$$j = -u(0) - u(1) = -\sum_{m=0}^{1} u(m).$$

The H function is $H(m) = -u(m) + \lambda(m + 1)[x(m) - \alpha u^2(m)]$ and

$$\frac{\partial H(m)}{\partial u(m)} = -1 - 2\alpha u(m)\lambda(m + 1); \quad \lambda(m) = \lambda(m + 1) = \lambda.$$

It follows from $\partial H/\partial u = 0$ that $u = -\lambda/2\alpha$ and the state equation becomes $x(m + 1) = x(m) - \lambda^2/4\alpha$. Application of the condition $x(2) = 4$ gives $\lambda = \pm 2(3\alpha)^{1/2}$. With $u = (3/\alpha)^{1/2}$ the minimum value of J is given by $\exp[-2(3/\alpha)^{1/2}]$.

This simple problem is easily solved by means of differential calculus. For example, if $x = u(0)$ and $y = u(1)$ then one has to minimize $J = \exp(-x-y)$ subject to $x^2 + y^2 = 6/\alpha$.

7.4 Multi-dimensional Optimization by Gradient Methods

Assume that $\phi = \phi(x_1, x_2, \ldots, x_n)$ and that each of the partial derivatives $\partial\phi/\partial x_i$, $i = 1, \ldots, n$ exists. It is desired to locate a local maximum or minimum of the function ϕ.

One way to proceed is to form each $\partial\phi/\partial x_i$, $i = 1, \ldots, n$ and set each derivative to zero. This procedure satisfies a necessary condition for a local optimum with the x's being the solution of a nonlinear system of coupled equations. There are some computer codes which can form the derivatives in an analytic manner and then solve the resulting system of equations. A recent synopsis of this area is given in the paper by Rall (1980).

The method which is developed in this Section is based on taking some path that will lead from an initial non-stationary point to a local optimum. The function ϕ increases along a direction s provided that $d\phi/ds > 0$. It is therefore reasonable to consider a particular path which optimizes $d\phi/ds$ at any given point within the region defined by the x's. By use of the chain rule for partial differentiation

$$\frac{d\phi}{ds} = \frac{\partial\phi}{\partial x_1}\frac{dx_1}{ds} + \frac{\partial\phi}{\partial x_2}\frac{dx_2}{ds} + \ldots + \frac{\partial\phi}{\partial x_n}\frac{dx_n}{ds} = \sum_{i=1}^{n} \frac{\partial\phi}{\partial x_i}\frac{dx_i}{ds} .$$

There is a constraint between ds and dx_i given by the Pythagorean theorem in the form

$$(ds)^2 = (dx_1)^2 + (dx_2)^2 + \ldots + (dx_n)^2 \text{ or } \sum_{i=1}^{n} \left(\frac{dx_i}{ds}\right)^2 = 1. \tag{7.7}$$

We now wish to optimize ϕ subject to this constraint. A method which is convenient is as follows. Form the Lagrangian function

$$L = L\left(\frac{dx_1}{ds}, \frac{dx_2}{ds}, \ldots, \frac{dx_n}{ds}, \lambda\right) = \sum_{i=1}^{n} \frac{\partial\phi}{\partial x_i}\frac{dx_i}{ds} + \lambda\left[\sum_{i=1}^{n}\left(\frac{dx_i}{ds}\right)^2 - 1\right]$$

and consider the derivatives dx_i/ds to be independent variables. These derivatives are the direction cosines between the tangent to s and the respective x_i axes. The partial derivatives of L with respect to dx_i/ds, $i = 1, \ldots, n$, are set to zero to give $\partial\phi/\partial x_i + 2\lambda\, dx_i/ds = 0$ or

$$\frac{dx_i}{ds} = -\frac{1}{2\lambda}\frac{\partial\phi}{\partial x_i}, \quad i = 1, \ldots, n,$$

since the Lagrange multiplier λ is not zero. Substitution of this result into the above constraint (7.7) gives the equation for λ:

$$\lambda = \pm\frac{1}{2}\left[\sum_{i=1}^{n}\left(\frac{\partial\phi}{\partial x_i}\right)^2\right]^{1/2} .$$

Hence

$$\frac{dx_i}{ds} = \pm \left[\sum_{j=1}^{n} \left(\frac{\partial \phi}{\partial x_j} \right)^2 \right]^{-1/2} \frac{\partial \phi}{\partial x_i} , \quad i = 1,\ldots,n,$$

which are the optimum values of the direction cosines. The rate of steepest ascent towards a local maximum of ϕ is given by taking the plus sign, whereas the rate of steepest descent towards a local minimum of ϕ corresponds to taking the negative sign.

If dx_i/ds is the derivative at $s = s_o$ then a numerical scheme can be constructed for which

$$x_i(s_o + h) = x_i(s_o) \pm h\left[\sum_{j=1}^{n} \left(\frac{\partial \phi}{\partial x_j} \right)^2 \right]^{-1/2} \frac{\partial \phi}{\partial x_i} , \quad i = 1,\ldots,n, \tag{7.8}$$

with h denoting the step-length. Here $x_i(s_o)$ is the first guess or estimate of x_i and the last equation provides a way of determining x_i at $s_o + h$. The derivatives $\partial\phi/\partial x_i$ can also be approximated numerically. When the plus symbol is selected in (7.8) then a path of <u>steepest ascent</u> is being constructed. A path of <u>steepest descent</u> is being developed when the minus symbol is chosen.

In optimal control theory a simple numerical method is based on (7.8). Define

$$K = h\left[\sum_{j=1}^{n} \left(\frac{\partial \phi}{\partial x_j} \right)^2 \right]^{-1/2} ,$$

and assume that K is a constant. For example, a steepest descent gradient method for the minimization of the Hamiltonian could be written as

$$\underset{\sim}{u}^{p+1}(k) = \underset{\sim}{u}^{p}(k) - K \frac{\partial H}{\partial \underset{\sim}{u}^{p}(k)} , \quad p = 0,1,\ldots \quad . \tag{7.9}$$

Assume that some estimate $\underset{\sim}{u}^{o}(k)$ is known then this last equation provides a means for obtaining a new estimate $\underset{\sim}{u}^{1}(k)$ for the control vector. In order to do the calculation some estimate of K is required, and this value is frequently selected by the investigator. For example, the calculations may be performed with K = 0.1 and the whole process repeated with K = 0.2, 0.3, etc., or some other sequence, until one gets a feel for the convergence of the process. In some cases it may be possible to obtain an explicit solution of the difference equation (7.9). Analysis of the stability of this solution as p increases frequently produces a restriction on the allowable values for K; see, e.g., Sage and White (1977, Chapter 10).

Intuitively one would think that the simple gradient method would converge rapidly. Unfortunately this is not the case and solution of many examples indicates that the steepest descent procedure tends to zigzag back and forth near the optimum, thus requiring many iterations.

A number of the above points are discussed in the following example.

Example 7.2: Analytical Solution

Minimize

$$J(U) = \frac{1}{2} \sum_{m=0}^{3} u^2(m)$$

subject to

$$x(m + 1) = x(m) + \alpha u(m), \; x(0) = 1, \; x(4) = 0,$$

where α is a positive constant. By inspection of the boundary conditions and the form of the state equation it is evident that the controls will turn out to be negative. The H function is

$$H(m) = \frac{1}{2} u^2(m) + \lambda(m + 1)[x(m) + \alpha u(m)].$$

Equations (7.5) and (7.6) give

$$\frac{\partial H(m)}{\partial u(m)} = u(m) + \alpha\lambda(m + 1) = 0;$$

$$\lambda(m) = \frac{\partial H(m)}{\partial x(m)} = \lambda(m + 1).$$

Hence $\lambda(m)$ is a constant, say λ, for $m = 0,1,2,3$. It follows that each value of the control is also a constant; $u(m) = -\alpha\lambda$. Now the state equation gives $x(4) = 1 - 4\alpha^2\lambda$, and application of the second condition $x(4) = 0$ gives $\lambda = 1/4\alpha^2$; also $u = -1/4\alpha$. Finally $x(1) = 0.25$, $x(2) = 0.5$, $x(3) = 0.75$. Since $\partial^2 H(m)/\partial u^2(m) > 0$ the values for $u(m)$ produce the minimum value $1/8\alpha^2$ for the performance criterion.

Solution by Gradient Method

By (7.9)

$$u^{p+1}(m) = (1 - K)u^p(m) - K\alpha\lambda$$

which has the solution

$$u^p(m) = C(1 - K)^p - K\alpha\lambda \sum_{j=0}^{p-1} (1 - K)^j,$$

with C some arbitrary constant. Stability of the growth of this solution requires that $|1 - K| < 1$ or $0 < K < 2$. If $K = 1$ then there is no need to be concerned about C and now $u^p(m) = -\alpha\lambda$, which is independent of the iteration number p and the stage number m.

An alternative argument is as follows. It is required to satisfy the condition $\partial H(m)/\partial u(m) = 0$ and hence it is reasonable to find the value $u^p(m)$ for which the $(p + 1)$th iterate is equal to the pth, or $u^{p+1}(m) = u^p(m)$. For the present example application of this equation gives $u^p(m) = -\alpha\lambda$.

One way to proceed with the numerical scheme is as follows. Guess u^o and compute the corresponding value J^o. Now reduce J^o by a certain percentage and find J^1, from which u^1 can be calculated. Continue in this manner. Table 7.1 shows some results for $\alpha = 0.25$ when $u^o = -4$ and a 10% reduction is made in the performance criterion. A list of values of x(4) needs to be compiled since reduction of the performance criterion by itself is not adequate. It is necessary to check on how close the

p	0	1	2	3	...	26	27
u	-4	-3.79	-3.6	-3.41	...	-1.02	-0.97
J	32	28.8	25.92	23.33	...	2.08	1.87
x(4)					...	-0.020	0.029

Table 7.1 The performance criterion is reduced by 10% at each new iteration level; p is the iteration number.

condition x(4) = 0 is being satisfied. As Table 7.1 shows convergence is slow. The results indicate that u lies within the closed interval (-1.02, -0.97). If the average of these two values is taken, i.e., u = -.0995, then the calculation of x(4) = 0.0050. Hence u now lies within the closed interval (-1.02, -0.995); and the average value this time is u = -1.0075. It is evident how to proceed to obtain u to greater accuracy. Note that our previous analytical solution gives u = -1.

Instead of reducing J by 10%, a reduction of 20% or 30% or some other percentage could have been made, with corresponding acceleration of convergence.

Another method is to guess several numerical values for the control and solve the state equation. After a few trial runs it should be possible to find an interval in which the control lies. An interpolation formula could be used to refine estimates of the control.

A quicker procedure is to employ a penalty function.

7.5 Gradient Method with Penalty Function

Some illustrative examples of the penalty function method are presented in this Section. Then follows a general synopsis of the approach.

Consider the same problem as in Example 7.2. By inspection of the minimization of the performance criterion then it appears that a value of the control which is zero should be chosen. However with zero control, solution of the state equation produces a value for x(4) which is different from zero.

A way to proceed is now outlined and depends on the penalty function concept.

The controls are to be determined such that the constraint x(4) = 0 is satisfied. Introduce into the performance criterion a penalty for violating this constraint. For example, let the new performance criterion be

$$J = \frac{1}{2} c[x(4)]^2 + \frac{1}{2} \sum_{m=0}^{3} u^2(m),$$

where the square of x(4) is introduced as one possible measure of how far away the constraint is from being satisfied. The quantity c is assumed to be some nonnegative constant and is often found by trial and error in numerical work. In addition to the equations obtained in the analytical solution of Example 7.2 there is the equation $\lambda(4) = cx(4)$, which comes from the application of (7.4).

Assume that u(m) is a constant u^o for each m value. The state equation gives $x^o(4) = 1 + 4\alpha u^0$ and now

$$\lambda^o(4) = (1 + 4\alpha u^o)c.$$

But there is no way of estimating $\lambda^o(m)$, $m = 0,1,\ldots,3$. Consider the situation when $\lambda^o(m)$ is set equal to $\lambda^o(4)$, then

$$\frac{\partial H}{\partial u^o} = \alpha c + (1 + 4\alpha^2 c)u^o.$$

The gradient method (7.9) is in the form

$$u^{p+1} = u^p - K[\alpha c + (1 + 4\alpha^2 c)u^p], \quad p = 0,1,\ldots .$$

When $u^{p+1} = u^p$ then

$$u^p = -\alpha c/(1 + 4\alpha^2 c), \quad p = 0,1,\ldots .$$

Thus every iterate is the same and this last equation provides the estimate for the control u. As $c \to \infty$ then $u \to -1/4\alpha$, in agreement with the result for u found previously. The effect of increase of c when $\alpha = 0.25$ in the last displayed formula is shown in the following table.

c	200	400	600	800	...	∞
u	-0.9804	-0.9901	-0.9934	-0.995		-1
x(4)	0.0196	0.0099	0.0066	0.0050		0
J	1.9608	1.9802	1.9867	1.9900		2

So long as x(4) is different from zero then the term $(1/2)cx^2(4)$ produces an additional contribution to the augmented performance criterion and therefore is a penalty. Consequently, a measure of the success of the penalty function method is to see how quickly the terminal value $x(4) = 0$ is being reached; see above table.

The main conclusion to be drawn from the present discussion is that the use of the gradient method with an appropriate penalty function for the solution of this two-point boundary-value pattern has considerably improved the speed of convergence in obtaining approximate values for the controls.

For the present problem it is also interesting to note that

$$u^{p+1} = [1 - (1 + 4\alpha^2 c)K]u^p - K\alpha c.$$

If u^{p+1} is forced to be a constant, independent of the iteration number p, then this last equation gives

$$K = \frac{1}{1 + 4\alpha^2 c}, \quad u^{p+1} = -K\alpha c = \frac{-\alpha c}{1 + 4\alpha^2 c}$$

and $K \to 0$ as $c \to \infty$.

Example 7.3:

Minimize

$$J(u) = \frac{1}{2} \sum_{m=0}^{3} u^2(m)$$

subject to

$$x(m + 1) = x(m) + \alpha m u(m), \; x(0) = 1, \; x(4) = 0.$$

This is a variable coefficient problem with solution

$$u(m) = -\frac{m}{14\alpha}, \quad x(m + 1) = x(m) - \frac{m^2}{14}, \quad \lambda = \frac{1}{14\alpha^2},$$

and minimum value of $J = 1/28\alpha^2$.

The numerical solution will be obtained using a gradient method with a penalty function. Construct a new performance criterion which now includes a penalty function:

$$J = \frac{1}{2} cx^2(4) + \frac{1}{2} \sum_{m=0}^{3} u^2(m).$$

Since the state equation has non-constant coefficients it is reasonable to guess values $u^o(1)$, $u^o(2)$ and $u^o(3)$ for the controls. Hence, on using (7.4),

$$\lambda^o(4) = cx^o(4) = c[1 + \alpha u^o(1) + 2\alpha u^o(2) + 3\alpha u^o(3)].$$

Also, assuming that $\lambda(m) \cong \lambda^o(4)$,

$$\frac{\partial H(m)}{\partial u^o(m)} = u^o(m) + \alpha m \lambda^o(4).$$

The gradient method (7.9) is now extended to accommodate vector quantities. Write

$$\begin{bmatrix} u^1(1) \\ u^1(2) \\ u^1(3) \end{bmatrix} = \begin{bmatrix} u^o(1) \\ u^o(2) \\ u^o(3) \end{bmatrix} - \begin{bmatrix} K_1 & 0 & 0 \\ 0 & K_2 & 0 \\ 0 & 0 & K_3 \end{bmatrix} \begin{bmatrix} \partial H(1)/\partial u^o(1) \\ \partial H(2)/\partial u^o(2) \\ \partial H(3)/\partial u^o(3) \end{bmatrix}$$

Define

$$\underset{\sim}{A} = \begin{bmatrix} 1+\alpha^2 c & 2\alpha^2 c & 3\alpha^2 c \\ 2\alpha^2 c & 1+4\alpha^2 c & 6\alpha^2 c \\ 3\alpha^2 c & 6\alpha^2 c & 1+9\alpha^2 c \end{bmatrix}$$

$$\underset{\sim}{u} = \begin{bmatrix} u(1) \\ u(2) \\ u(3) \end{bmatrix}, \quad \underset{\sim}{K} = \begin{bmatrix} K_1 & 0 & 0 \\ 0 & K_2 & 0 \\ 0 & 0 & K_3 \end{bmatrix}, \quad \underset{\sim}{C} = \begin{bmatrix} \alpha c \\ 2\alpha c \\ 3\alpha c \end{bmatrix}$$

then

$$\underset{\sim}{u}^1 = \underset{\sim}{u}^o - \underset{\sim}{K}(\underset{\sim}{C} + \underset{\sim}{A}\underset{\sim}{u}^o) = (\underset{\sim}{I} - \underset{\sim}{K}\underset{\sim}{A})\underset{\sim}{u}^o - \underset{\sim}{K}\,\underset{\sim}{C},$$

with $\underset{\sim}{I}$ denoting the identity matrix. After p iterations

$$\underset{\sim}{u}^{p+1} = (\underset{\sim}{I} - \underset{\sim}{K}\underset{\sim}{A})\underset{\sim}{u}^p - \underset{\sim}{K}\,\underset{\sim}{C}.$$

When $\underset{\sim}{y}^{p+1} = \underset{\sim}{u}^p$ then

$$\underset{\sim}{u}^p = -\underset{\sim}{A}^{-1}\,\underset{\sim}{C}$$

$$= \frac{-1}{1+14\alpha^2 c} \begin{bmatrix} 1+13\alpha^2 c & -2\alpha^2 c & -3\alpha^2 c \\ -2\alpha^2 c & 1+10\alpha^2 c & -6\alpha^2 c \\ -3\alpha^2 c & -6\alpha^2 c & 1+5\alpha^2 c \end{bmatrix} \begin{bmatrix} \alpha c \\ 2\alpha c \\ 3\alpha c \end{bmatrix}$$

$$= \frac{-\alpha c}{1+14\alpha^2 c} \begin{bmatrix} 1 \\ 2 \\ 3 \end{bmatrix}.$$

As c increases this approximation to the control vector improves, and as $c \to \infty$, $u^p(m) \to -m/14\alpha$, as found in the exact solution.

Example 7.4:

Minimize

$$J(u) = \frac{1}{2} \sum_{m=0}^{3} u^2(m)$$

subject to

$$x(m + 1) = x(m) - u(m)/[1 + u(m)], \; x(0) = 1, \; x(4) = 0.$$

The state equation is linear in x(m) and nonlinear in u(m). The analytic solution gives $1 + u(m) = \pm\lambda$. For $u(m) = -1 - \lambda$ then $\lambda = -4/3$, $u = 1/3$ whereas $u(m) = -1 + \lambda$ gives $\lambda = 4/3$, $u = 1/3$. Finally, $x(m + 1) = x(m) - 1/4$.

Use of a penalty function $cx^2(4)$ and the gradient method (7.9) produces

$$u^1 = u^o - K \frac{u^o}{(1+u^o)^2} [(1 + u^o)^2 - c + \frac{4cu^o}{1+u^o}].$$

If $u^1 = u^0$ then

$$(1 + u^o)^3 + 3(1 + u^o)c - 4c = 0.$$

This is a nonlinear (cubic) equation for u^o. Now a real solution of

$$z^3 + az - b = 0,$$

where $a \geq 0$ and b are real, is given by the expression

$$z = (A + B^{1/2})^{1/3} + (A - B^{1/2})^{1/3},$$

$$A = b/2, \quad B = b^2/4 + a^3/27.$$

Hence,

$$u^o = [2c + (4c^2 + c^3)^{1/2}]^{1/3} + [2c - (4c^2 + c^3)^{1/2}]^{1/3} - 1.$$

Some values of u^o calculated from this formula are shown in the following table:

c	100	1,000	10,000
u^o	0.325569	0.332545	0.333254

When the performance criterion is quadratic in the control variable and the state equation is linear in the same control variable, then the gradient method gives a linear equation for the pth iterate $u^p(m)$. However, if the control variable now occurs in a nonlinear manner in the state equation then the pth iterate $u^p(m)$ satisfies a nonlinear equation, which may require some numerical procedure to be used for its solution.

Many multistage optimization problems can be solved by analytical means. However there are a large number of two-point boundary-value problems which have a complicated structure; e.g., have variable coefficients, are nonlinear, or are combinations of these. For these multi-stage problems the difficulty is to find a numerical method which will guarantee that the terminal condition (usually a constraint on the state variable(s)) is being satisfied. One method that can be applied is to use the concept of the penalty function. (A discussion of the use of different types of penalty function is given in Dorny (1975, p. 538) for nonlinear optimization problems.) As the previous examples show, the idea is to introduce an additional portion (the penalty) into the performance criterion. A numerical method is devised for which the (p + 1)th estimate of the control is given in terms of the previous value. For an estimate of the control the state equation is solved and the performance criterion is evaluated. The process continues until some stopping requirement on the iteration is satisfied. A method of this type, using a penalty function, is sometimes referred to as an "unconstrained" problem because the reformulated problem with the new performance criterion does not have a terminal constraint. In the description of the illustrative examples the solution of the costate equation was elementary. For more complicated problems this can present a more difficult challenge. It is worthwhile noting that the inclusion of a penalty function into a problem does not necessarily guarantee improvement in the speed of convergence of a numerical procedure. See Example 7.6 where the penalty function method does not work.

Quintana and Davison (1970) introduced the "time-weighted steepest descent" method as an extension of the gradient method. They demonstrated that it has a rate of convergence which is significantly faster than the regular gradient method. An interesting application of this time-weighted steepest descent method in a complicated continuous time optimal control problem occurs in the work by Cherchas and Ng (1978). No one appears to have considered the application of this new method to discrete time optimal control problems.

7.6 A Numerical Scheme for a Nonlinear Problem

Each of the previous discrete time optimal control problems was able to be solved explicitly. In this section a nonlinear problem in the state variable is examined. A key feature in the solution is the role played by the costate equation. In the previous examples the special structure allowed for the costate variable to be a constant, a somewhat artificial feature.

Example 7.5:

Minimize

$$J = \frac{1}{2} \sum_{m=0}^{3} u^2(m)$$

subject to

$$x(m+1) = x^2(m)u(m) - x(m), \quad x(0) = 10, \quad x(4) = 1.$$

The additional complication in this problem is that conditions on the state variable are specified at the end-points.

The costate equation is

$$\lambda(m) = 2\lambda(m+1)u(m)x(m) - \lambda(m+1),$$

and $\partial H(m)/\partial u(m) = 0$ gives

$$u(m) = -\lambda(m+1)x^2(m). \tag{7.10}$$

This last equation allows for the control $u(m)$ to be eliminated from the state and costate equations, so that

$$x(m+1) = -\lambda(m+1)x^4(m) - x(m), \quad x(0) = 10, \quad x(4) = 1, \tag{7.11}$$

$$\lambda(m) = -2x^3(m)\lambda^2(m+1) - \lambda(m+1). \tag{7.12}$$

The following solution of the quadratic equation in $\lambda(m+1)$ is taken

$$\lambda(m+1) = \frac{-1 - [1 - 8\lambda(m)x^3(m)]^{1/2}}{4x^3(m)}. \tag{7.13}$$

(Later on in the discussion the other root will be considered.)

Careful inspection of the coupled equations (7.11) and (7.12) indicates that the key to the numerical solution lies in the determination of $\lambda(0)$. If $\lambda(0)$ is known then (7.12) can be used to compute $\lambda(1)$ and then $x(1)$ is found from (7.11), since $x(0)$ is prescribed.

Try to guess the shape of the curve drawn through the values of the state variables. Roughly speaking there are three possibilities between the end-points: (a) a straight line, (b) a bell-shaped curve, or (c) a U-shaped curve. The author used (a) to estimate $x(1)$ then (7.11) was used to determine $\lambda(1)$; $\lambda(0)$ was then computed from (7.12). This approach was unsuccessful but suggested that a closer approximation to $\lambda(0)$ could be obtained if (b) was assumed. Eventually $\lambda(0) = -0.002$ was picked, which then suggested that solutions be computed with the $\lambda(0)$ values as shown in the following tables:

$\lambda(0)$	$x(4)$
-0.01	2.13
-0.00988	0.2583

$\lambda(0)$	$x(4)$
-0.0095	-2.59
-0.009	< 0

It is evident from these values that $-0.01 < \lambda(0) < -0.00988$. The average of these two values is $\lambda(0) = -0.009940$, which gives $x(4) = 1.1074$. At this point in the calculation it is reasonable to use inverse linear interpolation and this gives $\lambda(0) = -0.0099324$ with $x(4) = 0.99785$; hence

$$-0.009940 < \lambda(0) < -0.0099324.$$

The minimum value of $J \approx 0.0495$. With the selection (7.13) each value of the costate variable is negative. Table 7.2 shows some approximate solutions calculated from $\lambda(0) = -0.0099324$.

$\lambda(1) = -0.0024925$,	$x(1) = 14.925$,	$u(0) = 0.24925$,
$\lambda(2) = -0.00069207$,	$x(2) = 19.413$,	$u(1) = 0.15416$,
$\lambda(3) = -0.00025431$,	$x(3) = 16.709$,	$u(2) = 0.095845$,
$\lambda(4) = -0.00022718$,	$x(4) = 0.99785$,	$u(3) = 0.063424$.

Table 7.2 Approximate solutions to Example 7.5.

Instead of (7.13) the other root of (7.12) is given by

$$\lambda(m + 1) = \{-1 + [1 - 8\lambda(m)x^3(m)]^{1/2}\}/4x^3(m). \tag{7.14}$$

For real values of the costate variable this last equation requires that $\lambda(0) \leq 1/8x^3(0)$. When $\lambda(0) = 1/8x^3(0)$ the values of the state variables oscillate about zero and $x(4) \approx 5.002$. As $\lambda(0)$ decreases away from $1/8x^3(0)$ then larger and larger swings in the values of the state variables occur. These oscillations become progressively larger as $\lambda(0)$ takes on increasing negative values. There is no approach to the terminal condition $x(4) = 1$ and consequently (7.14) is rejected in favor of (7.13).

It is interesting to note that the penalty function approach, in the form in which it was used earlier, is too cumbersome a procedure for numerical solution of the present problem. The reasons for this are demonstrated in the next example.

Example 7.6:

Consider the solution of the following problem by means of a penalty function. Minimize

$$J = \frac{1}{2} \sum_{m=0}^{1} u^2(m)$$

subject to

$$x(m + 1) = x^2(m)u(m) - x(m)$$

with

$$x(0) = 10 \text{ and } x(2) = a,$$

where $a = 19.4136186$. This example is a shortened version of the previous one.

For convenience write $x_o = x(0)$, $x_1 = x(1)$, $\lambda_o = \lambda(0)$, $u_o = u(0)$, etc. The state and costate equations are

$$x_1 = x_o^2 u_o - x_o, \quad x_2 = x_1^2 u_1 - x_1, \quad \lambda_o = (2u_o x_o - 1)\lambda_1,$$

$$\lambda_1 = (2u_1 x_1 - 1)\lambda_2.$$

From $\partial H/\partial u = 0$, $u_o = -\lambda_1 x_o^2$ and $u_1 = -\lambda_2 x_1^2$. By systematic elimination it is possible to produce a single equation for x_1. The last three equations give

$$u_o x_1^2 = (2u_1 x_1 - 1)u_1 x_o^2. \tag{7.15}$$

The second state equation gives

$$u_1 = \frac{a + x_1}{x_1^2} = \frac{a + x_o^2 u_o - x_o}{(x_o^2 u_o - x_o)^2}.$$

Elimination of u_o from (7.15) be means of the first state equation together with the expression for u_1 in terms of x_1 produces

$$(x_1 + x_o)x_1^5 = x_o^4(a + x_1)(2a + x_1), \tag{7.16}$$

which is a sixth order polynomial equation for x_1.

Define

$$y(x) = x^5(x + x_o)/x_o^4, \quad z(x) = (x + a)(x + 2a), \quad f(x) = y(x) - z(x).$$

Then

$$f(-a) > 0, \quad f(-x_o) < 0, \quad f(x_o) < 0, \quad f(2x_o) > 0$$

and hence there is a root of $f(x) = 0$ in $-a < x < -x_o$ and one in $x_o < x < 2x_o$. That these are the only real roots can be demonstrated by drawing the graphs of $y(x)$ and $z(x)$. With $x_1^o = 15$ as a guess for x_1 Newton's method produces a better estimate $x_1 = 14.92480659$ with $u_o = 0.2492480659$ and $u_1 = 0.154156894$.

Introduce a penalty function so that the performance criterion is now of the form

$$J = \frac{c}{2}\,[x(2) - a]^2 + \frac{1}{2}\sum_{m=0}^{1} u^2(m).$$

Then

$$\lambda(2) = c[x(2) - a] = c(x_1^2 u_1 - x_1 - a),$$

$$\lambda(1) = (2x_1 u_1 - 1)\lambda(2).$$

Also, $\partial H(m)/\partial u(m) = u(m) + \lambda(m + 1)x^2(m)$.

The simple gradient method (7.9), when $\underset{\sim}{u}^{p+1} = \underset{\sim}{u}^p$, gives

$$\begin{bmatrix} u_o^p \\ u_1^p \end{bmatrix} = -\begin{bmatrix} \lambda_1^p\, x_o^2 \\ \lambda_2^p (x_1^p)^2 \end{bmatrix} = -\begin{bmatrix} (2x_1^p u_1^p - 1)x_0^2 \lambda_2^p \\ \lambda_2^p (x_1^p)^2 \end{bmatrix}.$$

From the second of these equations

$$u_1^p = \frac{c(x_1^p)^2(x_1^p + a)}{1 + c(x_1^p)^4} \rightarrow \frac{x_1^p + a}{(x_1^p)^2} \quad \text{as } c \rightarrow \infty,$$

and the first, after some algebra, takes the form

$$(x_1 + x_o)x_1^5\left(1 + \frac{1}{cx_1^4}\right)^2 = x_o^4(a + x_1)\left(2a + x_1 - \frac{1}{cx_1^2}\right),$$

where the iteration number p has been omitted. For any finite value of c this last equation is a ninth order polynomial for x_1, which is more complicated than the sixth order polynomial in (7.16).

If more stages are considered, as in Example 7.5, then the proposed scheme for obtaining approximate solutions to the costate equation would appear to be less cumbersome than use of the present penalty function approach.

7.7 The Method of Conjugate Gradients

Instead of proceeding in the direction of steepest descent one may follow a different path which ultimately leads to the optimum in a fewer number of iterations. There are various ways of selecting the path. One is to use the method of conjugate gradients. A sequence of one-dimensional searches is carried out in directions, which are determined by the partial derivatives of the objective function (i.e., the function that is being minimized, or maximized).

The method of conjugate gradients was originally presented by Hestenes and

Steifel (1952) for solving the system $\underset{\sim}{A}\underset{\sim}{x} = \underset{\sim}{b}$ of linear albegraic equations. A subsequent extension was given by Fletcher and Reeves (1964). Lasdon et al. (1967) discussed the method in connection with optimal control problems. In the present Section some of the basic ideas of the conjugate gradient method are developed. The approach involves the minimization of the performance criterion J as a function of the control vector $\underset{\sim}{u}$, and the final algorithm uses the gradient $\partial J/\partial \underset{\sim}{u}$. However, in practice many algorithms utilize the gradient of the Hamiltonian.

Assume that the control vector $\underset{\sim}{u} = \underset{\sim}{\sigma}$ minimizes the performance criterion J. In the vicinity of this minimum assume that J can be written in the quadratic form

$$J(\underset{\sim}{u}) = J(\underset{\sim}{\sigma}) + \frac{1}{2}(\underset{\sim}{u} - \underset{\sim}{\sigma})^T \underset{\sim}{A}(\underset{\sim}{u} - \underset{\sim}{\sigma}),$$

where $\underset{\sim}{A}$ is a real, symmetric, positive-definite matrix consisting of second-order partial derivatives. Then its gradient is defined by

$$\underset{\sim}{G}(\underset{\sim}{u}) = \underset{\sim}{A}(\underset{\sim}{u} - \underset{\sim}{\sigma}). \tag{7.17}$$

An initial guess to the control vector is written as $\underset{\sim}{u}_o$. The step from the estimate $\underset{\sim}{u}_i$ to $\underset{\sim}{u}_{i+1}$ is expressed in the form

$$\underset{\sim}{u}_{i+1} = \underset{\sim}{u}_i + \alpha_i \underset{\sim}{p}_i, \quad i = 0,1,\ldots, \tag{7.18}$$

where α_i is a positive scalar and $\underset{\sim}{p}_i$ is a search vector. Repeated usage of this equation gives

$$\underset{\sim}{u}_n = \underset{\sim}{u}_{j+1} + \sum_{i=j+1}^{n-1} \alpha_i \underset{\sim}{p}_i,$$

for any j in $0 \leq j \leq n - 1$. Define $\underset{\sim}{G}_i = \underset{\sim}{G}(\underset{\sim}{u}_i)$ then

$$\underset{\sim}{G}_n = \underset{\sim}{G}_{j+1} + \sum_{i=j+1}^{n-1} \alpha_i \underset{\sim}{A} \underset{\sim}{p}_i. \tag{7.19}$$

Many one-variable problems in calculus involve the use of the first derivative. When more than one variable occurs a key role is played by the gradient vector. The gradient vector is normal to the surfaces of J = constant in the present problem. A central feature of the conjugate gradient method is the selection

$$\underset{\sim}{G}_{i+1}^T \underset{\sim}{p}_i = 0,$$

where, as usual, T denotes transpose. On combining the results of the last two displayed equations it follows that

$$G_n^T \underset{\sim}{p}_j = \sum_{i=j+1}^{n-1} \alpha_i \underset{\sim}{p}_i^T A \underset{\sim}{p}_j.$$

If the vectors $\underset{\sim}{p}_0, \underset{\sim}{p}_1, \ldots, \underset{\sim}{p}_{n-1}$ are A-conjugate, satisfying

$$\underset{\sim}{p}_i^T A \underset{\sim}{p}_j = 0 \text{ for } i \neq j,$$

then

$$G_n^T \underset{\sim}{p}_j = 0,$$

and therefore, since $\underset{\sim}{p}_0, \underset{\sim}{p}_1, \ldots, \underset{\sim}{p}_{n-1}$ form a basis, $G_n = 0$. Equation (7.17) now produces $\underset{\sim}{u} = \underset{\sim}{\sigma}$.

What has just been demonstrated is that the method of successive linear searches converges quadratically when using any set of A-conjugate directions. The minimum is located at the nth iteration, or earlier, if some of the α_i turn out to be zero.

How are the $\underset{\sim}{p}_i$ chosen? Arbitrarily set $\underset{\sim}{p}_0 = -G(\underset{\sim}{u}_0)$ and then write

$$\underset{\sim}{p}_{i+1} = -G_{i+1} + \beta_i \underset{\sim}{p}_i, \quad i = 0, 1, \ldots, n-1. \tag{7.20}$$

The background motivation for this selection is provided by Beckman (1960). From the A-conjugacy condition it is noted that $\underset{\sim}{p}_i^T A \underset{\sim}{p}_{i+1} = 0$. Replace $\underset{\sim}{p}_{i+1}$ in this last equation by its representation in the previous display so that

$$\beta_i = \underset{\sim}{p}_i^T A G_{i+1} / \underset{\sim}{p}_i^T A \underset{\sim}{p}_i. \tag{7.21}$$

Since A appears as a result of a particular expansion of the performance criterion it may not be easy to obtain its elements in practice. Happily, it is possible to derive an alternative expression for β_i that avoids the use of the matrix A. This final result for β_i is often quoted but the derivation is usually omitted. For the reader's benefit a derivation, which unfortunately is somewhat involved, is presented here. From (7.19) and the estimate $\underset{\sim}{u}_{i+1}$ given by (7.18)

$$G_{i+1} = G_i + \alpha_i A \underset{\sim}{p}_i. \tag{7.22}$$

But $\underset{\sim}{p}_i^T G_{i+1} = 0$, and therefore $\underset{\sim}{p}_i^T G_i + \alpha_i \underset{\sim}{p}_i^T A \underset{\sim}{p}_i = 0$, which gives

$$\underset{\sim}{p}_i^T A \underset{\sim}{p}_i = -(1/\alpha_i) \underset{\sim}{p}_i^T G_i.$$

Premultiply (7.20) by G_{i+1} to produce

$$G_{i+1}^T p_{i+1} = -G_{i+1}^T G_{i+1} + \beta_i G_{i+1}^T p_i,$$

which becomes, since the last term vanishes,

$$G_i^T p_i = p_i^T G_i = -G_i^T G_i.$$

The last three displays can be combined to produce the result

$$p_i^T A p_i = (1/\alpha_i) G_i^T G_i. \qquad (7.23)$$

On using (7.22)

$$G_{i+1}^T G_{i+1} = G_{i+1}^T G_i + \alpha_i G_{i+1}^T A p_i$$

$$= G_{i+1}^T G_i + \alpha_i p_i^T A G_{i+1},$$

since A is symmetric. Hence,

$$p_i^T A G_{i+1} = (1/\alpha_i)[G_{i+1}^T G_{i+1} - G_{i+1}^T G_i]. \qquad (7.24)$$

Now use (7.22) again to produce

$$p_{i-1}^T G_{i+1} = p_{i-1}^T G_i + \alpha_i p_{i-1}^T A p_i = 0,$$

by the selection of the p_i and the A-conjugacy condition. Rearrangement of the defining equation for p_{i+1} gives $p_{i-1} = (1/\beta_{i-1})(p_i + G_i)$ and premultiplication by G_{i+1}^T results in

$$G_{i+1}^T p_{i-1} = (1/\beta_{i-1})(G_{i+1}^T p_i + G_{i+1}^T G_i).$$

The left-hand side of this equation is zero by the previous display and the first term on the right vanishes because of the way in which the p_i are selected. Therefore,

$$G_{i+1}^T G_i = 0$$

and (7.24) simplifies to give

$$p_i A G_{i+1} = (1/\alpha_i) G_{i+1}^T G_{i+1}.$$

This last result together with (7.23) are now substituted into (7.21) to yield

$$\beta_i = (G_{i+1}^T \, G_{i+1})/(G_i^T \, G_i),$$

and, in this form, knowledge of the matrix $\tilde{A}$ is not required.

Almost all of the effort so far in the conjugate gradient method has been spent on the selection of the search vectors $\tilde{p}_i$. However nothing has been stated on how to determine the α_i which appears in the new estimate for $\tilde{u}_{i+1}$. One way to proceed is to substitute for $\tilde{u}_1$ into the performance criterion J, which will now be dependent on α_o. Minimize J with respect to α_o. Since $\tilde{u}_1$ is now known the other quantities of interest can be computed and the process repeated for the determination of α_1, and so on.

Earlier in this Chapter it was pointed out that, for certain continuous time optimal control problems, the minimization of the performance criterion subject to certain state equations and initial and boundary conditions was equivalent to the minimization of the "Hamiltonian". The assumption is now made that the H function can be expanded in a quadratic form similar to the expansion of the performance criterion. Define the gradient vector

$$\tilde{g}_i = g(\tilde{u}_i) = \partial H/\partial \tilde{u}_i,$$

then an algorithm for the conjugate gradient method can be written as follows:

(i) $\tilde{u}_o$ = arbitrary,

$\tilde{g}_o = \tilde{g}(\tilde{u}_o)$,

$\tilde{s}_o = -\tilde{g}_o$.

Select $\alpha = \alpha_i$ to minimize $J(\tilde{u}_i + \alpha_i \tilde{s}_i)$ with the iterative scheme

$$\tilde{u}_{i+1} = \tilde{u}_i + \alpha_i \tilde{s}_i,$$

$$\tilde{g}_{i+1} = g(\tilde{u}_{i+1}),$$

$$\beta_i = (\tilde{g}_{i+1}, \tilde{g}_{i+1})/(\tilde{g}_i, \tilde{g}_i)$$

$$\tilde{s}_{i+1} = -\tilde{g}_{i+1} + \beta_i \tilde{s}_i.$$

In the expression for β_i the bracket notation for a scalar product of two vectors is used. For example, if t_o and t_f are the initial and final times, respectively, then

$$(\tilde{g}_i, \tilde{g}_j) = \int_{t_o}^{t_f} \tilde{g}_i^T(t) \tilde{g}_j(t) dt.$$

It is not possible, in practice, to exactly perform the one-dimensional minimization of the performance criterion. A technique that has been tried with success is to increment the search direction until the objective function J starts to increase in values. Cubic interpolation is often suggested for locating the numerical minimum.

Lasdon et al. (1967) give a convergence proof of the above algorithm. However in his extensive review article, Polak (1973) p. 563, points out that their convergence proof is in error. For three examples of continuous time optimal control problems with no terminal conditions or inequality constraints Lasdon et al. (1967) show that the conjugate gradient algorithm produces numerical results at a much faster rate than ordinary gradient methods.

For multi-variable optimal control problems of the type outlined in Section 7.3 a conjugate gradient algorithm can be written in the following manner:

(i) Choose an initial guess for $\underset{\sim}{u}$; denote it by $\underset{\sim}{u}_o$.

(ii) With the value of $\underset{\sim}{u}_i$ and the initial data $\underset{\sim}{x}(0)$ use the state equation to compute the elements of the state vector $\underset{\sim}{x}_i$. Here i refers to the location in the iteration scheme which starts with i = 0.

(iii) From the estimates of $\underset{\sim}{u}_i$ and $\underset{\sim}{x}_i$ use the costate equation to calculate the multipliers $\underset{\sim}{\lambda}_i$.

(iv) Compute the gradient vector $\underset{\sim}{g}_i$ at $\underset{\sim}{u} = \underset{\sim}{u}_i$, $\underset{\sim}{x} = \underset{\sim}{x}_i$, and $\underset{\sim}{\lambda} = \underset{\sim}{\lambda}_i$, with

$$g_i = \left(\frac{\partial H(0)}{\partial u_i(0)}, \frac{\partial H(1)}{\partial u_i(1)}, \ldots, \frac{\partial H(N-1)}{\partial u_i(N-1)} \right),$$

indicating that there are N components.

(v) Determine the new conjugate direction $\underset{\sim}{s}_i$, also an N-vector, by

$$\underset{\sim}{s}_i = \begin{cases} -\underset{\sim}{g}_o, & i = 0, \\ -\underset{\sim}{g}_i + \beta_i \underset{\sim}{s}_{i-1}, & i \neq 0, \end{cases}$$

where $\beta_i = \langle \underset{\sim}{g}_i, \underset{\sim}{g}_i \rangle / \langle \underset{\sim}{g}_{i-1}, \underset{\sim}{g}_{i-1} \rangle$. The notation $\langle\ ,\ \rangle$ means that the inner product of the two N-vectors is formed.

(vi) Minimize the performance criterion J along the conjugate direction from $\underset{\sim}{u}_i$. The objective is to determine the non-negative scalar ψ that minimizes $J(\underset{\sim}{u}_i + \psi \underset{\sim}{s}_i; x(0))$.

(vii) Write $\underset{\sim}{u}_{i+1} = \underset{\sim}{u}_i + \psi \underset{\sim}{s}_i$ and return to step (ii) to commence the next iteration.

The major difficulty in the implementation of the algorithm, as stated, is in the need to calculate a good approximation to ψ.

Example 7.7:

Investigate the application of the conjugate gradient algorithm to the problem examined in Example 7.3 which, for $\alpha = 0.25$, gave the results

$$\underset{\sim}{u} = (-0.285714, -0.571429, -0.857142), \quad \lambda = 1.142857,$$

$$\underset{\sim}{x} = (1, 0.9285715, 0.6428570, 0.0000005), \; J = 0.571428.$$

In the first description of the algorithm the explicit representation for x(4) from the state equation is used; λ = constant. This allows for the performance criterion J to be expressed in terms of the multiplier ψ and its minimization can then be carried through analytically. Subscripts denote the position in the iteration. Now $\underset{\sim}{u}_1(m) = \underset{\sim}{u}_o(m) + \underset{\sim}{s}_o(m)\psi$ with

$$J_1(\psi) = \frac{1}{2}\, c\, x_1^2(4) + \frac{1}{2} \sum_{m=1}^{3} u_1^2(m),$$

$$x_1(4) = 1 + \alpha u_1(1) + 2\alpha u_1(2) + 3\alpha u_1(3).$$

By direct differentiation,

$$\frac{dJ_1(\psi)}{d\psi} = c\, x_1(4)\, \frac{dx_1(4)}{d\psi} + \sum_{m=1}^{3} u_1(m)s_o(m) = P + Q\psi,$$

where

$$P = \alpha c[s_o(1) + 2s_o(2) + 3s_o(3)][1 + \alpha u_o(1) + 2\alpha u_o(2) + 3\alpha u_o(3)] + \sum_{m=1}^{3} u_o(m)s_o(m),$$

$$Q = c\alpha^2[s_o(1) + 2s_o(2) + 3s_o(3)]^2 + [s_o(1)]^2 + [s_o(2)]^2 + [s_o(3)]^2 > 0.$$

Hence $\psi = -P/Q$ minimizes $J(\psi)$. Guess $\underset{\sim}{u}_o = (-0.2, -0.4, -0.7)$ and assume c = 1000. Then $\lambda_o(4) = 225$ and

$$\underset{\sim}{s}_o = -\underset{\sim}{g}_o = (-56.05, -112.1, -168.05) \equiv [s_o(1), s_o(2), s_o(3)].$$

With $\alpha = 0.25$ then $\psi = 0.01142$ and

$$\underset{\sim}{u}_1 = (-0.26398, -0.52802, -0.89191).$$

There is no difficulty in proceeding with the iteration for $\underset{\sim}{u}_2(m) = \underset{\sim}{u}_1(m) + \underset{\sim}{s}_1(m)\psi$. The new value of ψ which minimizes the performance criterion can be readily computed. Now continue with the algorithm until the desired degree of accuracy is achieved for the elements of the control vector.

When the differentiation of $J(\psi)$ is <u>not</u> performed analytically then the application of the algorithm is extremely difficult, as is now shown. As before, $\alpha = 0.25$, c = 1000 and $\underset{\sim}{u}_o = (-0.2, -0.4, -0.7)$ with $J_o = 25.66$ and $\langle g_o, g_o \rangle = 43{,}948.815$. Assume that the costate variable is a constant, which may change from iteration to iteration;

$\lambda_o = 225$.

Guess $\psi = 0.003$ then $\underset{\sim}{u}_1 = (-0.36815, -0.73630, -1.2041)$, $J_1 = 67.06$.

Guess $\psi = 0.002$ then $\underset{\sim}{u}_1 = (-0.3121, -0.6242, -1.036)$, $J_1 = 14.77$.

Guess $\psi = 0.001$ then $\underset{\sim}{u}_1 = (-0.2560, -0.5121, -0.8685)$, $J_1 = 0.9478$.

Let ψ continue to decrease then, when $\psi = 0$, $\underset{\sim}{u}_1 = \underset{\sim}{u}_o$ and $J_1 = 25.66$. Therefore consider the results for $\psi = 0.001$:

$$\lambda_1 = (1000)(0.0285625) = 28.5625,$$

$$<\underset{\sim}{g}_1,\underset{\sim}{g}_1> = 659.427,$$

$$\beta_1 = <\underset{\sim}{g}_1,\underset{\sim}{g}_1>/<\underset{\sim}{g}_o,\underset{\sim}{g}_o> = 0.0150044,$$

$$\underset{\sim}{s}_1 = -\underset{\sim}{g}_1 + \beta_1\underset{\sim}{s}_o = (-7.72557, -15.4511, -23.0749).$$

Write $\underset{\sim}{u}_2 = \underset{\sim}{u}_1 + \underset{\sim}{s}_1\psi$. Now choose ψ according to the equation

$$s_1(1)\psi = (p/100)u_1(1).$$

Comparison of the results of the calculations with $p = 6, 4, 3$ suggests that $p = 3$ and now

$$\underset{\sim}{x}_2 = (1, 0.935739, 0.672007, 0.00342475).$$

Hence,

$$\lambda_2 = 3.42475,$$

$$<\underset{\sim}{g}_2,\underset{\sim}{g}_2> = 4.57572,$$

$$\underset{\sim}{s}_2 = -\underset{\sim}{g}_2 + \beta_2\underset{\sim}{s}_1 = (-0.652751, -1.29213, -1.83723).$$

Write $\underset{\sim}{u}_3 = \underset{\sim}{u}_2 + \underset{\sim}{s}_2\psi$ and select $s_2(1)\psi = (p/100)u_2(1)$. With $p = 2$, 1 and 0.25 it is found that the smallest value of J (=0.572740) occurs in the results which come from using $p = 0.25$.

The new estimate of λ is $\lambda_3 = 1.272$. Write $\underset{\sim}{u}_4 = \underset{\sim}{u}_3 + \underset{\sim}{s}_3\psi$, where it is assumed that $s_3(1)\psi = (p.100)u_3(1)$. Values of J were obtained from $p = 0.25$, 0.125, 0.0625 and 0.3125, with the last value giving the smallest. Then follows the new estimate of λ, namely $\lambda_4 = 1.1145$. Also,

$$\underset{\sim}{g}_4 = (0.0208580, 0.0283710, -0.057464),\ <\underset{\sim}{g}_4,\underset{\sim}{g}_4> = 0.00454208,$$

$$\underset{\sim}{s}_4 = -\underset{\sim}{g}_4 + \beta_4 \underset{\sim}{s}_3 = (-0.0360514, -0.0555222, 0.0409899),$$

$$\underset{\sim}{u}_4 = (-0.257767, -0.528879, -0.893339), \; J = 0.572727,$$

$$\underset{\sim}{x}_4 = (1, 0.935558, 0.671119, 0.0011145).$$

The interesting feature in these displayed numbers is that the last component of $\underset{\sim}{g}_4$ has now become a negative quantity. This means that the third component of the control vector will decrease in size at the next iteration. Assume that $s_4(1)\psi = (p/100)u_4(1)$ and compute $\underset{\sim}{u}(5)$ for p = 0.5, 1, 2, 4, 6, 8, 10, 11, 11.5, and 12. The last three give

$$p = 11, \; \underset{\sim}{u}_5 = (-0.286121, -0.572547, -0.861100), \; J = 0.582168,$$

$$p = 11.5, \; \underset{\sim}{u}_5 = (-0.287410, -0.574532, -0.859635), \; J = 0.583223,$$

$$p = 12, \; \underset{\sim}{u}_5 = (-0.288669, -0.576517, -0.858170), \; J = 0.584332.$$

Compare the "exact" numerical results with these approximations. When p = 11 it is the third component of $\underset{\sim}{u}$ which is too large and its square contributed to J a value that is also too large. Further changes in ψ now increase the first two elements of $\underset{\sim}{u}$, while decreasing the third element and yet it is not at all clear that the "exact" numerical solution is contained within the last displayed results. If the strict numerical minimum of J is selected from the results for p = 0.5, 1, ... , 12 then it occurs for p = 2, with J = 0.572491, and the components of $\underset{\sim}{u}$ and $\underset{\sim}{x}$ are <u>still</u> not even correct to one significant figure.

There does not appear to be any point in continuing this example. The application of the conjugate gradient method to this simple multi-stage multivariable optimal control problem has not been successful. Instead of changing u(1) at each iteration one could have altered u(2) or u(3), but it is not at all evident from calculations performed by the author that this offers any improvement in convergence. Furthermore in this example no stopping criterion on the algorithm was implemented.

However one interesting "experimental" feature that is worthwhile noting is the following. After the first iterate of the algorithm the value of J corresponding to $\psi = 0.001$ was taken. From the vector $\underset{\sim}{u}_1$ the equation $u_1(1) + \alpha\lambda_1 = 0$ gives $\lambda_1 = 1.024$, which is close to the true value 1.143.

7.8 Discrete Dynamic Programming

In what has been described as a significant pioneering effort, Bellman (1957) introduced the area of dynamic programming. Five years later Bellman and Dreyfus (1962) published another book in the same area. Since the publication of these works many other books and scientific papers have been published dealing with extensions and applications in numerous fields. While a lot of attention has been paid to continuous time dynamic programming it turns out that there are many applications of the discrete time theory. Some of these are examined in this Section.

The objective is to minimize the performance criterion

$$J = \theta[x(N)] + \sum_{m=0}^{N-1} L[x(m),u(m),m],$$

subject to the first order state (or recurrence) relation

$$x(m+1) = f[x(m),u(m),m].$$

Here x(m) and u(m) are regarded as being scalar functions of the stage number m. The additive form of the performance criterion and the state equation give

$$\begin{aligned} J &= L[x(0),\ u(0),\ 0] + L[x(1),\ u(1),\ 1] + \ldots + \theta[x(N)] \\ &= L[x(0),\ u(0),\ 0] + L[f[x(0),\ u(0),\ 0],\ u(1),\ 1] + \ldots \\ &= J[x(0),\ u(0),\ u(1),\ \ldots\ ,\ u(N-1)], \end{aligned}$$

which indicates that it depends only on the initial state x(0) and the sequence of controls u(0), u(1), ..., u(N-1). Therefore, it follows that the optimal value of J, if indeed one exists, minimized with respect to u(0), u(1), ...,u(N-1) depends only on the initial state x(0). It is worthwhile emphasizing this dependence. To this end define

V(x,N) = value of the performance criterion over N stages using the optimal control starting from the initial state x(0) = x.

$$= \min_{u(0),u(1),\ldots,u(N-1)} J[x,\ u(0),\ u(1),\ \ldots,\ u(N-1)].$$

Since J is a purely mathematical function of its arguments x(0), u(0),...,u(N-1) the N minimizations can be performed in any arbitrary order. For example the minimization with respect to u(0) could be done last to give

$$V(X,N) = \min_{u(0)} \left[\min_{u(1),\ \ldots,\ u(N-1)} J \right].$$

However, the additive property of the performance criterion indicates that its first term L[x,u(0),0] is independent of u(1),...,u(N-1) and hence the inner minimization can be expressed as

$$\min_{u(1),\ldots,u(N-1)} J = L[x,u(0),0] + \min_{u(1),\ldots,u(N-1)} \{L[f[x,u(0),0],u(1),1] + \ldots\}.$$

On using the notation introduced in the definition of V(x,N) it is apparent that the second term in this last expression

$$\min_{u(1),\ldots,u(N-1)} \{L[f[x,u(0),0],u(1),1] + \ldots \} \equiv V[f[x,u(0),0],N-1].$$

It therefore follows that

$$V(x,N) = \min_{u(0)} \{L[x,u(0),0] + V[f[x,u(0),0],N-1]\}. \tag{7.25}$$

Equation (7.25) is the basic functional relation due to Bellman (1957); it relates the value V(x,N) for an N-stage process to the value for an (N - 1)-stage process. The particular structure of (7.25) makes it ideally suited for numerical implementation. If the quantity V(x,N) is known for some value of N then the recurrence relation (7.25) can be solved for successive values of N. For a single-stage process with N = 1 then the definition of V(x,N) provides the initial value for (7.25) as

$$V(x,1) = \min_{u(0)} L[x,u(0),0]. \tag{7.26}$$

In the language of dynamic programming the controls u(0),u(1),... are referred to as the decision variables. Restrictions on the decision variables can be of various types. For example one assumption might be that the current decision u(m) depends only on states up to x(m) and previous decisions with

$$u(m) = u(x(0),\ldots,x(m);\ u(0),\ldots,u(m-1)),$$

which is an example of a policy function. Optimal policies are at the heart of Bellman's principle of optimality: "An optimal policy has the property that whatever the initial state and initial decisions are, the remaining decisions must constitute an optimal policy with regard to the state resulting from the first decision."

Equation (7.25) is a mathematical statement of Bellman's principle of optimality. The functional relation states that the minimum cost for state x at stage q is found by choosing the control that minimizes the sum of the cost to be paid at the present stage and the minimum cost in going to the end from the state at stage q + 1, which results in applying this control. In practice the functional relation is solved backwards from the terminal stage to the initial stage; see Example 7.8.

When the state equations are linear in both the state and control variables and the performance criterion is quadratic in these variables then the dynamic programming equations have analytic solutions.

The extension to the case of multi-variable control problems is immediate:

$$V(\underset{\sim}{x},N) = \min_{\underset{\sim}{u}} \{L(\underset{\sim}{x},\underset{\sim}{u}) + V[\underset{\sim}{f}(\underset{\sim}{x},\underset{\sim}{u}), N-1]\},$$

and $\underset{\sim}{x}(m + 1) = \underset{\sim}{f}[\underset{\sim}{x}(m),\underset{\sim}{u}(m)]$.

Example 7.8:

A growing population of cells is assumed to obey the logistic equation $\dot{N}(t) = [a - bN(t)]N(t)$, a, b, constants. If $N(t)$ denotes the level of cells at time t then

$$N(t) = aN(t_o)\rho/[a + (\rho - 1)bN(t_o)], \ \rho \equiv \exp[a(t - t_o)].$$

At times $t_1,t_2,\ldots,t_{n-1}$ fractions $k_1,k_2,\ldots,k_{n-1}$ of the population are removed and at the final time t_n the remaining level of cells is taken. If $t_n - t_{n-1} = \ldots = t_2 - t_1 = t_1 - t_o$ determine the values of these fractions in order that the yield of cells taken is maximized. A detailed analysis of this problem was presented by Swan (1975).

This is an n-stage harvesting problem and can be solved by dynamic programming as follows. The maximum yield at stage n - 2 is determined by choosing the fraction value that maximizes the sum of the yield at the present stage and the maximum yield in going to the end from the state at stage n - 1, which results in applying this fraction value. In symbols,

$$y(n - 2) = \max_{k_{n-2}} [k_{n-2}N(t_{n-2}) + y(n - 1)].$$

Here the maximum yield at stage n - 1 is given by

$$y(n - 1) = \max_{k_{n-1}} [k_{n-1}N(t_{n-1}) + N(t_n)]$$

$$= \max_{k_{n-1}} \left[k_{n-1}N(t_{n-1}) + \frac{a(1 - k_{n-1})N(t_{n-1})\rho}{a + b(1 - k_{n-1})N(t_{n-1})(\rho - 1)}\right].$$

The expression within the square brackets is a continuous function of k_{n-1} $(0 \leq k_{n-1} \leq 1)$ and its local maxima and minima can be determined by differential calculus. There is a maximum for

$$k_{n-1} = 1 - a/bN(t_{n-1})(\rho^{1/2} + 1),$$

and hence, with this fraction value,

$$N(t_n) = \frac{a\rho^{1/2}}{b(\rho^{1/2} + 1)}, \quad y(n-1) = N(t_{n-1}) + \frac{a}{b}\frac{\rho^{1/2} - 1}{\rho^{1/2} + 1}.$$

It follows that

$$y(n-2) = \max_{k_{n-2}} \left[k_{n-2}N(t_{n-2}) + N(t_{n-1}) + \frac{a}{b}\frac{\rho^{1/2} - 1}{\rho^{1/2} + 1}\right].$$

The way to continue is evident: Determine $N(t_{n-1})$ in terms of k_{n-2} and $N(t_{n-2})$ and differentiate with respect to k_{n-2} to find $k_{n-2} = 1 - a/bN(t_{n-2})(\rho^{1/2} + 1)$ and $N(t_{n-1}) = a\rho^{1/2}/b(\rho^{1/2} + 1)$. Finally it is found that

$$k_1 = 1 - a/b(\rho^{1/2} + 1)N_1, \; k_2 = k_3 = \dots = k_{n-1} = 1 - \rho^{-1/2},$$

$$N_1 = N(t_1), \; N(t_2) = N(t_3) = \dots = N(t_n) = a\rho^{1/2}/b(\rho^{1/2} + 1),$$

and the maximum yield is

$$N_1 + (n-1)a(\rho^{1/2} - 1)/b(\rho^{1/2} + 1).$$

Example 7.9:

Use the technique of dynamic programming to solve Example 7.6.

In order to use dynamic programming in this problem it is necessary at the stages 0 and 1 to specify a range of values for each of u(0) and u(1). For example, see Table 7.3, u(0) is chosen to be 0.3, 0.25, 0.2, and 0.1 in turn. To the value of u(0) = 0.3 guesses to u(1) are made, namely 0.3, 0.25, 0.2 and 0.1. For each pair of values of u(0) and u(1) the state equation can be solved for x(2), and the value determined for the performance criterion J. The results of these calculations are shown in the upper portion of Table 7.3. They suggest that u(0) should be varied in the vicinity of 0.25 and u(1) should take increments between 0.1 and 0.2. Results are shown for u(0) = 0.251 and 0.249. Since it is required that x(2) = 19.4136186 it is reasonable to make the selections for u(0) and u(1) shown in the bottom portion of Table 7.3. To four significant figures the results are u(0) = 0.2492 and u(1) = 0.1542. The way to proceed to obtain greater accuracy is to further refine the values of the controls.

The dynamic programming solution to this problem has been obtained where J is being minimized and at the same time x(2) is at a value closest to its desired value of 19.4136186.

This example illustrates that there is a need for computer storage of many values. As the size of the program increases, to include a large number of stages and/or state and control variables, the storage problems can be of such a magnitude that present-day computers are unable to handle it. Such is the "curse of dimensionality". For this reason many investigators are happy to obtain sub-optimal control values from a computer solution in those situations where the determination of optimal controls is not within their reach.

u(0)	u(1)	J	x(2)	u(0)	u(1)	J	x(2)
0.3	0.3	0.09	100	0.25	0.3	0.076	52.5
0.3	0.25	0.076	80	0.25	0.25	0.062	41.2
0.3	0.2	0.065	60	0.25	0.2	0.051	30
0.3	0.1	0.05	20	0.25	0.1	0.036	7.5
0.2	0.3	0.065	20	0.1	0.3	0.05	0
0.2	0.25	0.051	15	0.1	0.25	0.036	0
0.2	0.2	0.04	10	0.1	0.2	0.025	0
0.2	0.1	0.025	0	0.1	0.1	0.01	0
0.251	0.15	0.04275	19.10	0.249	0.15	0.04225	18.4
0.251	0.152	0.04305	19.557	0.249	0.152	0.04286	18.845
0.251	0.154	0.04336	20.013	0.249	0.154	0.04286	19.289
0.251	0.156	0.04367	20.469	0.249	0.156	0.04317	19.736
0.251	0.158	0.04398	20.926	0.249	0.158	0.04348	20.177

u(0)	u(1)	J	x(2)
0.2491	0.1541	0.042899	19.3477
0.2491	0.1542	0.042914	19.3699
0.2491	0.1543	0.042930	19.3921
0.2492	0.1541	0.042924	19.3836
0.2492	0.1542	0.042939	19.4059
0.2492	0.1543	0.042955	19.4282

Table 7.3 Intermediate numerical values in the dynamic programming solution of Example 7.9.

The area of dynamic programming is so important that it is worthwhile presenting a separate bibliography of a number of books, which may be of interest.

Dynamic Programming - Selected Bibliography

Angel, E. and R. Bellman. 1972. Dynamic Programming and Partial Differential Equations. New York: Academic Press.

Aris, R. 1964. Discrete Dynamic Programming. New York: Blaisdell.

Bellman, R. 1957. Dynamic Programming. Princeton: Princeton University Press.

Bellman, R., and S.E. Dreyfus. 1962. Applied Dynamic Programming. Princeton: Princeton University Press.

Bellman, R., and R. Kalaba. 1965. Dynamic Programming and Modern Control Theory. New York: Academic Press.

Bertelè, U., and F. Brioschi. 1972. Nonserial Dynamic Programming. New York: Academic Press.

Boudarel, R., J. Delmas, and P. Guichet. 1971. Dynamic Programming and its Application to Optimal Control. New York: Academic Press.

Bertsekas, D.P. 1976. Dynamic Programming and Stochastic Control. New York: Academic Press.

Dan, S. 1975. Nonlinear and Dynamic Programming. New York: Springer-Verlag.

Dreyfus, S.E. 1965. Dynamic Programming and the Calculus of Variations. New York: Academic Press.

Dreyfus, S.E., and A.M. Law. 1977. The Art and Theory of Dynamic Programming. New York: Academic Press.

Hadley, G. 1964. Nonlinear and Dynamic Programming. Reading: Addison-Wesley.

Hinderer, K. 1970. Foundations of Non-stationary Dynamic Programming with Discrete Time Parameter. New York: Springer-Verlag.

Howard, R.A. 1960. Dynamic Programming and Markov Processes. Cambridge: The MIT Press.

Larson, R.E. 1968. State Increment Dynamic Programming. New York: American Elsevier.

Larson, R.E. and J.L. Casti. 1978. Principles of Dynamic Programming. New York: M. Dekker.

Nemhauser, G.L. 1966. Introduction to Dynamic Programming. New York: J. Wiley and Sons.

Norman, J.M. 1975. Elementary Dynamic Programming. London: E. Arnold.

Puterman, M.L. (editor). 1979. Dynamic Programming and Its Applications. New York: Academic Press.

Roberts, S.M. 1964 Dynamic Programming in Chemical Engineering and Process Control. New York: Academic Press.

Applications of dynamic programming in radiotherapy are presented in Sections 6.5 and 6.7.

Chapter 8

SOME OPTIMIZATION CRITERIA IN RADIOTHERAPY

8.1 Introduction

Earlier chapters in this book have focussed on features such as cell survival expressions, kinetic models, instantaneous cell kill and sophisticated methods such as optimal control theory in the implementation of fractionated therapy. The present chapter presents material which is aimed at dealing with strategy and treatment objectives in radiotherapy.

The clinician tends to make some assessment of the value of P_d, the probability of damage to normal tissues. That is, P_d is some measure of the probability of the possibility of a life-threatening injury such as hemorrhage or of an incapacitating injury or of some mutilating injury. Also, the clinician recognizes that there is some probability of cure of the tumor, P_c. If P_c and P_d are thought of as being functions of the radiation dose level D, then, intuitively, one expects that, as D increases, the ratio P_c/P_d will decrease in a monotonic manner. Current radiation treatment appears to depend on the assignment of a limit to the damage that can be tolerated. That is, most cancer radiotherapy is not directed to the production of a cancericidal effect but is delimited by some risk of damage. As Andrews (1978b) noted: "Is optimization, quite simply, merely the assignment of a limit of risk, of damage, P_d, and treatment to that limit?"

Part of the philosophy of this book is that optimization of human cancer radiotherapy is more than just treating to a preassigned bound on P_d. For example, in Chapter 6 the following optimization criteria were utilized in connection with fractionation therapy:

(1) Minimize the surviving fraction of tumor cells; see Sections 6.2 and 6.3.

(2) Maximize the surviving fraction of normal cells while reducing the final tumor size to less than one cell; see Sections 6.5 - 6.7.

Generally, it is easier to deal with a single criterion in an optimization procedure because one can understand the results. In contrast, the results from using several different criteria simultaneously may not be in a form which indicates that separate criterion contributing the most influence. An example of a composite criterion is given in (6.24).

However there is nothing in these earlier discussions which precludes the introduction of other criteria and some of these are examined in this Chapter.

To this author it is remarkable that the pioneering work by Cohen (1960) has been overlooked. This early paper, together with update, Cohen (1973a), provides a basis for computing the conditional probabilities of eradicating a given tumor or of causing an adverse reaction to sensitive normal tissue. He noted that there were relatively large standard deviations in a probit analysis of pooled data. Hopefully, when more uniform experimental or clinical data can be obtained, the efficiency of his computer program in an optimization procedure for radiation therapy can be improved.

It is interesting that Cohen's approach is essentially equivalent to the procedure developed by Moore and Mendelsohn (1972), and which has similarities with the material in Prewitt (1973). The basic idea in Moore and Mendelsohn's approach, which is not specifically restricted to radiation therapy, is to use a treatment characteristic curve, see Figure 8.4b, as a graphical method for summarizing the responses of normal and tumor tissue to therapy. For those treatment responses that are cumulative normal, the treatment characteristic curve, constructed by plotting the probit probability of tissue damage, is a straight line. The slope of this line is the ratio of the standard deviations of the two responses and whose position measures the relative sensitivity of the cancer and normal tissue. Treatment characteristic curves are examined in Section 8.2. A key feature of the work by Moore and Mendelsohn is that they suggested the scheme of Figure 8.10.

Their method also makes use of an expected loss function, which gives estimates of the effectiveness of therapy. If a simple change in algebraic sign is made in the equation involving the loss function (also known as the cost-benefit equation) then a benefit function (8.1) can be produced. The author preferred to discuss the material of this Chapter in terms of the benefit function because it sounds more optimistic than cost benefit or loss. Prewitt (1973) also refers to the benefit function.

The present Chapter presents some of the features of the benefit function and its unique maximization under experimentally (or clinically) constrained values of P_c and P_d.

The next section deals with some of the theoretical background concerned with therapeutic policy and strategy. Usually clinical trials do not produce information which can allow one to decide on the optimum usage of an old or new modality. This area is investigated in Section 8.3. Score functions and age response functions are evaluated for their potential usefulness in Section 8.4.

In Section 8.5 there are some observations on the comparison of optimization models.

Finally in Section 8.6 there is a brief discussion of the complication probability factor method as a means for selecting radiation treatment plans.

8.2 Therapeutic Policy, Strategy and Tactics

It is interesting that in 1972 Prewitt independently of Moore and Mendelsohn presented papers with a certain amount of similar content and concerned with radiotherapy optimization. Their contributions are examined in this section.

Prewitt (1972) in her approach to optimal radiotherapy introduces the following three phases:

(i) A full explanation of the radiotherapeutic intent.

(ii) Optimizing treatment protocol on the basis of contemporary models for the growth kinetics and radiobiology of normal tissues and tumors.

(iii) Optimizing implementation and delivery of the best radiation treatment protocol using the available therapy equipment.

She designates each of these in turn by therapeutic policy, therapeutic strategy and therapeutic tactics.

Introduce the following symbols and terminology. Let P_c = probability of cure of the tumor, P_d = probability of tissue destruction. The specification of numerical values to the probabilities of the outcomes of treatment P_c and P_d leaves the investigator to interpret them in terms of some decision criterion or value judgment. The probability of cure is assumed to be the probability that no tumor cells survive irradiation. One may need to settle for less and after irradiation some tumor cells may survive. Associated with this tumor control will be some other probability, p_c. Frequently both probabilities are assigned the same symbol, but for clarity they will be kept distinct in this Chapter.

i) Therapeutic policy

Consider a situation for a prescribed course of treatment in which the probability of cure $P_c > 1/2$ and the probability for tissue damage $P_d < 1/2$ suggests that the plan of treatment is beneficial and may be classified as being conservative. However the classification, as exemplified by Fig. 8.1(a) does not take into consideration concurrent tumors and tissue effects, which could modify the probability ranges.

A better approach is to introduce the concept of a benefit function b(T), which measures the expected therapeutic value for each treatment plan T.

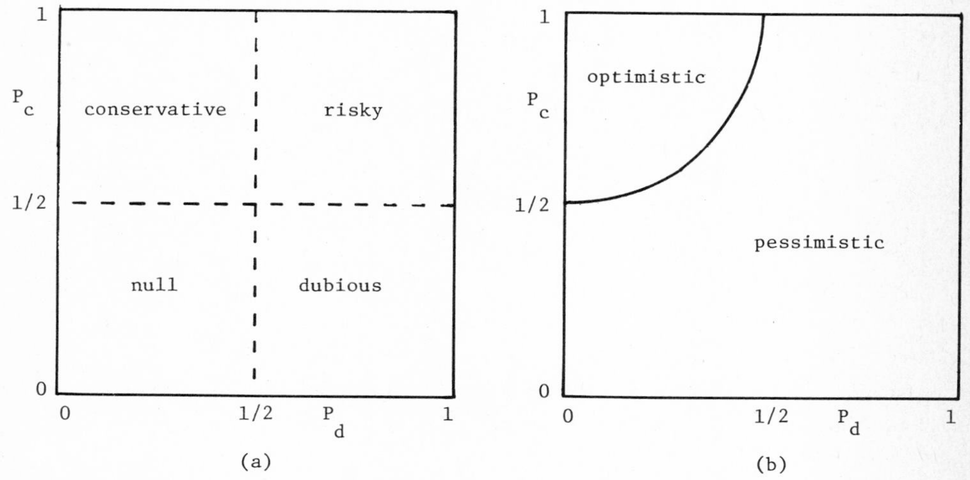

Figure 8.1(a) Probabilistic criteria on curability and vulnerability
(b) Therapeutic benefit criterion

In terms of the independent conditional probabilities P_c and P_d:

$$\begin{aligned} b(T) = a_1 &\text{ (prob. of cure)(prob. of no tissue damage)} \\ &-a_2 \text{ (prob. of cure)(prob. of tissue damage)} \\ &-a_3 \text{ (prob. of no cure)(prob. of no tissue damage)} \\ &-a_4 \text{ (prob. of no cure)(prob. of tissue damage)} \\ &= a_1P_c(1 - P_d) - a_2P_cP_d - a_3(1 - P_c)(1 - P_d) - a_4(1 - P_c)P_d, \\ &= -a_3 + (a_1 + a_3)P_c + (a_3 - a_4)P_d + (a_4 - a_1 - a_2 - a_3)P_cP_d, \end{aligned} \tag{8.1}$$

where $a_1 \geq 0$, $a_2 \geq 0$, $a_3 \geq 0$ and $a_4 \geq 0$ are utilities or penalties or costs ascribed by the therapist to the possible outcomes. One can assign numerical values to the weights a_i, $i = 1,\ldots,4$, to accommodate a selection of treatment goals. If there is some threshold value b_o then those treatment plans for which b(T) exceeds b_o are said to have an optimistic prognosis and all others have a pessimistic prognosis; see Figure 8.1b. During any one day physicians involved in radiation therapy make a number of clinical decisions. What (8.1) requires is that the difficult selection of numerical values associated with these decisions be made. The weights a_i, $i = 1, \ldots, 4$, will almost certainly depend on the type and location of the cancer as well as how far it has progressed with or without other therapy such as surgical intervention or chemotherapy. The assignment of weights can be expected to vary from physician to physician. These difficulties do not preclude an examination of the consequences of considering an expression like (8.1).

When $P_d = 0$ and $P_c = 1$ this corresponds to the best possible outcome; $b = a_1$. The other extreme (the worst outcome) occurs when $P_d = 1$ and $P_c = 0$; $b = -a_4$.

For example it is reasonable to think of b(T), or simply b, as a parameter and rewrite (8.1) as

$$P_c = \frac{b + a_3 + (a_4 - a_3)P_d}{a_1 + a_3 - \gamma P_d}, \tag{8.2}$$

where

$$\gamma = a_1 + a_2 + a_3 - a_4. \tag{8.3}$$

Note that b and γ can be positive, zero or negative; also $0 \leq P_c \leq 1$, $0 \leq P_d \leq 1$.

Regard P_c as an ordinate and P_d as an abscissa. Then it is straightforward to examine the behavior of the curves given by (8.2). One has

$$\frac{dP_c}{dP_d} = \frac{b\gamma + a_2a_3 + a_4a_1}{(a_1 + a_3 - \gamma P_d)^2}, \quad \frac{d^2P_c}{dP_d^2} = \frac{2(b\gamma + a_2a_3 + a_4a_1)\gamma}{(a_1 + a_3 - \gamma P_d)^3},$$

indicating that the curvature depends on the sign of γ. Assume now that $a_3 = a_2$.

Consider the situation when $\gamma > 0$. Let X, $0 < X < 1$, be the value of P_d when

$P_c = 1$ then (8.2) gives

$$b + a_3 = (a_1 + a_3)(1 - X) > 0.$$

Therefore, when $P_d = 0$, $P_c = 1 - X$. For a threshold value $b_o = \gamma/4$ and $P_d = 1/2$ then P_c calculated from (8.2) is also one half, which indicates that those treatment plans with better than even odds for uncomplicated cure are optimistic and all others are pessimistic. Some typical curves at equal benefit values are presented in Figure 8.2a.

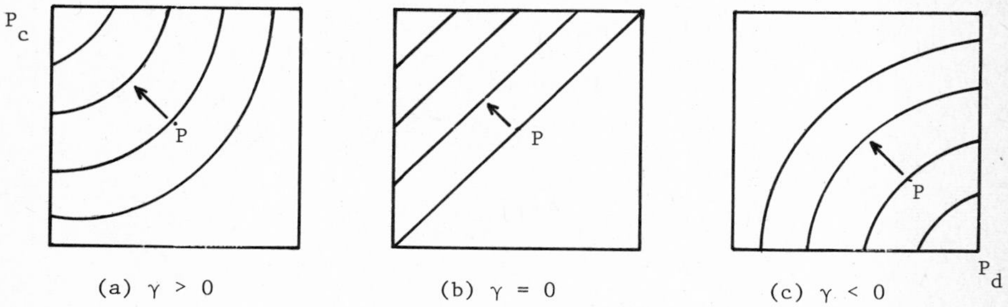

(a) $\gamma > 0$ (b) $\gamma = 0$ (c) $\gamma < 0$

Figure 8.2 Iso-benefit contours based on (8.2). The curves given in (a) and (c) and the lines in (b) are symmetrical about the line $P_c = 1 - P_d$, because of the assumption that $a_3 = a_2$. Note that P is the point (1/2,1/2). The arrow indicates the direction of increase of b; γ is defined by (8.3).

When $\gamma = 0$ then (8.2) reduces to the equation of a straight line. Consider the case when $P_d = P_c = 1$ then $b = -a_2$ (since $a_3 = a_2$) and the equation of the line reduces to $P_c = P_d$. This line and some others are shown in Figure 8.2b.

Now consider the situation with $\gamma < 0$, or $a_4 - a_2 > a_1 + a_3 > 0$, and let Y, $0 < Y < 1$, be the value of P_c when $P_d = 1$. Then (8.2) gives $b + a_3 = -(a_4 - a_2) \times (1 - Y) < 0$. Hence a typical curve must intersect the P_d axis at $P_d = 1 - Y$. The point (1/2,1/2) lies on the curve with $b_o = \gamma/4$ (<0). Some iso-benefit contours are shown in Figure 8.2c.

Prewitt (1973) assumes that $a_1 \geq a_2 \geq a_3 \geq a_4 \geq 0$, but there does not appear to be any motivation for this selection.

Write $a_1 = C_1$, $a_2 = C_3$, $a_3 = C_2$ and $a_4 = C_4$, then (8.1) takes the form

$$L(T) = -b(T)$$

$$= C_2 - (C_1 + C_2)P_c + (C_4 - C_2)P_d + (C_1 + C_2 + C_3 - C_4)P_cP_d, \quad (8.4)$$

which is the cost-benefit equation given in Moore and Mendelsohn (1972). The C's are interpreted as costs associated with the particular form of therapy. Note that their probability of tumor ablation (P_a) is equivalent to the symbol P_c used here. The quantity $-b(T)$ is now interpreted as an expected loss, $L(T)$, for some treatment T.

ii) Therapeutic strategy

Earlier, Figure 5.4 demonstrated some iso-effect curves for a mammary carcinoma. For the upper portion of Figure 5.4 the intersections of ordinates with the two iso-effect curves could be represented by sigmoid dose-effect functions which describe the separate probabilities of tumor control and of the reaction on normal tissue. This leads to curves of the type shown in Figure 8.3. For low biological dosage the

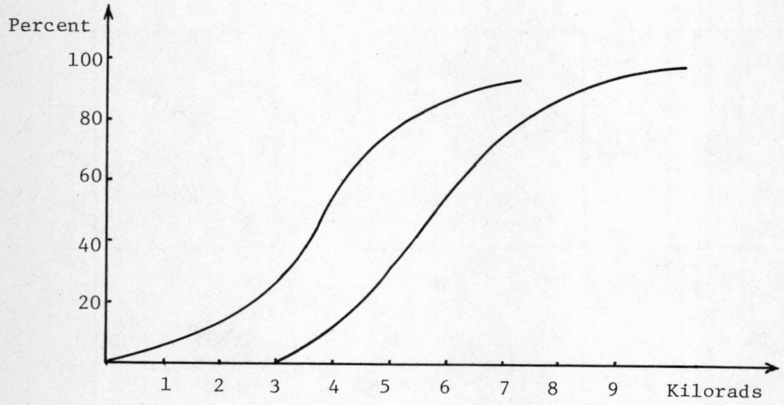

Figure 8.3 Computed dose-response curves for cure of mammary cancer and onset of severe skin reactions. Cohen (1973a), with permission.

chance of tumor reduction and risk of damage to normal tissue is small. At high dosage levels there is a definite decrease in tumor size but at the expense of irreparable injury to normal tissue. In between these two extremes there is some maximum probability of uncomplicated cure and occurs at some intermediate dose level.

Cohen (1960) proposed a way in which the fractionation scheme could provide the largest effective separation of the two response curves (Figure 8.3) and thereafter identify an "optimal" dose for that fractionation process. His idea was to use simple dose-time-volume relationships and therapeutic ratios. He assumed that the "optimal" treatment was that one which gave the largest ratio between the skin tolerance limit and tumor lethal dose. In a later paper, Cohen (1973a), he presents a block diagram for a computer algorithm. The object of the computer program is to compute the conditional probabilities (of eradicating a given tumor or of causing an adverse normal tissue reaction). The approach makes use of probit analysis; Finney (1971).

Moore and Mendelsohn (1972) suggested that the conditional probabilities of tumor and normal tissue responses could be combined to produce a treatment characteristic function (see Figure 8.4b), which offered the promise of more realistic optimization procedures.

That the two approaches by Cohen and Moore and Mendelsohn are essentially the same follows because the therapeutic ratio consists of a ratio of doses and so depends on the horizontal separation of the two response curves (Figure 8.3), while conditional probabilities depend on the vertical separation of corresponding points on the same two curves.

The effect of treatment level on the responses of normal and cancer tissue is assumed to be as shown in Figure 8.4a; Moore and Mendelsohn (1972). Two sigmoid treatment-response curves occur if it is assumed that the function chosen (e.g. log dose) gives paired cumulative normal responses. The shapes of the sigmoid curves are determined by their means (μ_c and μ_d) and standard deviations (σ_c and σ_d). Moore and Mendelsohn combine the two dose-response curves into a single treatment characteristic curve, as shown in Figure 8.4b. Let X denote some treatment level. Then, by the

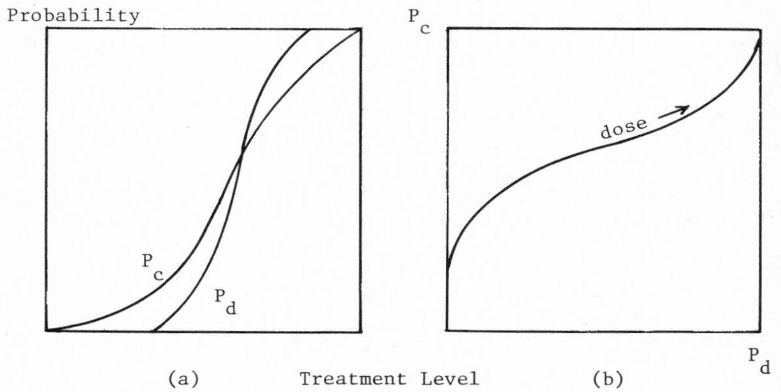

Figure 8.4 (a) Treatment response curves. Here P_c is the probability of cure and P_d is the probability of tissue damage. These curves indicate the differential radiosensitivity between the tumor and normal tissues, under the assumption of a homogeneous class of patients.
(b) Treatment characteristic curve showing P_c as a function of P_d for the treatment response curves of (a). Note that the variation of the mean dose to a vital organ is a function not only of the mean dose to the tumor, but also of the geometric restrictions on the placement of the irradiating beam of particles.

cumulative normal assumption,

$$P_c = F\left(\frac{X - \mu_c}{\sigma_c}\right), \qquad P_d = F\left(\frac{X - \mu_d}{\sigma_d}\right),$$

where F is the cumulative normal distribution function. The latter equation is solved for X to give

$$X = \sigma_d F^{-1}(P_d) + \mu_d,$$

where $F^{-1}(P_d)$ is the normal deviate of P_d and the notation F^{-1} means the function inverse to F. The equation of the treatment characteristic curve is now given by substitution for X in the first equation:

$$P_c = F\,[\,\frac{\sigma_d}{\sigma_c} F^{-1}\,(P_d) + \frac{\mu_d - \mu_c}{\sigma_c}\,].$$

By the probit transformation

$$F^{-1}(P) = \text{Probit}\,(P) - 5.0$$

and hence

$$[\text{Probit}\,(P_c) - 5)] = \frac{\sigma_d}{\sigma_c}\,[\text{Probit}\,(P_d) - 5] + \frac{\mu_d - \mu_c}{\sigma_c}\quad ,$$

which is a linear equation. This means that any pair of cumulative normal treatment-response curves can be reduced to a straight line on a probit-probit graph. For example, two data points, such as P_c and P_d from two treatment series at different doses, uniquely determine a treatment characteristic curve and provide estimates of σ_d/σ_c and $(\mu_d - \mu_c)/\sigma_c$. By examination of more data points it is possible to test for linearity, which, if verified, supports the assertion that the treatment responses in fact are cumulative normal.

The full range of therapeutic response of a homogeneous group of patients to a particular type of treatment is presented in the dose-response curves. The modality of treatment may be irradiation or chemotherapy. It is useful to keep in mind that the dose-response curves, a treatment characteristic curve or a probit treatment characteristic curve are equivalent representations of the same phenomenon.

In order to make judgments about the relative quality of different protocols or to determine the best treatment level within any one protocol these curves must be combined with the benefit function b(T) given in (8.1).

As noted earlier in the discussion of Figure 8.3 there is some (unique) maximum probability of uncomplicated cure and would correspond to the point P on curve (i) in Figure 8.5. This curve is a manifestation of the empirical constraints which delimit the possibilities for P_c and P_d. Therefore the greatest benefit to be derived from the therapy is also associated with P. Accordingly there must be a benefit curve given by (8.2), which is <u>tangential</u> to curve (i) at P. This benefit curve is designated by the label (ii) in Figure 8.5. Therapy optimization occurs at P and is thus determined jointly by the tangency of the constraint and benefit curves.

For convenience, designate curve (i) by the equation

$$P_c = g(P_d). \tag{8.5}$$

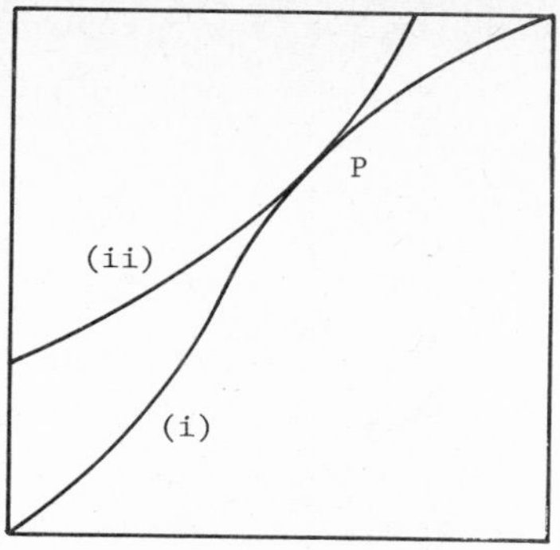

Figure 8.5 The benefit curve is given by (ii). Curve (i) arises as a consequence of the empirical constraints on P_c and P_d. The curves are tangential at P, the point at which therapy optimization occurs.

At P, the curves given by (8.2) and (8.5) must have equal ordinates, i.e.

$$\frac{b + a_3 + (a_4 - a_3)P_d}{a_1 + a_3 - \gamma P_d} = g(P_d),$$

and equal slopes, with

$$\frac{\gamma b + a_2 a_3 + a_4 a_1}{(a_1 + a_3 - \gamma P_d)^2} = g'(P_d).$$

On using these results form the expression

$$\gamma g(P_d) + a_4 - a_3 = \frac{\gamma b + a_2 a_3 + a_4 a_1}{a_1 + a_3 - \gamma P_d} = (a_1 + a_3 - \gamma P_d)g'(P_d).$$

This means that

$$(a_1 + a_3 - \gamma P_d)dP_c = (\gamma P_c + a_4 - a_3)dP_d, \tag{8.6}$$

which is equivalent to db = 0, the necessary condition for the function b to have a local turning point. Equation (8.6) is used in the illustrative example in the next subsection when the benefit function is maximized.

In her discussion on strategy, Prewitt (1973) suggests that stochastic processes are important in describing tumor survival and tissue damage. In a treated lesion tumor cure is equated with the removal of all tumor cells and so P_c, the probability of cure, is thus the probability that no tumor cells survive irradiation. However, as is known in practice, one often has to settle for control of the tumor. This means that P_c becomes the probability that, at worst, a number of tumor cells survive. These tumor cells are incapable of sustained growth. A number of mathematical results are given in the last portion of her presentation on strategy.

It is of interest to explore some of the consequences of the possibility of being able to maximize the benefit function and this is investigated in the next subsection.

iii) Therapeutic optimization

a) The benefit function

The purpose of this subsection is to select some hypothetical data and examine some of the specific details of the optimization of treatment. Here optimization is to be understood as the maximizing of the benefit function (8.1) under constraints on the probabilities P_c and P_d.

The following example provides an opportunity for discussion of a number of points in connection with the benefit function and the constraint relation between P_c and P_d. Let $a_1 = a_2 = a_3 = 1$ and $a_4 = 1.133975$ then (8.1) becomes

$$b = -1 + 2P_c - 0.133975\ P_d - 1.866025\ P_c P_d. \qquad (8.7)$$

Assume that P_c and P_d depend on the radiation dose D in the manner

$$P_c = 1 - \exp(-D^2/K_1),\ K_1 = 5.56978 \times 10^4\ (\text{rad})^2, \qquad (8.8)$$

$$P_d = [1 - \exp(-D^2/K_2)]^2,\ K_2 = 4.46664 \times 10^4\ (\text{rad})^2. \qquad (8.9)$$

The shapes of the curves given by these last two equations are of the type shown in Fig. 8.4a. Elimination of D^2 between these equations gives the constraint relation between P_c and P_d, namely,

$$P_c = 1 - [1 - (P_d)^{1/2}]^k,\ k = K_2/K_1, \qquad (8.10)$$

and the shape of the curve given by this equation is similar to (i) in Fig. 8.5.

From (8.10) it is easy to obtain dP_c/dP_d and hence (8.6) now takes the form

$$(2 - \gamma P_d)\,\frac{k}{2}\,\frac{[1 - (P_d)^{1/2}]^{k-1}}{(P_d)^{1/2}} = \gamma\,\{1 - [1 - (P_d)^{1/2}]^k\} + 0.133975,$$

with $\gamma = 1.866025$, which is the equation for the abscissa of the turning point. Numerical solution of this equation gives $P_d = 0.350000$. Hence (8.10) gives $P_c = 0.512352$. The benefit function, as a function of the dose D, has a local maximum for D = 200 rads. Some other values of b are given in Table 8.1. In Fig. 8.6 the expected value of the benefit is plotted as a function of P_c on the lower scale and

D	P_c	P_b	b
0	0	0	-1
50	0.043893	0.002963	-0.912854
100	0.164346	0.040237	-0.689038
150	0.332330	0.156602	-0.453435
200	0.512352	0.350000	-0.356809
250	0.674413	0.567342	-0.441167
300	0.801281	0.751119	-0.621150
∞	1	1	-1

Table 8.1 Numerical values of the benefit function (8.7) when the assumptions (8.8) and (8.9) are used. There is a maximum for b(D), when D = 200 rads.

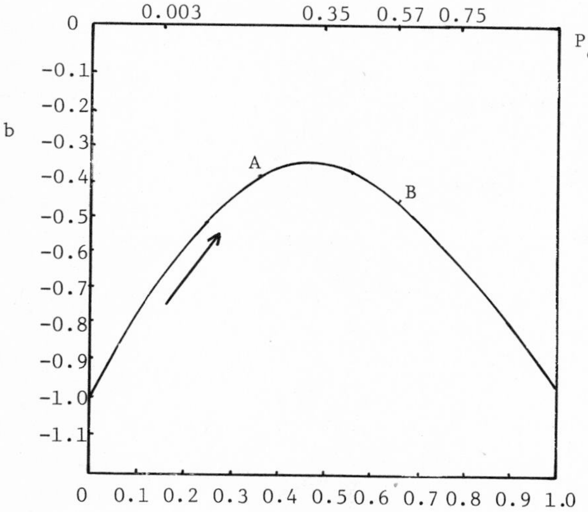

Figure 8.6 Expected benefit for the expressions given by (8.7) - (8.9); see text for details. The arrow indicates the direction of increase of the dosage.

P_d on the upper scale.

One way in which information of the type represented by Fig. 8.6 can be utilized is provided by the following hypothetical situation. Two hundred patients are assumed to have a common disease and are divided into two groups. Both groups are under the same therapeutic protocol save that those in group A are given a smaller radiation dose than those in group B. After a number of years the results are as shown in Table 8.2.

It is of interest to know the relative effectiveness of the treatment for each group as well as the "best" combination of P_c and P_d for this type of treatment.

Group	Patient totals	No. with cures	No. with damage
A	100	40	21
B	100	65	57

Table 8.2 Hypothetical case

Assume that the data points lie on and define the treatment and probit treatment curves, which in turn are expressed by equations (8.8) and (8.9). It follows that values of P_c and P_d can be determined from these formulae. Let the weights be chosen so that the benefit function is given by (8.7). Then the expected benefit for group A with $P_c = 0.40$ and $P_d = 0.21$ is computed from (8.7) as $b = -0.385$, for group B, $P_c = 0.65$, $P_d = 0.57$ and $b = -0.468$. These values of b respectively correspond to the points A and B in Fig. 8.6. Inspection of the figure indicates that group A incurred a greater benefit from the therapy than group B and that the optimum therapy lies between the two. The precise location of the optimum is given by the line of values in Table 8.1 corresponding to D = 200 rads.

Now consider the following changes in the values of the weights. Assume that $a_1 = 1$ (unchanged from its previous value), $a_2 = 0.85$ (approximately the same as before), $a_3 = 2.2$ (approximately doubled) and $a_4 = 0.40$ (approximately one third of its previous value). The new benefit function is

$$b = -2.2 + 3.2\ P_c + 1.8\ P_d - 3.65\ P_cP_d, \tag{8.11}$$

with the key feature being a significant increase in the value of the weight a_3. Assume that P_c and P_d also satisfy the constraint (8.10). Figure 8.7 shows the benefit function (8.7) together with the new one given by (8.11). Intuitively, one would have expected that the increase in the weight a_3 would give rise to a benefit function which lay beneath the one given by (8.7). That this is so is demonstrated in Fig. 8.7. A treatment based on (8.11) is less desirable than one based on (8.7). The new benefit function has a maximum value of -0.415625 when $P_c = 0.691686$, $P_d = 0.592034$ and D = 256 rads.

Figure 8.7 presents benefit functions corresponding to two levels of effect. The important point to keep in mind here is that a minimum requirement for the determination of "optimal" effectiveness, since this is not known in advance, is the investigation of at least two levels of effect. Further discussion of this point in connection with clinical trials is presented in Section 8.3. As is evident from the earlier discussions there is no difficulty (in principle) in obtaining information from the benefit function, when its weights are known.

A discussion, similar to the above, but involving the cost-benefit equation

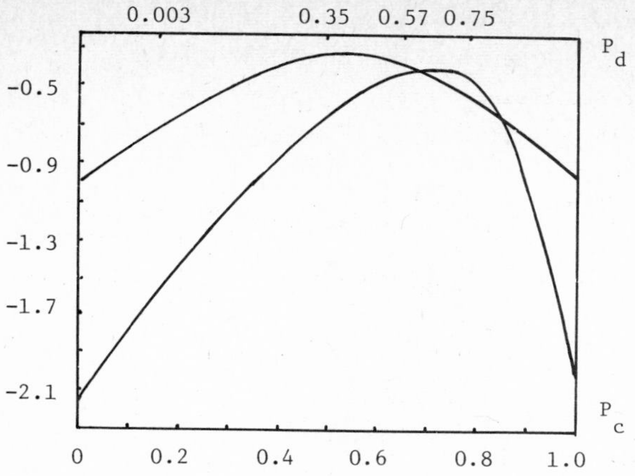

Fig. 8.7 Hypothetical studies involving the benefit functions (8.7), the upper curve, and (8.11), the lower curve.

(8.4) is given in the paper by Moore and Mendelsohn (1972).

(b) The criterion $p_c(1 - P_d)$

A primary consideration in radiation therapy is to control the growth of the tumor while minimizing the effects of damage on critical normal tissue. Control and damage are independent of one another and depend only on prognostic and therapeutic factors. One might specify that tumor control be defined as no recurrence of the tumor for five years or as no death due to cancer for at least five years. Also the definition of damage to normal tissues could be the necrosis or death due to normal tissue damage (including organs) within five years.

These comments suggest that one should seek to maximize the probability of control and no damage. Define

$$p_c = \text{probability of control.}$$

Since control and damage are independent then the objective would be to maximize

$$B(T) = p_c\,(1 - P_d), \tag{8.12}$$

where $1 - P_d$ represents the probability of no tissue damage. The quantity B(T) depends on the treatment plan T and is a benefit function. In fact, if it is assumed that the probability of control is the same thing as the probability of cure, with $p_c = P_c$, then (8.12) is just the first term associated with the weight a_1 which led to the benefit function (8.1).

The maximization of (8.12) is proposed by Hethcote (1978), who noted that D. Herbert and J.R. Andrews had also proposed using it in radiotherapy optimization.

Assume that p_c and P_d depend on some quality of therapeutic importance, such as the dose D. Then p_c and P_d will be monotonic increasing functions of D. Since $1 - P_d$ will be a monotonic decreasing function of D the graphs of p_c and $1 - P_d$ will intersect indicating that there will be a local maximum of the product $p_c(1 - P_d)$; see Fig. 8.8.

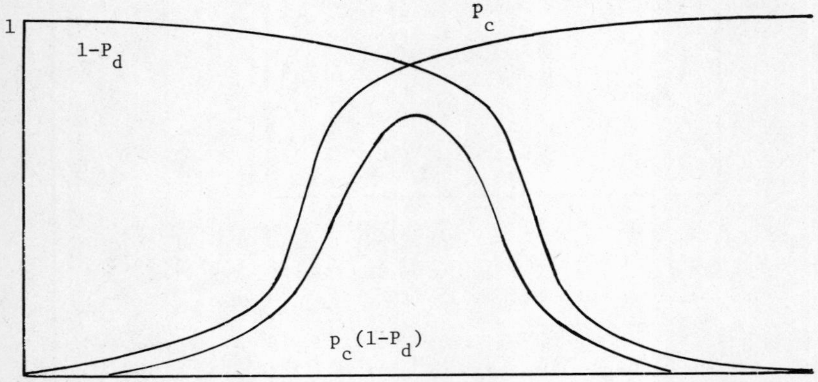

Figure 8.8 General behavior of the product $p_c(1 - P_d)$; p_c = probability of tumor control, P_d = probability of damage to normal tissues.

A specific example may be of interest. Assume that p_c is given by the right-hand side of (8.8) and that P_d satisfies (8.9). Some values of p_c and $1 - P_d$ can be produced from Table 8.1. The following table shows some other values in the vicinity of the maximum value of the product $p_c(1 - P_d)$:

D	p_c	P_d	$1 - P_d$	$p_c(1 - P_d)$
217.6	0.572636	0.427154	0.572846	0.328032

Note that a good approximation to the value of D corresponding to the location of the maximum can be obtained by plotting p_c and $1 - P_d$ as functions of D. The maximum occurs when $p_c = 1 - P_d$.

8.3 Optimization and Clinical Trials

A typical organization of a clinical trial is shown in Fig. 8.9. Traditionally there has been no focus on this approach to determine whether the optimum use is being made of either the old or the new modality. As a consequence, the study, as usually performed, is unable to produce the optimum use of either. One of the highlights in the paper by Moore and Mendelsohn (1972) is that they suggested the scheme of Fig. 8.10. They make the important point that, for each treatment modality, one

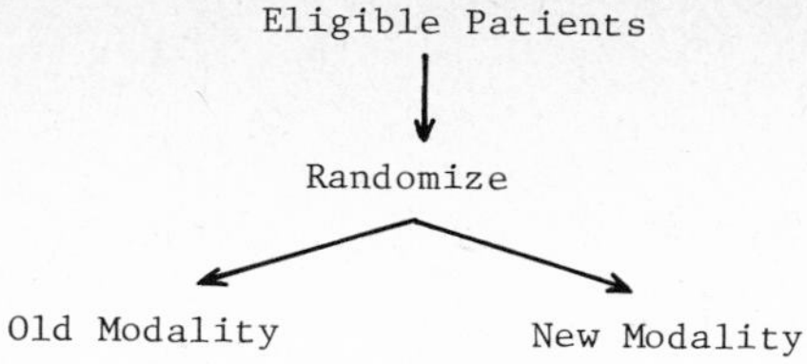

Figure 8.9 Schematic of a typical clinical trial.

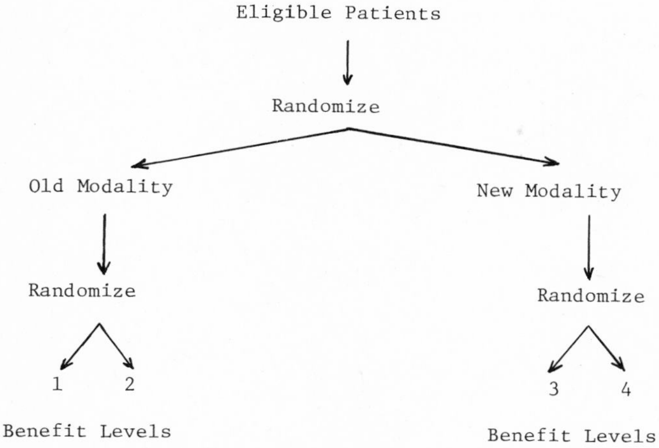

Figure 8.10 Possible organization of clinical trial for investigating optimal treatment therapies (Moore and Mendelsohn (1972); Andrews 1978b)).

should investigate at least two levels of effect. For example, corresponding to the levels 1 and 2 in Fig. 8.10 points are deduced which allow for the construction of an appropriate treatment characteristic curve. Repeat the construction for the levels 3 and 4. Now construct various benefit functions and compare them. To date no one has apparently carried through such an investigation.

One major reason for the lack of implementation of the Moore-Mendelsohn approach is the problem of standardization of measurements in all of the prognostic and therapeutic factors. Tumor stage, type and location as well as the patient's age, sex and health are examples of prognostic factors. The type of radiation applied to the tumor and normal tissues, dose rate, fractionation scheme, etc., provide information on therapeutic factors. When standardization of measurements can be improved there will follow a significant improvement in radiotherapy optimization. A similar statement is made by Cohen (1973a).

Hethcote (1978) examines relevant prognostic and therapeutic factors. He suggests that the most relevant prognostic factors are the number of fractions K and total dose D. If only K and D are used to describe the therapy then this implies that repair of sublethal damage is regarded as the most important radiobiological effect. The following list is suggested as relevant therapeutic factors:

(i) Regeneration or repopulation of tumor cells and normal tissue cells between irradiations. The overall time T (or time between doses T/K) is a variable which tries to incorporate this therapeutic factor.

(ii) Reoxygenation of the hypoxic cells in a solid tumor. This is an area of considerable importance. A mathematical tumor model incorporating hypoxic cells is presented in Section 6.4. Recently Denekamp et al. (1977) suggested that there was between 12 and 20 percent estimated proportion of hypoxic cells in a human tumor.

(iii) One effect of irradiation on cells is that they experience a radiation-induced synchronization of their progress through the cell cycle.

8.4 Score Functions and Age Response Functions

A pioneering effort to optimize X-ray treatment plans by computer judgment was introduced by the Scottish group of Hope and coworkers who suggested the score function approach; Hope et al. (1965, 1967). The score function represented the first systematic attempt to quantitate the number of desirable attributes of radiation treatment plans and to incorporate them into an objective function amenable to numerical optimization.

Basically the score function concept attempts to provide a means for the evaluation of a particular treatment plan in terms of six empirical criteria:

(i) gradient of dose across the tumor,
(ii) dose to tumor relative to the maximum incident dose,
(iii) total dose,
(iv) shape conformity of treated area relative to chosen treatment area,
(v) dose to radiosensitive or vulnerable healthy regions,
(vi) dose to regions with possible direct extension or spread by the lymphatic system.

For an individual treatment plan the approach takes these six features and quantitates them in a nonlinear manner in a polynomial, which provides a single summary score (or figure of merit). Components of the score are given by (i) dose gradient score, (ii) tumor dose score, (iii) total dose score, (iv) shape score, (v) vulnerable dose score, and (vi) entry point score. Each of these scores are complicated functions of the basic controllable treatment variables and generally uncontrollable radiobiological parameters.

Traditionally the score function was used in the review and comparison of suggested treatment plans. Suggestions have been proposed for the implementation of the score function approach on a digital computer. One major difficulty with such an implementation is that there is no guarantee that the particular score function used would be capable of reproducing therapists' judgments. Also it is not evident that all the important radiobiological variables and any intuitive guidelines are adequately, if at all, taken into account.

Criticisms of the score function approach include the following: Radiobiological phenomena at the cell and tissue level are not represented by score function criteria. A uniform dose gradient is usually assumed to be the optimal case for all tumors, yet there is no evidence in support of this. For example one would intuitively anticipate that a non-uniform dose gradient would be "more optimal" for those tumors which are known to possess spatial gradients of both cell density and radiosensitivity. It has been noted, during the study of actual score function behavior, when there is a variation in treatment delivery variables such as relative beam positions, that there is the existence of multiple local optima with different absolute scores. What this means is that the inherent mathematical properties of the score function preclude unequivocal determination of the unique globally optimal treatment plan. This ambiguity is undesirable.

Age Response Functions

There is considerable interest in exploiting differences between specific normal and malignant cell populations. One possible way of doing this was presented by Steward and Hahn (1971), who suggested the use of age response functions. These age response functions are computed from experimental age response functions.

The action of a therapeutic agent such as X-irradiation or drugs influences the cycling cells' response, which is determined by their physiological age. For example, for He La cells exposed to X-irradiation one can count the colonies surviving an exposure at various times after cell synchrony induced by mitotic selection. This leads to the experimental age response function--a histogram of survival fraction versus hours after collection. An approximation to the fractional survival of the colonies as a function of time, i.e., the experimental age response function, is given by

$$S(t) = 1 - \prod_{j=1}^{N} (1 - s_j)^{x_j(t)} ,$$

where N is the number of age intervals S(t) and s_j represent the experimental and calculated age responses respectively, $x_j(t)$ is the average number of cells in the age interval j at time t. Note that $x_j(t)$ is not necessarily an integer. This equation gives the survival probability of the colony of average multiplicity whose cells are distributed over the age intervals according to the predictions of the model. Trial and error variations in s_j can eventually approximate the experimentally produced S(t) as close as possible. A number of illustrative examples of this procedure are presented in Steward and Hahn's paper.

They considered a differential kill by X-irradiation of one cell line over another on the basis of the difference of their age responses. The age response for

He La cells was taken with allowance made for cell multiplicity and desynchrony. For the other cell line they took data reported in the literature for the age response of mouse L cells. Twenty doses of 300 rads were given. Dose in this context refers not to an actual dose but to a prescribed value in their numerical simulations. Each subsequent dose was given between 10 and 20 hours after the previous one. They calculated the ratio of the survivals of the two cell lines when the spacing for each dose, within the 10 hour interval, was chosen at random. This ratio was also found when the spacing was "optimized".

Their conclusion is that there is a definite cell killing enhancement of the one cell line over the other when there is an "optimum" timing of the sequential 300 rad doses. However it is not clear what technique was actually utilized to "optimize" the spacing of doses, and so one is left wondering how the optimum timing was arrived at. The remaining portions of their paper deals with the use of the age response function to cancer chemotherapy. Steward and Hahn suggest that their technique may be of more direct relevance to the chemotherapy of some of the leukemias. This feature is discussed at length in their paper.

8.5 Comparison of Models Used in Optimization Procedures

The material in the earlier sections of this chapter dealt with the benefit function and probability of cure. Also considered was a procedure for optimizing clinical trials. The score function approach was briefly discussed. A further report on its use in treatment plans is in Section 9.2.

In this section the optimization approaches by Graffman and coworkers are investigated.

A cell kinetic approach to optimizing dose distribution in radiation therapy is introduced by Graffman et al. (1975). They introduce (compare Section 1.4) the concept that there is a "goodness of treatment" which can be mathematically represented by the equation

$$C = \exp[-\int S^K \zeta \, dv],$$

where C is the probability that no tumor cells survive the irradiation, ζ is the local tumor cell density, K is the number of fractions, and the integration is taken throughout the region containing tumor tissue. The surviving fraction S is represented by (2.1). To approximate a bronchial carcinoma ellipses are used for the outline of the lungs and the patient contour. The tumor is divided into an inner region of constant cell density and an outer region in which the tumor cell density decreased in a sigmoid manner from the center of the tumor. In each tumor region there are assumed to be two distinct subpopulations of cells--one hypoxic and the other euoxic. Calculations are performed for the total "curability function" which is the product of the curabilities for the subpopulations. Plots of the curability function (as ordinate) versus the beam weight for the posterior field (as abscissa) indicate that the resultant curves are unimodal in shape, i.e. appear to have a solitary maximum. Also, there is an optimum setting of the posterior beam angle and width of the posterior field.

The more recent work of Graffman et al. (1979) is now examined.

A simplification of the Fischer (1971a) tumor model was proposed by Hethcote and Waltman and discussed in detail in Section 6.5; it is used by Graffman et al. (1979). The parameter values which are chosen are the same as those in problem 1 in Section 6.5, excepting that the initial size of the tumor L(1) is taken to be 3.9 x 10^9 cells, and hence $\mu \approx 0.256 \times 10^{-9}$. The number of fractions K = 30 and D(1) = D(2) = ... = 200 rads. Equation (6.19), with $t - \gamma D(i)$ replaced with the maximum of 0 or $t - \gamma D(i)$, is then used to show that, with this fractionation scheme, the tumor is reduced to one surviving cell.

Instead of (2.1) the shoulderless survival expression $S = \exp(-D/D_o)$ is then used in the calculations corresponding to those described in the previous paragraph. On comparing the results with those obtained when (2.1) is used one can obtain the characteristic doses and extrapolation numbers that correspond to a calculated variance in curability which is less than 0.01.

The Kirk CRE formula (6.1) was applied to a fully oxygenated tumor population of initial size 10^{10} cells. It is assumed that there is one irradiation per day. Characteristic dose and extrapolation numbers exist that allow for the prediction, based on using the shoulderless survival expression, of a constant curability under those conditions that give a constant CRE value.

Unfortunately Eq. (7) in Graffman et al. (1979) contains the quantity S_i in the numerator. The correct expression, compare (5.13), does not have S_i.

8.6 The Complication Probability Factor

Earlier in Section 8.2 it is assumed that the treatment response curves are of a sigmoidal shape. An analytical expression, the cumulative normal, can be fitted to clinical data in order to obtain estimates of the means and standard deviations. This appears to be a reasonable approach since many of the clinical data points appear to fall on a sigmoid-shaped curve. It is possible to compare different treatment plans and determine the therapeutic optimum, and this was shown earlier in this chapter.

However some recent work replaces the treatment response curves with linear approximations and uses them in radiotherapy optimization treatment planning schemes. This approach is now examined.

A recent paper on the complication probability factor, p, is by Dritschilo et al. (1978), who assume that it follows a sigmoid-shaped curve when plotted against dose, and is linearly dependent on treatment volume. Application of these assumptions to a single type of healthy tissue gives

$$p = \sum_D p_D v_D,$$

where v_D is the total volume of healthy tissue irradiated at the dose level D, and p_D is the probability per unit volume that this dose creates damage to the tissue.

In order to calculate p Walbarst et al. (1980a) cover the area of interest with a grid (designated by them as a "voxel ensemble"). The voxels with labels k = 1,..., j - 1 are assumed to contain tumor whereas k = j,...,M contain healthy tissue. Then

$$p = \sum_{k=j}^{M} p_k v_k, \tag{8.13}$$

where the kth element, of volume v_k, receives a local dose d_k and p_k is the corresponding local probability of complications density. It is convenient to take each v_k to be the same volume v. Clinical data provide points on a graph of p_k versus d_k. Wolbarst et al. (1980a) assume that it is possible to fit a straight line through these data and hence they are able to approximate p_k in (8.13) by linear functions. This is done by writing

$$p_k \equiv p(d_k, r) = \begin{cases} (d_k - d_r)m_r, & d_k > d_r, \\ 0, & d_k \leq d_r, \end{cases} \tag{8.14}$$

where different tissue regions are parameterized by r; r = 1,2,..., and r = r(k). The threshold dose for the tissue type of region r is d_r and the quantity m_r is a measure of the increase in probability of complications per unit of volume and dose.

Assume that the local dose d_k is generated by external beams of given dose (i.e. the dose at maximum buildup for one field) X_i, i = 1,2,..., then the ith beam contributes $A_{ki}X_i$ to the dose in the kth voxel, and the total dose there is

$$d_i = \sum_i a_{ki}X_i, \; a_{ki} \geq 0. \tag{8.15}$$

Hence, on combining (8.13) and (8.14) with (8.15),

$$p = v \sum_{k=j}^{M} m_r(k) \, [\sum_i a_{ki}X_i - d_{r(k)}], \; d_k > d_{r(k)}, \tag{8.16}$$

and p = 0 for $d_k \leq d_{r(k)}$.

In addition, there are the constraints

$$\sum_i a_{ki}X_i \geq d_T, \; k = 1,\ldots,j - 1,$$

$$\sum_i a_{ki} X_i \leq d^*_{r(k)}, \quad k = 1,\ldots,M.$$

The first constraint ensures that the tumor receives the prescribed tumor dose d_T, whereas the second is a mathematical statement that restricts any voxel from receiving more than a clinically predetermined region-specific critical dose $d^*_{r(k)}$.

A Fortran program for the implementation of (8.16) is described by Wolbarst et al. (1980b) and some results are given in Wolbarst et al. (1980a).

Chapter 9

THE OPTIMIZATION OF EXTERNAL BEAM RADIATION THERAPY

9.1 Introduction

The purpose of the present chapter is to consider some practical techniques for optimizing external beam radiation therapy.

The clinical objective is to deliver as great a dose of radiation to the tumor as possible with minimal damage to surrounding vulnerable normal tissues. Yet how can this be achieved, since the macroscopic distribution of external beam radiotherapy to tumor cells generally is the same as that to normal cells? The increase in beam energy of the ionizing radiation plays a significant role in modern treatment. Attention is being placed on improving the ratio

$$\frac{\text{integral (or total tissue) dose}}{\text{tumor dose}} .$$

When the value of this ratio is "low" then this implies that there is a selective localization of irradiation to the tumor. Undesirable irradiation effects on normal tissues are enhanced when this ratio is "high". It is possible to select a nominal value for this ratio (say unity) and then obtain values for the ratio when other energies and types of radiations are utilized. Considerations of the values of ratios of this type (together with other evaluations) leads to variations of the distribution of doses in irradiated tissues which frequently entail the usage of orthovoltage (200 keV) and megavoltage (31 MeV) X-rays, and megavoltage (10-35 MeV) electrons. Some advantages of the use of million electron volt electrons include the following:

(i) More efficient tumor treatment, since depth doses are better.

(ii) Decrease in radiation sickness since there is less side scatter.

(iii) More uniform dosage available.

(iv) There is only slight radiation dermatitis.

These physical ways of modifying the dose are fundamental to the response and recovery of the irradiated tissue. As more sophisticated equipment is developed, built and used in radiation therapy to provide many beams with different particles and energies, it becomes a significant challenge to determine if the macroscopic distribution of the radiation dose is being optimized. This is a problem in applied radiophysics and is not examined in this book.

Instead, the material in this chapter comes in the category of optimization of response, a problem in applied radiobiology.

In Section 9.2 a brief outline is presented of some of the traditional approaches for treatment plans. The amount of tedious work involved in the construction of appropriate plans was enormous. The pioneering efforts by Tsien (1955) heralded the onset of the wave of computer technology and applications to automated treatment planning. Some of the papers which deal with the automation of treatment planning are also considered in Section 9.2. One just needs to visit a patient treatment using radiation oncology to be overwhelmed by the barrage of modern computer technology used during the preparation of patients for treatment and also during actual treatment. The prospects for even more esoteric technological advances leading to improved therapy equipment are shown in the brief article by Boone et al. (1976).

Separate from the advances being made in computer technology the analysis of linear programming problems was being undertaken. With the advent of computers the solutions of many linear programming problems were being tackled by implementation of the revised simplex method. As the dimensionality and complexity of the linear programming problems increased it became necessary to develop more efficient computer algorithms for their solution. These algorithms are readily available for current digital computers. A brief introduction to linear programming is presented in Section 9.3. Apparently a completely different and superior method of dealing with linear programming problems has recently appeared in the work of a Russian, Khachian; see Kolata (1979). His work is examined in detail by Gacs and Lovasz (1979) and Delsarte (1980). Initial responses suggest that implementation of the Khachian algorithm will provide a powerful basis for the numerical solution of linear programming problems.

Investigations by the author indicate that the first published work dealing with the application of linear programming to radiation treatment planning appears to be from the Soviet Union; see Klepper (1966). Subsequent Russian work appears in the papers by Klepper (1967, 1969), Sinitsyn (1968a, b), and Polyakov (1978). However, it appears that the work by Bahr et al. (1968), and Jameson and Trevelyan (1969), provided the impetus for a number of subsequent investigations in the West. Some of this work is examined in Section 9.4 and deals with applications to treatment plans for whole bladder lesions, supplemented beam therapy to intracavitary radiation treatment, and a treatment plan for the cancer of the esophagus. Also included are plans for treating a brain tumor. A brief introduction is included for the use of linear programming in the determination of the number and coordinates of centers of rotation of beam sources.

Section 9.5 deals with the optimal beam configuration for a dose distribution which provides the best "least-squares fit" to a prescribed tumor contour, when there are limiting doses at nearby vulnerable sites.

Section 9.6 deals with a procedure for estimating and diagramming cumulative biological effects resulting from various fractionation schemes used in external beam radiotherapy.

9.2 Some Approaches for Treatment Plans

In the early sixties the following description applied to a typical irradiation treatment plan:

(i) First obtain a contour of the appropriate cross-section of the patient's body and then draw it onto transparent paper.

(ii) Localization of the tumor is found from a combination of physical examination and radiographs and then drawn in its proper location on the paper. Other important normal structures such as the spinal cord are also drawn.

(iii) Decide on the size of the lethal dose to the tumor which spares critical adjacent normal tissues.

(iv) Deliver a number of beams through the body so that they intersect at the location of the malignancy. The reason for this is that since the effects of radiation are additive it is possible to increase the dose at the tumor while other locations have smaller doses.

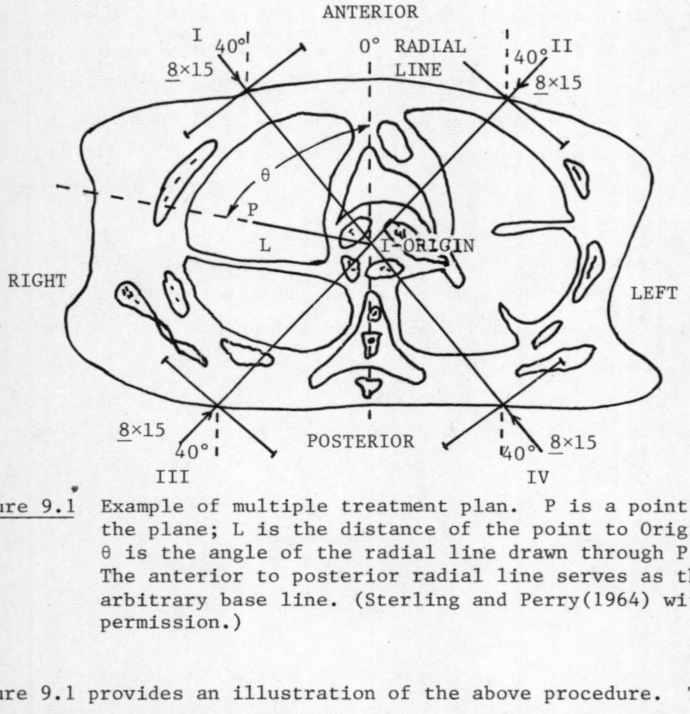

Figure 9.1 Example of multiple treatment plan. P is a point in the plane; L is the distance of the point to Origin I; θ is the angle of the radial line drawn through P and I. The anterior to posterior radial line serves as the arbitrary base line. (Sterling and Perry(1964) with permission.)

Figure 9.1 provides an illustration of the above procedure. The patient had a carcinoma of the esophagus and was to be treated with Cobalt 60, i.e. ^{60}Co, teletherapy; the skin to source distance was 80 cm and there were four 8 x 15 cm fields. The fields were to enter at angles of 40° to the vertical. At any point in the region of interest the total dose is the sum of the contributions from each treatment field at that point.

How can one determine values of the combined doses for an adequate number of points in the treatment field in order to evaluate a treatment plan and assess the effect of the treatment on the tumor, the neighboring area and specific critical tissues?

It was thought that optimization of the therapy to the patient depended on a knowledge of (a) an appropriate combination of a number of beams, (b) portal sizes, (c) angles of entry, and (d) the contribution of each beam to total dose that results in maximum dosage to the tumor and minimum radiation elsewhere.

Up to 1964 (at least) the methods of calculation of dose that were available were based on interpolations by hand from graphs. For a specific treatment plan the configuration of beams were copied onto large sheets of paper and different colors were employed to identify the different beams. The dose value at any required point would be obtained by the radiologist by interpolating between the dose values of the nearest isodose curves. It is evident that this method suffers from the deficiencies of being inaccurate, tedious and slow.

Tsien (1955) developed the first computer method to automatically sum doses from contributing beams in a simple convergent field. Thereafter, computer applications in radiation therapy made it possible for the physician to plan and replan each individual treatment. Also, different conditions of treatment and patterns of doses could be studied.

Sterling and Perry (1964) indicated that the dose C at any point on the central axis of a beam from any Cobalt 60 portal size was adequately represented by the mathematical expression

$$\log C = 2.044 - 0.36D + (0.013D - 0.0056)\log(A/P), \tag{9.1}$$

where

$$A/P = \text{(area/perimeter) of the field}$$

$$D = \text{vertical depth of the field.}$$

They also deduced that

$$P = f(\rho)C$$

gives the value of any off axis point regardless of field size. The ratio ℓ/L is the mirror image of the cumulative normal probability function:

$$f(\rho) = k = 1 - \frac{1}{\sqrt{2\pi}\sigma}\int_{-\infty}^{\ell/L} \exp\left[\frac{(\ell/L - \mu)^2}{2\sigma^2}\right] d\ell \tag{9.2}$$

with $\mu = 1$ and $\sigma = 0.17$. On using (9.1) - (9.2) it is possible to calculate the percent depth dose at any point in the field. Although these formulae apply to a Cobalt 60 source at 80 cm source to skin distance one can calculate the dose distributions from other energy sources equally well.

For a more recent perspective on a method for calculating doses in the treatment field see, e.g., McDonald et al. (1976).

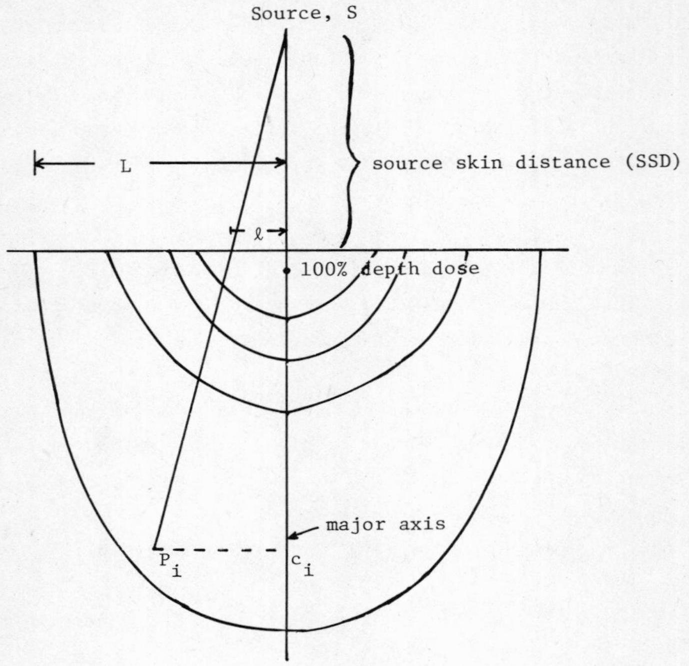

Fig. 9.2 Beam geometry; L = 1/2 length of field and ℓ = distance between major axis and line P_iS at the surface.

As indicated at the beginning of this section, the selection of a treatment plan for multiple beam therapy may require the preparation of drawings of the isodose distribution formed by the superimposed beams. Considerable time is involved in producing a carefully drawn plan, especially when allowance is made for patient curvature. How interesting and useful it would be if a large number of plans could be evaluated in sequence. After each result the beam settings could be altered, the new plan examined, and as a consequence improved plans could be discovered.

A start in this direction is provided by Worthley and Cooper (1967). They describe the mathematical background to a generalized parametric model for the behavior of external beams of X-rays incident upon tissue. The means by which their approach can be extended to calculate appropriate percentage depth doses in the presence of arbitrary skin contours and internal contours of arbitrary dose density are also provided. In a subsequent paper, Cooper and Worthley (1967) applied their mathematical model to practical two-dimensional radiotherapy planning. Corrections are made for obliquity of the incident beam on the tissue surface and passage of the X-rays through inhomogeneous tissue.

A novel facility for automating treatment planning is described by Holmes (1970). A rho-theta position transducer is used to digitalize patient contours, isodose charts and other line drawings. This information is combined with a novel computer system known as the Programmed Console, which is designed to calculate and display isodose distributions from multiple external beams. This system comprises a small digital computer, an input/output unit utilizing a magnetic card reader and writer, a display oscilloscope, and the position transducer or plotter for digitalizing patient contours and isodose charts. The patient contour and other areas of interest are traced and this information is entered into the computer. Also entered is information on the number of selected radiation beams with their desired size, orientation, and strength. The input device is provided with controls, which allow the operator to vary the position, angle, and source-to-skin distance of each beam. At a given point within a patient contour radiation intensities are produced from a method of mathematically representing beam doses. The particular representation selected is a table of doses spaced at points throughout the region of usable beam. At the beam source originate fan lines which are freely positioned in order to be close together in those regions of rapid dose change such as the penumbra. Depth lines are parallel to the surface and equally spaced. The fan lines and dose lines intersect and located at their points or intersection are the dose values. All this information is used by a computer program that is used in the calculation of the radiation dose distribution, which would result from the application of the selected radiation beams on the patient's contour. An oscilloscope displays the resultant isodose lines and, if needed, a hard copy of the display can be obtained. If the isodose plot is not satisfactory the operator changes the values of the input variables (number of beams, their size, orientation, etc.) and the process is repeated.

Holmes describes the programs for use with the Programmed Console and provides some illustrative test cases of various isodose contours.

Prior to this computer work by Holmes isodose plots were hand calculated. Therefore the considerable time spent on deriving these plots has been significantly reduced. The technique described by Holmes is not one for the optimization of radiation treatment planning. The beam strength of each of the external radiation beams is preselected and the resultant dosage distribution within the patient contour is examined for acceptability. This means that the therapist needs to perform an educated guess as to the correct beam strength necessary from each of the many differently oriented beams to produce the desired dosage at various external points, while keeping the dosage at neighboring vulnerable tissues at "minimum" levels. In short, this is a trial and error procedure.

Further discussion on the work by Holmes is presented in Section 9.4 in connection with the optimization technique described by Hodes.

During the last ten years dramatic progress has been made in the automation of treatment planning. In the short space available here some of the papers in this area are referred to.

An example of a particularly versatile computer system is given by Weinkam and Sterling (1972). Their radiation treatment planning (RTP) system is designed to give the radiotherapist and radiophysicist maximum versatility in calculating and displaying dose distribution throughout the irradiation of a three-dimensional target volume in a patient. This system can compute dose distributions for treatment plans involving either fixed or moving beams. There are many other features in their system and the interested reader is referred to their paper for the details.

Van de Geijn(1972a) considers the digital computer simulation of two- and three-dimensional dose distributions. This is done via the introduction of "patient models" and computer oriented beam models. His paper has a useful bibliography. An extension of his work on the computer program for dose distribution in high energy photon beam energy is in van de Geijn (1972b).

A survey of a number of typical computer-assisted methods in radiation treatment planning is given in van de Geijn (1975). It is apparent from this paper that much refinement of computer programs has occurred. The last part of van de Geijn's paper raises the matter of optimization in relation to true individual patient planning. In this connection he notes that an interactive computing system is required if one is interested in three-dimensional optimization of a treatment technique for an individual patient.

More recently, Khan and Lee (1979) present material on a computer algorithm for use in electron beam treatment planning.

In Section 8.3 there is a brief discussion of the score function approach of Hope and coworkers. An extension of this procedure is presented by Van der Laarse and Strackee (1976). The following is a list of their score functions:

(i) Dose delivery to tumor relative to incident dose.
(ii) Equality of dose delivery to target area.
(iii) Dose to vulnerable regions.
(iv) Integral absorbed dose.
(v) Obliqueness of the beam entries to the patient contour.
(vi) Mutual beam positions.

The total score consists of forming a weighted sum of these different score functions. A number of programs are available which they need for a particular treatment plan. Of special note is their list of four main criticisms of their score function approach and the reader is referred to their paper for specific details. Their approach, however, has merit as shown in the following example. They took three combinations of beam incidence directions for three fields, two wedges for each beam, and two beams with equal weights. This leads to comparison of 1,536 different dose distributions. It is interesting to note that, in just about all the situations considered, the computer-generated optimum treatment plan is as good as, or improves on that which is produced by a radiotherapist.

Another extension of the score function approach by Hope and coworkers is provided in the paper by Cooper (1978), who proposed the minimization of a "treatment evaluation function". This function is the weighted sum of two quantities E_1 and E_2, which contain treatment parameters such as wedge filter angle, the angle of incidence of the external beam, point of beam entry, relative weighting and beam width for each field. In particular a measure of tumor dose uniformity is given by

$$E_1 = \frac{1}{Pd_o^2} \sum_{j=1}^{P} \left[\sum_{i=1}^{n} w_j D_{ij} - D_o \right]^2 , \tag{9.3}$$

where

P = number of sample points taken over the tumor,

$D_{i,j}$ = percentage depth dose at the jth point from the ith field,

n = number of treatment fields,

d_o = average percentage depth dose to the tumor,

$$= \frac{1}{P} \sum_{j=1}^{P} \sum_{i=1}^{n} w_i D_{ij} . \tag{9.4}$$

The tissue damage function is

$$E_2 = (1/RS) - 1, \tag{9.5}$$

where

S = cell survival fraction at the end of radiation treatment

R = recovery factor for these cells for this treatment.

What variations in the various treatment parameters will result in improvement to a particular plan? Cooper examines the evaluation of all derivatives of the treatment function with respect to all the treatment parameters. He suggests that the treatment evaluation function be minimized in order to gain insight into parameter variations.

This paper is one of the few in the important area of variation of treatment parameters.

9.3 Linear Programming

Many breakfast cereals have lists of the vitamin content, mineral content, carbohydrate content etc. on the side of the package. Apart from Government regulations, this information is provided as an aid to individuals who are interested in having a balanced diet. Suppose that a person wishes to determine from a given number of food products the lowest cost diet that satisfies the minimum requirements for a balanced diet. This is an example of a problem whose solution can be obtained by a systematic procedure known as linear programming.

Another example is provided in the determination of an overall objective, which is to maximize the growth of capital in a portfolio of stocks and bonds so as not to exceed prescribed degrees of risk. This problem can be formulated and solved using the techniques of linear programming, a fact that is well-known to many money managers.

It seems unfortunate in some ways that most of the original work in dealing with linear programming problems was done for military purposes during the second world war. In the general upsurge of intellectual pursuit in the fifties it was noted that many types of problems could be cast into the mathematical framework of what is called linear programming. An interesting historical perspective is given by one of the key first investigators--Dantzig (1970). A useful introductory book with lots of examples is that by Wolfe (1973). The book by Gass (1975) is also useful. There are many books in this area but most tend to be too theoretical and dry. A particularly clear exposition is by Noble (1969), whose approach is developed in this section.

What is a linear programming problem? Generally speaking, one seeks to maximize or minimize a <u>linear</u> sum of quantities having cost (or weight) coefficients subject to a finite number of <u>linear</u> inequality constraints. Techniques for solving for the unknowns rely on linear algebra. Significant progress in the size and scope of linear programming problems that could be handled was made with the developments in the digital computer. The situation at the present time is such that one can use well-tried and tested computer algorithms to obtain numerical solutions to rather formidable linear programming problems. There is now an extensive literature on the applications and theory of linear programming together with extensions of it to such areas as nonlinear programming.

With the simplicity of usage of computer algorithms, without requiring an extensive background in mathematics, it was natural then to anticipate that linear programming would be used in radiation treatment planning and therapy.

The basic mathematical formulation and simplex method of solutions is developed in this section. Then, in the next section, some of the applications of linear programming in radiotherapy are examined.

Consider the following linear programming problem:

<u>Objective</u>: Maximize $J = 7w_1 + 10w_2$.

<u>Constraints</u>:

$$w_1 + 2w_2 \le 80,$$
$$w_1 + w_2 \le 70,$$
$$2w_1 + w_2 \le 90,$$
$$w_1 \ge 0,\ w_2 \ge 0.$$

The simplex method of solution of this problem is now described. First, one introduces slack variables w_3, w_4 and w_5 in order to convert the inequalities into equalities:

$$\left.\begin{aligned} w_1 + 2w_2 + w_3 \qquad\qquad &= 80 \\ w_1 + w_2 \qquad + w_4 \qquad &= 70 \\ 2w_1 + w_2 \qquad\qquad + w_5 &= 90 \end{aligned}\right\} \tag{9.6}$$

Because of the signs of the inequalities the slack variables must be positive and now

$$w_i \geq 0, \; i = 1,\ldots,5.$$

The problem is to determine w_i, $i = 1,\ldots,5$ in order to maximize

$$J = 7w_1 + 10w_2. \tag{9.7}$$

Equations (9.6) constitute a system of three equations in five unknowns, with rank 3. This means that if two of the variables are arbitrarily assigned then, in general, it is possible to solve for the remaining variables. Simply assign the value zero to two of the variables. For example select $w_1 = w_2 = 0$ in (9.6) so that

$$w_3 = 80, \; w_4 = 70, \; w_5 = 90,$$

which is called a basic solution; variables other than those that are set to zero are referred to as basic variables. The value of J corresponding to this basic solution is $J = 0$. Either w_1 or w_2 can be taken to have a positive value. Since $J = 7w_1 + 10w_2$ it is appropriate to select w_2 for this purpose so that an increase of w_2 by one unit increases J by 10 whereas, if w_1 has an increase of one unit, J increases by only 7 units. Therefore increase w_2 while retaining w_1 at its value of zero. This change in the value of w_2 increases J, and forces a reduction in w_3, w_4 and w_5 in order to retain the equalities in (9.6). Since w_1 still has the value zero, (9.6) gives

$$\left.\begin{aligned} w_3 &= 2(40 - w_2) \\ w_4 &= 70 - w_2 \\ w_5 &= 90 - w_2 \end{aligned}\right\} \tag{9.8}$$

The quantities w_3, w_4 and w_5 must be non-negative and w_2 cannot be increased indefinitely. The first equation in (9.8) implies that $w_2 \leq 40$, the second implies that

$w_2 \leq 70$ and the third $w_2 \leq 90$. The maximum permissible value of w_2 is the smallest of these numbers. Hence a new basic feasibility solution, using (9.6), is given by

$$w_1 = 0,\ w_2 = 40,\ w_3 = 0,\ w_4 = 30,\ w_5 = 50.$$

The word feasible refers to any solution of (9.8) that also satisfies $w_i \geq 0$. Also, the new basic variables are w_2, w_4 and w_5. The value of J is now

$$J = 7w_1 + 10w_2 = 400, \tag{9.9}$$

which is greater than the previous value of zero. This completes the first step in the simplex method of solution.

Only one of the basic variables w_3, w_4, w_5 occurred in each of the equations (9.6) and this is the reason why it is so straightforward to write (9.8). This suggests that adjustments be made so that each of the new basic variables w_2, w_4 and w_5 occurs in only one equation. By inspection of (9.6) it is apparent that this is possible by using the first equation to eliminate w_2 from the second and third equations. The result is

$$\left.\begin{aligned} w_1 + 2w_2 + w_3 \qquad\qquad &= 80 \\ w_1 \qquad - w_3 + 2w_4 \qquad &= 60 \\ 3w_1 \qquad - w_3 \qquad + 2w_5 &= 100 \end{aligned}\right\} \tag{9.10}$$

Now introduce the nonbasic variables w_1 and w_3 into J, by using the first equation in (9.6), so that (9.7) becomes

$$J = 400 + 2w_1 - 5w_3. \tag{9.11}$$

Note that $w_1 = w_3 = 0$ and $J = 400$ as it should be. The advantage of this last displayed expression for J over (9.9) is that it clearly illustrates what happens when w_1 or w_3 increases. Inspection of (9.11) indicates that w_1 must now be varied, keeping w_3 equal to zero. Equations (9.10) give

$$w_2 = (1/2)(80 - w_1),$$
$$w_4 = (1/2)(60 - w_1),$$
$$w_5 = (1/2)(100/3 - w_1).$$

Since w_2, w_4 and w_5 cannot be negative these equations indicate that w_1 cannot exceed 80, 60, 100/3, respectively, and the selection of 100/3 is now the greatest allowable value of w_1. It follows that the new basic feasible solution is given by

$$w_1 = 100/3,\ w_2 = 70/3,\ w_3 = 0,\ w_4 = 40,\ w_4 = 40/3,\ w_5 = 0. \tag{9.12}$$

The new basic variables are w_1, w_2 and w_4, and using the same reasoning as before, rearrangements of the system of equations (9.10) are made in order to assure that each of these appears in only one equation. To achieve this, eliminate w_1 from the first and third equations in (9.10) by means of the third:

$$\left.\begin{aligned} w_2 + (2/3)w_3 \qquad - (1/3)w_5 &= 70/3 \\ w_3 - 3w_4 + \qquad w_5 &= -40 \\ w_1 \qquad - (1/3)w_3 \qquad + (2/3)w_5 &= 100/3 \end{aligned}\right\} \tag{9.13}$$

Elimination of w_1 from (9.12) using the last equation produces

$$J = (1400 - 13w_3 - 4w_5)/3 \quad .$$

Alteration of w_3 or w_5 through positive values can only decrease J, and thus no further improvement is possible. The results in (9.12) are therefore the optimal solution to the problem. A feasible solution that also maximizes J is referred to as an optimal feasible solution. This completes the second step in the simplex method and for the present problem it is also the final step.

The purpose of the above steps is to provide an elementary understanding of the simplex method. For theorems on the theory of this method for solving linear programming problems the reader is referred to the books listed earlier in this Section.

However, it is worthwhile interpreting the above steps of the simplex method in terms of row operations on matrices.

Express (9.6) and (9.7) in the array

$$\begin{matrix} J & & w_1 & w_2 & w_3 & w_4 & w_5 & \\ 0 & \Bigg[& 1 & 2 & 1 & 0 & 0 & 80 \\ 0 & & 1 & 1 & 0 & 1 & 0 & 70 \\ 0 & & 2 & 1 & 0 & 0 & 1 & 90 \\ 1 & & -7 & -10 & 0 & 0 & 0 & 0 \; \Bigg] \end{matrix} \tag{9.14}$$

The previous discussion started by changing w_2 since a unit change in w_2 would produce a greater change in J than a unit change in w_1. With reference to the matrix (9.14) choose the column with the most negative number in the last row. The step following (9.8) consists of dividing the first three elements in the last column of (9.14) by the corresponding elements in the second column and selecting the row which corresponds to the smallest of these three positive numbers. This is the first row.

Thereafter, the method proceeds with the elimination of w_2 from the second and third equations in (9.6). In the language of matrix algebra pivot on the (1,2) element in (9.14) and reduce the second, third and fourth elements to zero as in a Gauss-Jordan procedure. This yields (dropping the column for J, since it does not change)

$$\begin{bmatrix} 1 & 2 & 1 & 0 & 0 & 80 \\ 1 & 0 & -1 & 2 & 0 & 60 \\ 3 & 0 & -1 & 0 & 2 & 100 \\ -2 & 0 & 5 & 0 & 0 & 400 \end{bmatrix} \tag{9.15}$$

The first three rows give (9.10) and the last row must be interpreted as $J - 2w_1 + 5w_3 = 400$, which is (9.11).

As in the previous paragraph now locate that column which contains the most negative number in the last row of (9.15). Now divide each of the first three elements in the last column of (9.15) by the corresponding element in the first column, and select the smallest positive number among the results. This is the third with value of 100/3. Next pivot on the (3,1) element in (9.15) and use the standard Gauss-Jordan procedure to produce

$$\begin{bmatrix} 0 & 3 & 2 & 0 & -1 & 70 \\ 0 & 0 & 1 & -3 & 1 & -40 \\ 1 & 0 & -1/3 & 0 & 2/3 & 100/3 \\ 0 & 0 & 13/3 & 0 & 4/3 & 1400/3 \end{bmatrix}$$

The first three rows are equivalent to (9.13) and the last row is interpreted as

$$J + (13w_3 + 4w_5)/3 = 1400/3.$$

Since the elements in the last row are all positive this means that J cannot be increased further.

It is possible to present a geometrical perspective on the linear programming problem which has just been solved by the simplex method. The problem is to

$$\text{maximize} \quad J = 7w_1 + 10w_2,$$
$$\text{subject to} \quad w_1 \geq 0,\ w_2 \geq 0,$$

and

$$w_1 + 2w_2 \leq 80,\ w_1 + w_2 \leq 70,\ 2w_1 + w_2 \leq 90. \tag{9.16}$$

In this last display the expression $w_1 + 2w_2 = 80$ is the equation of a straight line in the (w_1,w_2) plane; see Figure 9.3.

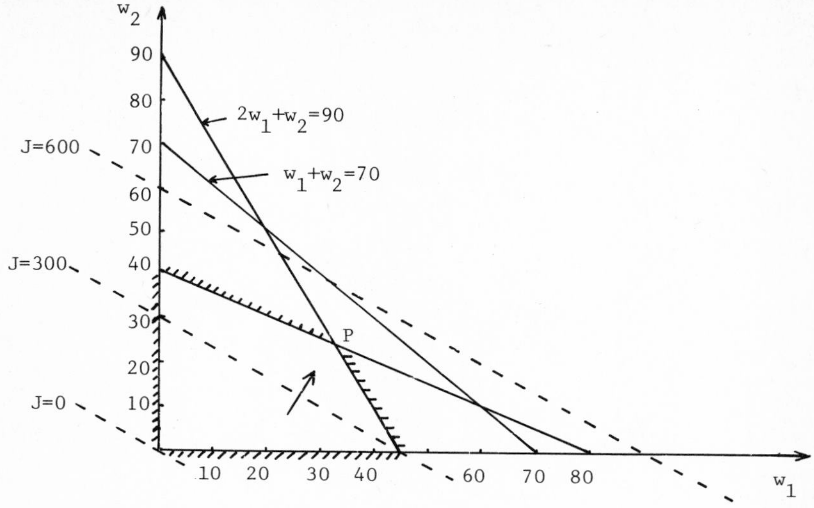

Figure 9.3 Geometric point of view.

The inequality $w_1 + 2w_2 \leq 80$ means that the point (w_1,w_2) must be beneath the straight line. Similarly, the other two inequalities in the last display define half-planes in which the permissible points (w_1,w_2) must lie. The constraints $w_1 \geq 0$ and $w_2 \geq 0$ indicate that (w_1,w_2) is restricted to the first quadrant. It is apparent that the inequalities confine the point (w_1,w_2) to the shaded polygonal region in Figure 9.3. The straight line $7w_1 + 10w_2 = J$ can be superimposed on the figure. For example, for $J = 0, 300, 600$ the corresponding straight lines are shown as the parallel dashed lines in Figure 9.3. The maximum J is obtained by proceeding as far as possible in a direction perpendicular to these lines in the direction of the arrow without leaving the admissible region. Eventually the point P is reached which is the intersection of

$$w_1 + 2w_2 = 80, \quad 2w_1 + w_2 = 90,$$

that is, $w_1 = 100/3$, $w_2 = 70/3$, and is the same result as obtained by the simplex method. The maximum value of J is 1400/3, as before.

The geometrical point of view indicates that two of the equations in (9.16) are strict equalities and one is an inequality. If slack variables are introduced two of these will be zero and one nonzero. Hence the solution is a basic feasible solution with three nonzero variables. The corners of the polygonal figure correspond to the basic feasible solution.

The above example is straightforward. In linear programming there are a number of special situations and simple illustrations of these are now presented.

(i) Non-unique optimal solutions

Objective: Maximize $J = 2w_1 + 4w_2$.

Constraints: $w_1 + 2w_2 \leq 8$, $2w_1 + w_2 \leq 10$,

$w_1 \geq 0$, $w_2 \geq 0$.

The special feature about this example is that the right-hand side of the expression for J is a linear multiple of one of the constraints. A geometrical picture is easily constructed. The maximum value of J is 16. There are an infinite number of (finite maximum) feasible solutions that satisfy the given problem.

(ii) No obvious feasible solution

The inequalities may be such that the origin of coordinates does not lie in the admissible region. Therefore the assumption that $w_1 = w_2 = 0$ does not lead to a feasible solution.

(iii) Contradictory constraints

This situation is self-evident from the title.

(iv) Unbounded solutions

The inequalities may be arranged in such a manner that any sufficiently large values of w_1, w_2 will satisfy the constraints.

A full discussion of the use of matrix methods for handling problems of this type (i)-(iv), and also the special case of degeneracy, is given, for example, in Noble (1969, pp. 173-180).

In numerical work on a digital computer the revised simplex algorithm is frequently utilized for linear programming problems. However, this procedure is not investigated here.

9.4 Linear Programming and Radiation Treatment Planning

The technicalities involved in the treatment of a patient with parallel opposing fields does not present as great a complication as a treatment plan in which several multiple arrangements are to be utilized. In order to obtain isodose lines at an angle different from 90° to the axis of a radiation beam wedge filters are introduced. A wedge filter is a radiation filter so constructed that its thickness or transmission characteristics vary continuously or in steps from one edge to the other. For a number of types of radiation treatment wedge filters are used to increase the uniformity of the dose. An illustration of the use of wedges in a hypothetical treatment plan is shown in Figure 9.4.

Before continuing it is worthwhile obtaining a perspective on the concept of optimization in radiotherapy with externally applied radiation beams. The work by Holmes (197), see Section 9.2, represents a significant milestone in the development of treatment plans, for his computer technique replaced much of what was done previously by hand. Once a procedure gets automated and is in operation for some time it is natural to think of ways in which optimization can be used to further improve the procedure. For example, after the isodose distribution is determined the therapist examines it for treatment plan attributes such as maintaining a sufficient dosage to the tumor, providing a minimal integral dose, no hot spots and so on. Yet, for a multibeam plan, how does the skilled therapist choose how strong each radiation field should be in order to achieve the desired effects? Can a technique for a radiation therapy treatment plan be produced in which the therapist assigns desired dosages at selected points within the treatment area of interest and then derive the number, orientation and strength of the radiation beams? One such optimization technique is linear programming, which provides a mathematical framework for a first attempt at dealing with questions of this type.

With the advent of advances in linear programming and digital computers it was natural that at some point in time someone would suggest their combination in tackling the problem of the optimization of dose. To many investigators in clinical radiotherapy the appearance of mathematics into the discussion of treatment plans may appear to be puzzling. After all, what relevance does all this mathematical abstraction have for clinical investigations? Biological sciences, in general, and the medical sciences in particular, have not experienced the same kind of impact and contributions that mathematics has made in physics, chemistry, engineering. Consequently it is interesting to note the introduction of the technique of linear programming into a basic radiological area--treatment planning. Depending on one's point of view it was fortunate or unfortunate that the basic work appeared to have been published in the Soviet Union. The pioneering efforts appear to have been made by Klepper (1966, 1967, 1969) and subsequently by Sinitsyn (1968a, b). These papers are in Russian. It does not seem to be apparent whether their work is still not understood, or if it has been superseded by work in the West by Bahr et al. (1968), Hodes (1974), Bourgat et al. (1974), McDonald and Rubin (1977), for example. However, in his paper, Orr (1972) noted the following in connection with Klepper's work:

> Klepper began by regarding his uniformity, shape, and vulnerability criteria as constraints with limiting values. His objective function was the integral dose which was to be minimized.
>
> The approach turned out to be of no value, so the objective function was altered to include shape and vulnerability as linear relationships. The uniformity criterion was retained as a constraint. This method was partially successful but the linearity imposed on the other criteria allowed undesirable local maxima which had to be adjusted manually.

For many of the linear programming problems that have been considered in radiology the objective is to deliver a lethal dose to the tumor with maximum dose concentration at the center of the tumor. To this objective are adjoined various constraints such as limiting the local dose to neighboring tissues and to vulnerable regions. In particular the objective function to be minimized often is a linear function of nonnegative beam weights or relative intensities (corresponding to short term exposure to radiation). The constraints consist of linear inequalities in the beam weights and correspond to limiting the dosage at selected points in the target. At this stage the problem is in the framework of linear programming and its solution can be readily determined. Adjustments to the constraints may need to be made because nonfeasible solutions (see the mathematical discussion in Section 9.3) may occur. Other objectives and constraints are possible and, so long as they are linear, the problem is easily solved on a digital computer. There is no requirement that the investigator need know anything of the details of the techniques for solving linear programming problems. The solution of the linear programming problem is the <u>best</u> solution to the problem in the manner in which it is formulated.

Literature in the West often refers to the work of Bahr et al. (1968) in connection with the (first) contribution of the method of linear programming to radiation treatment planning. The same material was given in a lecture to the Radiological Society of North America in Chicago, Illinois, Nov. 25 - Dec. 1, 1967. The work by Gallagher (1967) does not appear to have been published.

Bahr et al. (1968) consider the application of linear programming to planning the spatial dose map for a whole bladder lesion. The main point of their paper is to demonstrate that, in principle, the therapist need only provide a contour exhibiting areas of anatomical interest with the requirements for dosages in preassigned areas. Implementation of the linear programming algorithm on a digital computer is then straightforward. Their approach is now described in greater detail.

Let s^1 and s^3 respectively denote the cross-sectional areas of the heads and necks of the femurs, and let s^2 denote the cross-sectional area of the rectum. The target of the beam is the neoplastic area, which is surrounded by an area designated the "collar". A mosaic equivalent of the patient contour and boundaries of the above areas is now constructed. Superimposed on the mosaic equivalent is a system of squares; each square has length of side equal to 1 cm. The following notation is introduced:

$a_i^k \equiv$ the dose in kilorad in the square A^k by virtue of the ith unit treatment vector.

The unit treatment vector is defined by Bahr and coworkers and includes such features as the specification of area and shape of entrance portal, the source-skin distance associated with the uncorrected isodose map in question. This isodose map is for the direction of 90°, and is superimposed on the drawing of the patient's cross-sectional area.

They selected 72 distinct entries, spaced at 5° intervals about the contour of the patient, the central axis of each intersecting in common at a point at the approximate geometric center of the tumor region. As objective they chose to minimize, J, the integral dose over vulnerable regions, where

$$J \equiv J(W_1,\ldots,W_{72}) = \sum_{i=1}^{72} W_i(s_i^1 + s_i^2 + s_i^3),$$

and W_i, $i = 1,\ldots,72$ represent beam weightings.

The interpretation of W_i' as the weighting factor of the ith field means, physically, that this is the dose in kilorads to be delivered to the ith field at the classical 100 percent point. Since these weightings are nonnegative quantities, there are the constraints

$$W_i \geq 0, \; i = 1,\ldots,72.$$

In addition there are the following constraints on the radiation dose.

1. Tumor dose requirement:

$$\sum_{i=1}^{72} W_i \,(\text{target})_i \geq 6.0 \text{ kilorads},$$

$$\sum_{i=1}^{72} W_i (T_{max})_i \geq 6.0 \text{ kilorads}.$$

Here, the word target refers to the dose in the region of the tumor and $(T_{max})_i$ is the dose in kilorads in the grid square at the geometrical center of the treated region due to the ith field.

2. Anatomical dose requirements:

(a) the anatomy proper

$$\sum_{i=1}^{72} W_i s_i^1 \leq 3.0, \quad \sum_{i=1}^{72} W_i s_i^2 \leq 3.0, \quad \sum_{i=1}^{72} W_i s_i^3 \leq 3.0,$$

(b) tumor "collar"

$$\sum_{i=1}^{72} W_i a_i^k \leq 6.0 \text{ kilorads}, \; k = 1,2,3.$$

3. Upper bound

The dose at the 100 percent point of any entry is not to exceed 7.0 kilorads.

The objective function is linear and the constraints are also linear. Mathematically, there is a linear programming problem for the determination of the beam weightings. There are 28 constraint equations in the "collar" and 3 constraint equations in the anatomy proper, and so, in the appropriate hyperplane, for this over-determined mathematical problem, it is noteworthy than Bahr and coworkers were able to locate the extreme tangency point. (For the problem with geometric solution in Figure 9.3 the extreme tangency point is P.) In fact it is well to keep in mind that solutions (if they exist) to linear programming problems are always stated in terms of the extreme points in the associated hyperplane. Bahr et al. (1968) present a summary of their computer solution to the mathematical optimization problem. They indicate that this gives the solution to the posed problem of determining an optimized spatial treatment plan, and this is shown in Table 9.1

Angles of entry selected by L.P.		Weighting, W, by L.P.	W_iA_i (rads)	Area	
i = 6	25°	$W_6 = 4.637$	$W_6A_6 = 4637$	Target	$6000 \geq 6000$
i = 30	145°	$W_{30} = 3.627$	$W_{30}A_{30} = 3627$	T_{max}	$6003 \geq 6000$
i = 47	230°	$W_{47} = 2.698$	$W_{47}A_{47} = 2698$	Collar	$6000 \leq 6000$
i = 48	235°	$W_{48} = 0.057$	$W_{48}A_{48} = 57$	s^1	$1878 \leq 3000$
Dose bound (100% point) $4637 \leq 7000$ rads				s^2	$1552 \leq 3000$
				s^3	$1261 \leq 3000$

Table 9.1 Linear programming (L.P.) solution to provide a treatment plan for a whole bladder lesion. Area refers to dosages in rads to areas under constraint; s^1 (≡ left head and neck of femur), s^3 (≡ right head and neck of femur) and s^2 (≡ rectum). (Bahr et al. (1968), with permission.)

The effect of lowering the dose constraint on the "collar" region is examined by Bahr and coworkers and they find that there is an increase in dose uniformity.

Although linear programming is an extremely useful optimization approach care is needed in using it in radiotherapy planning. The extreme points solution generally violates the (usually) desired treatment characteristics of dose uniformity. Therefore this aspect of linear programming fundamentally opposes one of the therapeutic goals in treatment planning.

It is now evident that the paper by Bahr et al. (1968) was the forerunner to a number of attempts to utilize techniques like linear programming as an aid to the development of better treatment plans. A synopsis of their work appears in Bahr et al. (1970).

Jameson and Trevelyan (1969) seek the optimum lateral position of a double wedge filter which will produce a dose distribution across the pelvis, and having maximum and minimum values set by the radiotherapist. This problem arose in the context of using external beam therapy as a supplement in the treatment of gynecological conditions with intracavitary radium. The solution is obtained via the application of linear programming.

There appears to be a gap of five years in the literature in the West until the work of Hodes (1974) and Bourgat et al. (1974) appeared.

The linear programming solution is in terms of values at the extreme points of a many-sided polygon and this often opposes the fundamental approach in treatment planning--the production of a uniform dose across the target area. If this difficulty is kept in mind, then a technique such as linear programming could be used as an aid to the radiotherapist. Therefore it is natural to expect that any proposed usage of linear (or nonlinear) programming should proceed as an interactive effort between the radiotherapist and the computer. This is one of the key purposes in the system proposed by Hodes (1974). He produces seven steps in the interactive protocol between the operator/therapist and the computer. There are a number of similarities between these steps and the corresponding ones when using the programmed console, Holmes (1970), described in Section 9.2. However there are a number of differences between some steps in Hodes' procedure and those in Holmes'. For example, in Step 2, the operator can set the beam angles at a single direction, with different sizes and/or wedges. The operator can enter the sizes, including wedges, for each beam. Also, in contrast to the programmed console, field strengths are not entered. It is this capability of setting the dosage constraints directly on the cathode ray tube that strengthens Hodes' approach.

Figure 9.4 shows the plotter output of an actual 4-beam treatment plan. The outline of a brain tumor is shown off center in the cross section of a patient's head. The sizes and wedges of the four fields are shown together with the isodose pattern superimposed on the cross section. There are two left and right 10 x 10 cm-fields and two 8 x 10 cm anterior and posterior wedge fields. The first objective is to minimize the integral dose within the tumor. (Note that this can be compared to the work of Bahr et al. (1968), and Bourgat et al. (1974), who minimize the integral dose over an area.) Thereafter, Hodes seeks to minimize the maximum deviation at selected points to achieve uniformity. The linear constraints are of the type shown in Figure 9.5. Although the coefficients in Figure 9.5 come from a simulation of the system, in the implementation of Hodes' approach these would be obtained automatically. The w's represent the four field strengths. The $0.85w_1$ in the first line indicates that Point a receives 85% of field 1 in rads. Each of the numerical coefficients were obtained from hand-eye measurements to determine the percentage contribution from a given field at a given point. An isodose pattern for the field was placed over the cross-sectional contour at the proper position and angle, and then the dosage was estimated at the point of interest. Note that the integral dose is a linear function of the field strenghts.

Linear programming is used for the determination of the field strengths, which, in turn, are then used with the programmed console to produce an isodose pattern. Inspection of this isodose pattern suggests changes in limits, beams, etc. for the

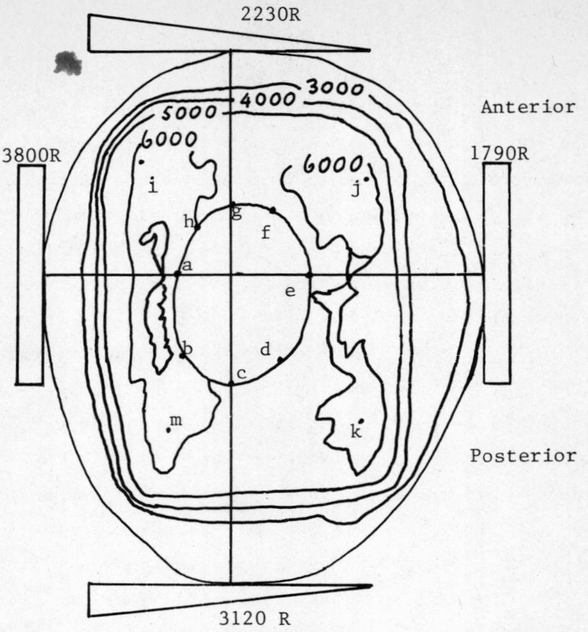

Figure 9.4 Isodose plot of original treatment plan for a brain tumor. The points a to h were first selected as limit points. The integral dose is 8.9 x 10^6 g/rad. (Hodes (1974), with permission.)

Point a: $0.85w_1 + 0.53w_2 + 0.37w_3 + 0.32w_4 \le 6000.$

Point b: $0.82w_1 + 0.54w_2 + 0.33w_3 + 0.38w_4 \le 6000.$

Point c: $0.72w_1 + 0.61w_2 + 0.35w_3 + 0.44w_4 \le 6000.$

Point d: $0.67w_1 + 0.67w_2 + 0.40w_3 + 0.44w_4 \le 6000.$

Point e: $0.65w_1 + 0.72w_2 + 0.47w_3 + 0.39w_4 \le 6000.$

Point f: $0.69w_1 + 0.66w_2 + 0.53w_3 + 0.32w_4 \le 6000.$

Point g: $0.75w_1 + 0.60w_2 + 0.50w_3 + 0.30w_4 \le 6000.$

Point h: $0.83w_1 + 0.55w_2 + 0.43w_3 + 0.29w_4 \le 6000.$

Center: $0.75w_1 + 0.62w_2 + 0.42w_3 + 0.36w_4 \ge 6000.$

Figure 9.5 Linear constraints; compare Figure 9.4.

next iteration of linear programming.

The solution is shown in Figure 9.6 and comparison of this plan with that of Figure 9.4 is favorable. It is seen that there is little difference in the tumor dose distribution and there are large differences in field strengths from the original

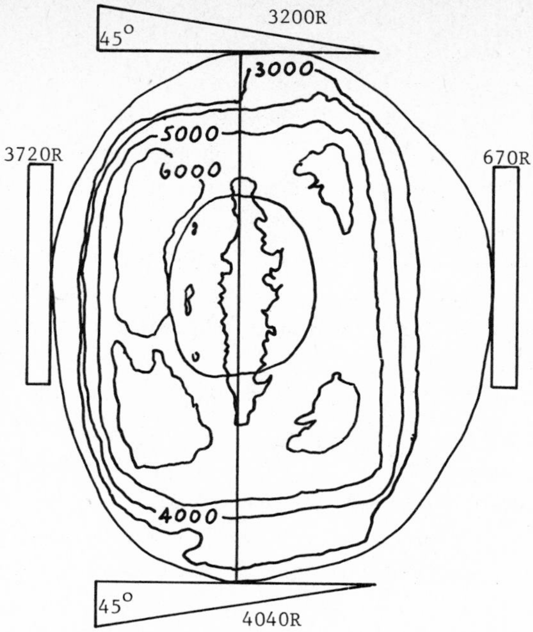

Figure 9.6 Isodose plot of solution to linear programming problem which minimizes the integral dose subject to the constraints at points a - h and the center in Figure 9.4. Integral dose is 8.8×10^6 g/rad. (Hodes (1974), with permission.)

plan.

Hodes now considers the situation with both wedge fields and regular fields leading to a total of ten fields in the four directions. To apply at least 6000 rads around the tumor he sets lower bounds of 6000 at each of the eight points a - h in Figure 9.4, and simultaneously, an upper bound of 6000 at each of the same eight points as before. This means that any solution to the constraints would have a dosage of exactly 6000 rads at all eight points. When the contributions from two or more fields would be superimposed the four points j, k, l, m in Figure 9.4 are selected with a dose limitation at each of them of 6000 rads. At the first attempt the algorithm fails to solve the linear programming problem and hence some of the dosage limits need to be relaxed. The interactive feature of the investigation continues in an iterative fashion through the seven steps of the protocol. Therein lies the strength of the interactive protocol. Finally the integral dose is of the order of 8.6×10^6 g/rad, a significant improvement over the original plan. Unfortunately this number was typed as 3.6×10^6 on p. 194 of the journal article and the corrected number was supplied to the author by Dr. Hodes in a personal communication.

The interactive protocol led to the selection of four fields including a wedge field at the right as well as at the anterior and posterior locations. Thus, Hodes' method can lead to previously unconsidered improvements.

A chest retreatment plan is briefly discussed in Hodes' paper.

It is interesting to note that Hodes is concerned with trying to overcome the deficiencies of the linear programming approach. Furthermore a patent has been granted, Hodes (1976), on his extension of the programmed console.

Bourgat et al. (1974) consider the following application of linear programming in the computer optimization of Cobalt 60 treatment planning. The outline of the patient's cross-section, tumor extent, and vulnerable tissues are superimposed on a two-dimensional square mesh. They wish to determine the non-negative beam weights that minimize the sum of doses delivered to vulnerable organs, or, in mathematical terms, minimize J, where

$$J \equiv J(w_1,w_2,\ldots,w_N) = \sum_{i=1}^{N} w_i \ (D_i^1 + D_i^2 + \ldots + D_i^q).$$

Here N denotes the number of beams, w's are the beam weights and q is the number of organs to be protected. There are three major constraints:

1. The dose over each tumor must be at least as large as some prescribed value D_T, i.e.

$$\sum_{i=1}^{N} w_i \ D_i^T \ (j) \geq D_T.$$

2. The dose over each mesh of vulnerable tissue must be less than a preassigned value D_K, i.e.

$$\sum_{i=1}^{N} w_i \ D_i^k \ (j) \leq D_K,$$

for j = 1,...,p and k = 1,...,q, where p is the number of beams to the qth vulnerable region.

3. Dose over entry mesh on beam axis must not exceed a prescribed level. This statement can be expressed in the form

$$\sum_{i=1}^{N} w_i \ D_i \ (j) \leq D_e, \ j = 1,\ldots,N.$$

The quantity $D_i(j)$ is the dose delivered by beam i at the point of entry on the axis of beam j. (That is, the depth dose at the jth point from the ith field.) The mathematical problem associated with the minimization of the linear objective function J together with the three linear constraints and $w_i \geq 0$ is a linear programming problem.

Bourgat and coworkers apply their procedure to devise a treatment plan for cancer of the esophagus. For example, the three constraints are of the form

Dose to tumor $\leq$ 6000 rads;

Dose to lungs < 2000 rads;

Dose to spinal cord < 4000 rads.

Those beams which contribute less than five percent to the treatment are eliminated from their final results.

The procedure implemented by Bourgat and coworkers is a straightforward application of linear programming to the optimization of radiation treatment planning. It appears from their work that it does not have the interactive capability contribution of Hodes (1974) whose work appeared a few months before that of Bourgat et al.

In fixed field radiation therapy some points on the outside of the tumor may receive a dose equal to or larger than the target dose. When rotational therapy is utilized it is possible to produce a dose per fraction outside the tumor which is relatively lower. Experience indicates that rotational therapy appears to be very useful in the treatment of small tumors with circular cross-section.

Many contours of patients' cross-sectional areas are elliptical in appearance. The dose distribution in conventional radiation therapy with high energy photons has an approximately elliptical high dose region with its major axis perpendicular to that of the patient's cross-section. In general this dose distribution does not coincide with the desired treatment volume. This led to the use of various methods (such as partial arcs with or without wedges) for shaping the high dose region. Unfortunately this can lead to hot spots outside the target volume and the potential for adverse effects can increase. When the center of the tumor is not located near the center of the patient, or when significant heterogeneities occur within the cross-section being treated, the center of the high dose region will not coincide with the axis of rotation. During a course of rotation therapy, such difficulties may be partly overcome by allowing both the field size and the dose rate to vary, as a function of gantry angle. Since there are linear accelerators which have the capacity to automatically change field size and dose rate this led Mantel et al. (1977) to propose an application of linear programming for the optimization of rotation therapy. The field size and dose rate are called controls.

Mantel et al. (1977) are concerned with the achievement of a dose distribution which is uniform to within a specified tolerance in the target volume and reduces the dose and adverse biological effects outside of the target volume. They wish to compare the automatic controls obtained by a standard method and by an optimization method. To demonstrate the usefulness of their approach comparisons are made of the effects of these controls on a treatment plan for cancer of the urinary bladder.

Their standard method is based on Weinkam and Sterling (1972) and computes field size by projecting the specified target area and sets the dose rate in each field in a way that seeks to maintain a uniform dose distribution to the target. Their optimization method uses linear programming and is set up as follows. Consider a cross-sectional area of the patient in which is drawn the outline of the tumor region, with a center C. Construct radial lines at 10° intervals drawn from C so that $P_o, P_1, \ldots, P_{35}$ designate the points of intersection of these 36 lines with the target boundary. On these lines, and at a distance d from C, points $M_o, M_1, \ldots, M_{35}$ are placed so that each M-point lies further out on the radial line than does a corresponding P-point. The field widths $W_o, W_1, \ldots, W_{35}$ are assumed to be chosen beforehand and the common field height h is also specified. Introduce the notations that $D_c, D_o, \ldots, D_{35}$ and $\overline{D}_o, \overline{D}_1, \ldots, \overline{D}_{35}$ respectively denote the dose values at the points $C, P_o, P_1, \ldots, P_{35}$ and $M_o, M_1, \ldots, M_{35}$. Also introduce the set of dose rates $R_o, \ldots, R_{35}$. Since the W's and the height h are fixed the dose values depend only on the dose rates.

It is reasonable, as a first clinical objective, to require that the dose rates be selected in such a manner in order to make the doses at each point $P_o, \ldots, P_{35}$ exceed some specified fraction α of the dose at the center C. The dose at the center of the target is assumed to be equal to the prescribed dose D_p. Expressed in mathematical terms these statements become

$$D_i \geq \alpha\, D_c,\ i = 0, \ldots, 35;\ D_c = D_p.$$

The fraction α is referred to as a "uniformity criterion" and has values of 0.90 or 0.95.

The second clinical objective is to minimize radiation exposure to healthy tissue, under the assumption that the target already includes a sufficient safety margin. One way to attempt to achieve this is to minimize the greatest dose at any point outside the target. If the points chosen for this are $M_o, M_1, \ldots$ then it is required that

$$\overline{D}_i \leq y,\ 0 \leq i \leq 35,$$

and the mathematical objective seeks to minimize y.

Mantel et al. indicate that the dose distribution obtained using dynamic rotation is superior to the dose distribution from conventional rotation. There is a decrease of dose to critical organs, a lack of hot spots and there is greater conformity of the high dose region to the shape of the target volume. It is interesting to note that this implies that there is an increase in the target dose to non-target dose ratio. Both techniques give the same integral doses. However a further improvement is obtained with the use of optimized rotation relative to dynamic rotation. There is a resultant decrease in the integral dose and considerable improvement in the target dose to non-target dose ratio. Furthermore the use of optimization produces a decrease in dose to the critical organ and an improvement in dose uniformity.

There are a number of technical innovations which are employed in current treatments of tumors by external beam irradiation. One of these involves rotation of a beam source along a circle which is located in a plane that is perpendicular to the axis of the patient's body. The location of the center of the circle with respect to the table (on which the patient is supported) can be altered by a parallel movement of the table in which the center is not moved from a specified plane.

Consider a single beam of radiation, directed at an angle ψ, having a width d and a center ξ. Define

$a_i(\xi,\psi,d) \equiv$ dose per second at the ith point of a square grid superimposed on the irradiated cross-section.

Let each point on this grid be associated with a physician's interpretation so that "+" designates desirability and "-" is undesirability of radiation, and with a weight c_i, which is a reflection of its clinical significance (or merit). Let α and β respectively denote the sets of indices which correspond to the points associated with the signs "+" and "-". Then the total dose rates over these sets are given by

$$\omega = \sum_{i\varepsilon\alpha} a_i(\xi,\psi,d), \quad \nu = \sum_{i\varepsilon\beta} a_i(\xi,\psi,d).$$

These equations and similar terminology are introduced in a recent application of linear programming in radiology research described by Polyakov (1978). One problem is concerned with the determination of the number and coordinates of centers of rotation of the sources. The linear programming problem involves the minimization of a linear combination of the ζ_k, $k = 1,\ldots,M$, where M is the number of beams and $\zeta = \omega/\nu$. A second problem deals with the selection of angular directions of the irradiation and of beam dimensions, and is cast in terms of integer linear programming. The final linear programming problem deals with the selection of the irradiation time.

An application of linear programming in intracavitary brachytherapy for carcinoma of the cervix is presented by Tai and Maruyama (1979). Their objective is to determine the optimal dose distribution for a given number of radioactive sources under the constraints of delivering an adequate dose to the appropriate tumor volumes while not exceeding normal tissue tolerance to other organs. Numerical results of their computer program are presented for a patient with cervical carcinoma which required four ^{137}Cs sources in the tandem and one in each of the two ovoids. Graphs are also given of the isodose rate distribution. Their computer program (available upon request) is easily adapted to deal with the situation when ovoids are not considered and when sources other than ^{137}Cs are used. Earlier, clinical, approaches to the optimization of dose in the radiation therapy of cervix carcinoma are described by Maruyama et al. (1976).

A survey of numerical mathematics in some medical problems is given by Bestehorn et al. (1979). They describe a situation of external beam therapy in which the source of radiation moves along one or more orbits around the patient. An optimization problem is formulated in which the objective function to be minimized is the total time of irradiation, subject to the constraints that there be a required minimal dose and a greatest dose at every point of the body. Linear programming is used as the method of solution of the problem. Two figures show results of their approach to the irradiation of a kidney tumor.

To conclude this section the work of Renner et al. (1979) is noted. While they did not deal with external beam therapy they did consider the application of a zero-one integer variable programming problem to the medical problem of deciding how many radioactive seeds to implant and how to attempt to distribute them.

The previous examples in this section illustrate some of the approaches involving linear programming as an optimization tool.

It is worthwhile keeping in mind that, as a first attempt at modeling many problems in radiation therapy, the linear programming approach has much in its favor. In other words one should not regard linear (or nonlinear) programming as the analytical technique to use, but rather one should keep its potential usefulness in mind as an aid to solving certain problems. The more complicated the problem the greater is the computer cost. However these costs should be offset by a reduction in physician and/or physicist time and by a decrease in the dose to critical organs with a corresponding reduction in adverse effects involving normal tissues.

Linear programming gives the solution at the extreme points and thus is in opposition to one of the goals in the treatment planning, namely, the requirement of dose uniformity.

The selection of the minimization of the integral dose as an appropriate criterion is open to question. No treatment parameters appear in this criterion and therefore it is insensitive to changes in their values. For a particular tumor dose, the criterion depends mainly on the anatomy of the patient. There needs to be more input into the formulation of linear (and nonlinear) programming models on implementing the needs of the clinician. Also, time-dose fractionation is not included in these models.

One consequence of these criticisms is that various investigators decided to use more clinically representative terms for the objective function. An improvement in this direction is the usage of quadratic programming, and this is investigated in the next section.

9.5 Optimization of External Beam Radiation Therapy Using Nonlinear Programming

In the previous section the method of linear programming is presented in connection with the minimization of a linear objective function subject to certain linear constraints. When a nonlinear objective function or nonlinear constraints occur the previous approach ceases to apply and a different method, based on nonlinear programming, needs to be utilized. A special class of nonlinear programming problems occurs when the objective is a quadratic function and the constraints are linear, namely, a quadratic programming problem. Historically, special procedures were developed for the solution of quadratic programming problems. However techniques are now available which not only can handle quite general nonlinear problems but can deal with the special case of a quadratic programming problem.

Before examining some of these problems in radiology some background information is first presented.

A mathematical statement of a quadratic programming problem is the following:

$$\underline{\text{Objective}}: \quad \text{Maximize } J = \sum_{j=1}^{n} c_j x_j + \sum_{k=1}^{n} \sum_{j=1}^{n} d_{kj} x_k x_j .$$

$$\underline{\text{Constraints}}: \quad a_{i1}x_1 + a_{i2}x_2 + \dots a_{in}x_n - b_i = 0, \; i = 1,\dots,m.$$

The c_j, a_{ij}, and d_{kj} are constants and generally $d_{kj} = d_{jk}$. Additional constraints may be that $x_j \geq 0$, $j = 1,2,\dots,n$.

In the fifties investigators such as Beale and Wolfe developed algorithms specifically tailored to the solution of quadratic programming problems. Hadley (1964, Chapter 7) gives a complete discussion of these problems and of Wolfe's algorithm based on the simplex method. A number of his applications are to problems in econometric theory, as indeed are the main topics of Boot (1964). Bracken and McCormick (1968) give various applications of quadratic programming. The current approach is to consider quadratic programming as a special case of nonlinear programming, in which the objective function together with the constraint equations have general nonlinear terms. The books by Himmelblau (1972) and Gottfried and Weisman (1973) give the flavor of the theoretical approach as well as providing the reader with a number of worked examples. More recent discussions on quadratic programming are in the books by Kuester and Mize (1973) and Daellenbach and George (1978).

There are two essentially distinct processes involved in the treatment planning stage of radiation therapy. One of these is the initial clinical planning stage involving considerations of the combined treatment modes, fractionation scheme, localization of the tumor and extent of its spread, required lethal dose to the tumor and tolerance doses for neighboring normal tissues. The second planning stage involves physical planning for the development of a treatment plan which gives a good approximation to some preferred dose distribution, consistent with the limitation imposed by the available facilities. The difficulty, in practice, is that the clinical data is inadequate to completely specify a preferred distribution. This forces the investigator to restrict attention to the specification of doses on some contour or at certain points, together with limiting doses within some volume.

Redpath et al. (1975) and McDonald and Rubin (1977) used an approximation to the preferred distribution which is based upon a comparison of doses at discrete points. (This is discussed in greater detail later in this section.)

Some details on dosimetry calculations are now presented.

Consider a plane circular polar coordinate system (ρ,ϕ). The introduction of an axial coordinate z extends this to a cylindrically-polar coordinate system (ρ,ϕ,z). If all radiation beams have their central axis in the plane $z = 0$, so that all beams have the same z-dimension and there is no drastic variation in patient thickness as z varies through the target region, the resulting dose distribution will be approximately cylindrical. The central plane $(z = 0)$ two dimensional dose distribution will be representative of the distribution away from that plane within the target region. Points outside the target volume, which receive significant doses of Cobalt 60 gamma rays and medium to high energy X-rays, usually occur within one or more of the treatment fields. Any scattered radiation, which is generally insignificant, reaches those points lying outside of the treatment fields. It therefore follows that those points with z-coordinates in the ranges greater than d or less than -d do not receive significant doses, provided all beams have coplanar central axes and equal z-dimensions of 2d cm. Under these conditions two-dimensional dosimetry should be an adequate representation of the actual three-dimensional situation.

Define the quantity $F(\rho,\theta)$ as the off-axis factor:

$$F(\rho,\theta) = D(\rho,\theta)/D_o,$$

where $D(\rho,\theta)$ is the dose at the point (ρ,θ) and D_o is the dose at the origin. Here the beam direction is towards the origin along the ray given by $\theta = 0$. It therefore follows that the dose at (ρ,θ) from a beam with dose D_o at the origin in tissue and directed towards the origin along the ray at angle ψ is given by

$$D(\rho,\theta,\psi) = F(\rho,\ \theta - \psi)D_o.$$

In this equation the quantity $F(\rho,\ \theta - \psi)$ is the off-axis factor at the point $(\rho,\ \theta - \psi)$ for a beam of the same energy and field size directed at the same origin along the ray with angle ψ. For example, if there are N beams with designations $i = 1,2,\ldots,N$ and orientations ψ_i and doses at the origin D_{oi}, the net dose at any point (ρ,θ) is given by

$$D(\rho,\theta) = \sum_{i=1}^{N} F(\rho,\ \theta - \psi_i)D_{oi}. \tag{9.17}$$

For each beam energy and field size the magnitudes of the off-axis factors are independently obtained and can be found from fixed source-axis distance isodose charts. From either the tissue-air ratio (or the tissue-maximum ratio) and the beam exposures in air with or without backscatter it is possible to determine the value for the dose D_o. Tables of the tissue-air ratios and tissue-maximum ratios are available for a number of energies and field sizes once the origin depth of tissue along the beam axis is known. Hence one can calculate the dose $D(\rho,\theta)$.

The total dose at the point (ρ,θ) from a number of beams 1,2... is provided by summing their respective doses at (ρ,θ):

$$D_{total}(\rho,\theta) = D_1(\rho,\theta) + D_2(\rho,\theta) + \ldots .$$

Each of these partial doses is proportional to the exposure of its corresponding beam and so the total dose at any point is a linear combination of the exposures of all the incident beams.

Redpath et al. (1975) refer to clinical studies which support the contention that there should be uniformity of dose distribution throughout the tumor. This feature plays a central role in their development of a mathematical model whose principle objective is the attainment of the uniform dose criterion. They choose to minimize the variance of the doses to preselected points within the tumor. The unknown beam weights occur in a quadratic manner in the mathematical expression (the objective function) for the variance. Limiting doses at certain points in the tumor provide linear constraints on the weights. The minimization of the quadratic objective function subject to the linear constraints can be considered as a representative problem in the area known as quadratic programming. Some of the features of this formulation and development are now presented together with selection of some treatment plans suggested by the method.

Define

$D_{p,i}$ = depth dose to the point p from the field designated by i with associated weight w_i.

Then, if a particular wedge arrangement for the treatment plan is assumed, the dose to any point p, namely D_p, is produced by the formula [c.f. (9.17)]

$$D_p = \sum_{i=1}^{N} D_{p,i} w_i, \tag{9.18}$$

with N denoting the number of fields.

Let $\overline{D}$ represent the average dose to k points within a tumor. By definition, the variance of the doses to these k points is given by the expression

$$v = \sum_{i=1}^{k} (D_i - \overline{D})^2,$$

which, by (9.18) can be rearranged in the form

$$v = \frac{1}{2} \sum_{i=1}^{N} \sum_{j=1}^{N} Q_{ij} w_i w_j. \tag{9.19}$$

At a number of points, j = 1,...,M, in the target volume the limiting doses to vulnerable tissues must not be exceeded. In symbols this statement takes the form

$$\sum_{i=1}^{N} a_{ij} w_i \leq b_j, \quad j = 1,2,\ldots,M. \tag{9.20}$$

One objective might be the following: Minimize the variance (9.18) or (9.19) of the doses to a selected set of points in the target volume so that the constraints imposed by (9.20) are satisfied. The expression (9.19) is quadratic in the weights and (9.20) is linear. In mathematical terms the weights are the solution of a quadratic programming problem. The radiotherapy plans considered by Redpath et al. (1975) and McDonald and Rubin (1977) involve the solution of quadratic programming problems of the type just formulated. Whereas Redpath et al. chose the sample points to be scattered throughout the tumor volume, McDonald and Rubin weighted the deviation of the real dose relative to the dose preferred in order to compensate for distortions arising from the choice of locations of the various sample points.

Equations (9.18) - (9.20) are utilized by Redpath et al. (1975) in their computer application to external beam radiation therapy. Details of a patient's outline are entered using an analogue tracing device attached to the computer. The treatment planner then superimposed the outline of the tumor. They have a planning program available, which automatically takes the previous information and assigns special (sample) points within the tumor. As noted earlier in this section these sample points are used in connection with the quadratic programming technique. From the point of view of the planner all that is needed is the setting up of the required beam arrangement and the typing of a single key to activate the quadratic programming algorithm. Within seconds the resulting treatment plan is available for visual inspection. Should undesirable regions of high dose appear in this plan then constraint points may be allocated and a return to the computation of a new plan is made. This process can be repeated as many times as desired. For each plan the treatment planner is provided with the standard deviation of dose over the tumor, since this is a more useful indication of uniformity, should the number of sample points in the tumor be changed. Redpath et al. (1975) provide verbal descriptions of their FORTRAN subroutines.

Many radiation treatments have field direction and size determined at the time of treatment simulation. Once the size of the target area has been satisfactorily established the determination of the optimum field width is straightforward. That is the point of view taken by Redpath and coworkers in the determination of weights of optimization methods. In a related paper, Redpath et al. (1976) present several applications of weight only optimization using quadratic programming. For example, Figure 9.7 shows a treatment plan for carcinoma of the bladder using three beams. Redpath and coworkers also present treatment plans for carcinoma of the hard palate and for carcinoma of the lung. More recent work is in the prepublication stage, Redpath (1980).

The criterion used is related to the "least-squares fit" that is often used in parameter estimation problems, see, e.g. Bracken and McCormick (1968).

The same type of criterion is used by McDonald and Rubin (1977) whose work is now examined. Although their mathematical formulation of the treatment planning problem gives rise to a quadratic programming problem it turns out that one can obtain its solution by direct appeal to a technique involving Lagrange multipliers. Their objective is to determine an optimal beam configuration which allows adequate

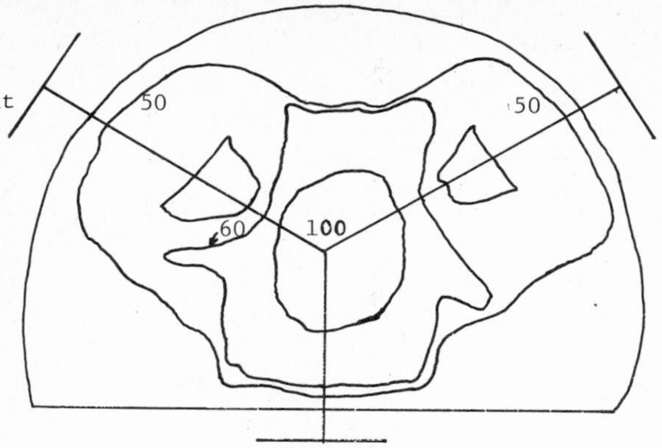

Figure 9.7 A treatment plan for carcinoma of the bladder. (Redpath et al. (1976), with permission.)

dose to the tumor subject to limitations on the dose at neighboring vulnerable tissues. They develop a FORTRAN program for the optimization in which a maximum of 72 co-planar beams could be utilized with up to 4 different field sizes directed towards a common axis from 18 different directions. Typical computer run times are between 10 and 30 minutes.

McDonald and Rubin consider first the case of a parallel-opposed treatment arrangement. The exposures of the opposed beams are the only variable quantities and there is no optimization with respect to beam orientation, field size, or beam energy. Two Cobalt 60 beams are parallel-opposed with intervening tissue thickness of 20.0 cm. For each beam the field size is 6 x 6 cm with source-axis distance each of length 80 cm to a point, the origin, which is a distance of 8 cm from the anterior surface. The origin is labelled C; see Figure 9.8. The anterior periphery of the tumor (point A) is 3.0 cm anteriorly from C and the posterior periphery (point B) is 2.0 cm posteriorly from C. The selection of critical points is as follows: C, a point E 5.0 cm anterior to C, and a point D 4.0 cm posterior from C. At these points the limiting doses are respectively chosen to be 110, 110 and 80 rads. The preferred dose to the tumor boundary is selected to be 100 rads. The label 1 refers to the anterior beam and 2 refers to the posterior beam.

Define the quantities X and Y as the doses in tissue at C due respectively to beam 1 alone and beam 2 alone. Then the doses at the sample points A and B are given by

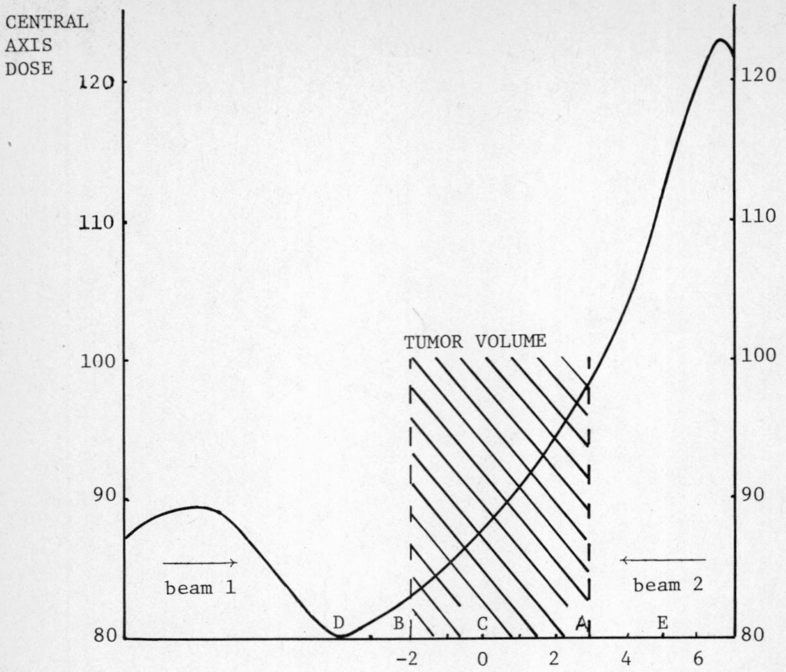

Figure 9.8 The central axis dose distribution for the one-dimensional optimization problem. See text for details. (McDonald and Rubin (1977), with permission.)

$$D_A = 1.28X + 0.78Y, \tag{9.21}$$

$$D_B = 0.85X + 1.18Y, \tag{9.22}$$

where the coefficients of X and Y are the respective off-axis factors extracted from a source-axis distance isodose chart for Cobalt 60, 6 x 6 cm, and 80 cm source-axis distance (Table 9.2). The doses X and Y differ from the exposures of beams 1 and 2 by the factors of the respective tissue air ratios. A quadratic programming problem for the determination of X and Y can be constructed in the following manner.

Let k denote the total number of sample points on the periphery of the tumor. Then in terms of the notation of (9.17)

$$v_i = \left[\sum_{n=1}^{N} \sum_{j=1}^{k} F_n(\rho_i, \theta_i - \psi_i) D_{oj,n} - D \right]^2 \tag{9.23}$$

Point	Beam 1	Beam 2
A	1.28	0.78
B	0.85	1.18
C	1.00	1.00
D	0.72	1.40
E	1.52	0.67

Table 9.2 Off-axis factors at points A, B, C, D, E in Figure 9.8.

is a least squares deviation from the preferred dose D, taking into consideration that there are N beams. To compensate for distortions due to irregular spacing of sample points along the contour a weight w_i associated with each sample point is included. Thus the expression for a weighted deviation from the preferred dose is given by

$$v = \sum_{i=1}^{k} w_i v_i. \tag{9.24}$$

The application of (9.23) to the present problem, since k = 2, for a preferred dose of 100 rads at A and B, gives

$$V = (D_A - 100)^2 + (D_B - 100)^2,$$

and at the same time the right-hand side of this expression defines V. Substitution of (9.21) and (9.22) into V, which now depends on the two variables X and Y, gives

$$V = (1.28X + 0.78Y - 100)^2 + (0.85X + 1.18Y - 100)^2. \tag{9.25}$$

This function $V = V(X,Y)$ is convex and differentiable. There is a global minimum of V at the point where $\partial V/\partial X = \partial V/\partial Y = 0$, or, equivalently,

$$2.3609X + 2.0014Y = 213.0,$$

$$2.0014X + 2.0008Y = 196.0.$$

These equations possess the solution X = 47.20, Y = 50.74, which are the values of the axis doses from beams 1 and 2. These values, however, are obtained in the absence of any other constraining equations. Such additional constraints arise by limiting the doses at the critical points C, D, and E. On using the off-axis factors in Table 9.2 the corresponding constraints are as follows:

$$\text{point C:} \quad X + Y \leq 110,$$

$$\text{point D:} \quad 0.72X + 1.40Y \leq 80,$$

$$\text{point E:} \quad 1.52X + 0.67Y \leq 110.$$

Accordingly the optimization problem requires that (9.25) be minimized subject to these last three constraints and $X \geq 0$, $Y \geq 0$. This is a quadratic programming problem, since V is quadratic in X and Y and the constraints are linear in these variables.

In the absence of these constraints the dose values fail to satisfy the constraint at the point D. The way to proceed is to introduce an additional variable λ, which is referred to as a Lagrange multiplier, and consider the following optimization problem. Optimize the function V(X,Y) subject to the inequality constraint at the point D. On letting the inequality at the point D become active, form the (Lagrangian) function

$$u(X,Y) = V(X,Y) + \lambda(0.72X + 1.40Y - 80)$$

then $\partial u/\partial X = 0 = \partial u/\partial Y$ give the necessary conditions for u(X,Y) to have an extremum at an interior point. That is,

$$2.3609X + 2.0014Y + 0.72\lambda = 213.0$$

$$2.0014X + 2.0008Y + 1.40\lambda = 196.0$$

$$0.72X + 1.40Y = 80.$$

For more background information on this usage of the Lagrange multiplier in optimization problems see Gottfried and Weisman (1973, pp. 49-56). This last set of equations has the solution $X = 68.107$, $Y = 22.116$, and $\lambda = 11.029$, and satisfies all the constraints except at the point E.

Now let the constraint at the point D be inactive and the inequality at the point E be active. The solution of the resulting set of equations violates the inequality at the point D.

Having used these inequalities in turn now let them both be active. Form the function

$$t = V + \lambda(0.72X + 1.40Y - 80) + \mu(1.52X + 0.67Y - 110),$$

where λ and μ are Lagrange multipliers. The necessary conditions for an extremum are

$$\partial t/\partial X = 2.3609X + 2.0014Y - 213 + 0.72\lambda + 1.52\mu = 0,$$

$$\partial t/\partial Y = 2.0014X + 2.0008Y - 196 + 1.40\lambda + 0.67\mu = 0,$$

$$\partial t/\partial \lambda = 0.72X + 1.40Y - 80 = 0,$$

$$\partial t/\partial \mu = 1.52X + 0.67Y - 110 = 0.$$

These last two equations possess the solution X = 61.01, Y = 25.77 which satisfy the constraint at the point C. Since V is a sum of squared quantities, and all the constraints are satisfied, then the optimization problem is now solved. The values (61.01, 25.77) respectively denote the doses at the origin in tissue which give the distribution that best fits the preferred contour while simultaneously satisfying the constraints. It is interesting to note that these optimal values for X and Y are determined from the inequality constraints and not from the equations resulting from setting the partial derivatives of V to zero. Finally, the exposures per beam at 80 cm source-axis distance are

$$D_1 = X/0.736 = 83 \text{ rads}, \quad D_2 = Y/0.580 = 44 \text{ rads},$$

where the numbers in the denominators are the appropriate tissue air ratios.

Figure 9.9 shows an application of the procedure just described to obtain a treatment plan for a centrally-located brain tumor. McDonald and Rubin also present treatment plans for the optimal dose distribution for (1) a laterally-located brain tumor, (2) an asymmetrical posteriorly-located brain tumor, (3) a tumor of the larynx, and (4) a centrally-located tumor in the thigh. All beams are Cobalt 60 γ-rays. For each of these applications the treatment planner is given a two-dimensional contour of the patient at the tumor level. In the plane of this contour is superimposed the outline of the tumor boundary and the locations of neighboring vulnerable tissues. The preferred dose to the tumor periphery and the limiting doses to the vulnerable tissues are also added. The origin is fixed within the tumor volume and is always taken to be a critical point. There the limiting dose is taken as 110% of the preferred dose at the tumor boundary in order that the variation over the tumor volume does not exceed 10% (approximately) above the periphery tissue. In these applications each radiation field is shown by a bar of width proportional to the field width at the origin, and displaced outwardly along the beam axis. Alongside each field is written the optimal exposure (with backscatter) at the origin. The isodose contour with value equal to the preferred tumor periphery dose is given along with a few typical isodose curves such as 90%, 70% and 50% of maximum dose. The origin, the point with the greatest dose, and other points of interest are shown. Figure 9.9 is representative of a display with this information.

The last example in this section involves moving strip therapy using a minicomputer.

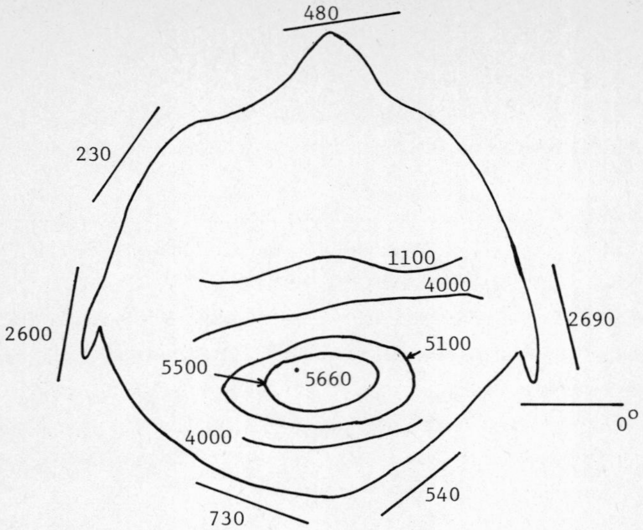

Figure 9.9 Optimal dose distribution and beam configuration for a centrally-located brain tumor. All beams are Cobalt 60 λ-rays with field sizes of 5 x 5 cm, with the exception of the anterior beam which is 4 x 5 cm. The source-axis distance for each beam is equal to 80 cm. The maximum dose is 5660 rads, and there is about a 3% variation across the tumor. (McDonald and Rubin (1977), with permission.)

There are a number of difficulties encountered in irradiating the entire abdomen with large open fields for tumors that originate within the pelvis or abdomen. Radiation intolerance is often manifested by taking blood counts. There is patient intolerance as indicated by nausea, vomiting and diarrhea. Furthermore, the maximum dose administered using open fields is 3000 rads in 4-6 weeks and this reduces the antitumor effect.

In the early 1940's the moving-strip technique, developed at Manchester, England, was developed. This technique was utilized by Delclos et al. (1963) in an attempt to diminish the difficulties in irradiating the abdomen. However there are three effects which together can introduce large variations in dose throughout the treatment volume:

(i) nonuniformity of dose because of local maxima located at the junction between strips and minima located at the center of each strip,

(ii) a decrease in dose near the upper and lower ends of the treatment volume,

(iii) nonuniformity of dose because of the variation in patient thickness over the treatment volume.

Smoron (1972) introduces strip-staggering as an approach for minimizing (iii). Fazekas and Maier (1974) present a comparison of the open-field and moving-strip techniques. With the moving-strip technique the patient tolerates the treatment better and there is the delivery of a more biologically effective dose. Yet the five year survival rates obtained with each technique are identical. A more recent account of the moving-strip technique is in Dembo et al. (1979).

In order to minimize effects (i) and (ii) Leavitt et al. (1975) develop a least squares procedure for the dose minimization at selected points. Their approach is similar to that presented in the work of Redpath and coworkers, and McDonald and Rubin discussed earlier in the present section. The radiation is from a Cobalt 60 source.

The weight associated with each beam W_i is set to 100% initially. The dose contribution of the ith beam to the jth point of interest can be computed and stored as the element D_{ij} of the dose-contribution matrix. By definition,

$$\text{the total dose at the interest point } j = \sum_i W_i D_{ij} = DX_j, \text{ say.}$$

Let the dose at a selected normalization point (such as the central interest point on the midline) be denoted by DX_{jc}. Now form the weighted sum of the squared deviation of doses at the selected interest points from the dose at the selected normalization point

$$v = \sum_j \left[\frac{1}{\Delta DX_j} (DX_j - DX_{jc}) \right]^2 .$$

The optimization problem now becomes the following: Minimize the variance of the doses to prescribed points within the tumor. Note that the (unknown) beam weights occur in a quadratic manner in the objective function v. Leavitt and coworkers use a one-dimensional search conducted along the direction of steepest descent (see Section 7.4 and equation (7.8)). In particular, if W_p denotes the pth estimate of W then (7.8) provides a scheme for producing the next estimate at p + 1, namely

$$W_{p+1} = W_p - hK_p,$$

where h is the distance moved in the direction of search. The quantity

$$K_p = \frac{\partial v}{\partial W_p} \Big/ \left[\sum_{j=1}^{N} \left(\frac{\partial v}{\partial W_j} \right)^2 \right]^{1/2},$$

where N is the number of beams. When a minimum is obtained in the direction of steepest descent, a new direction of search is investigated by comparing

(a) the derivatives of v with respect to the new beam weights

with (b) the previously determined derivatives of v with respect to the old beam weights.

Now conduct a one-dimensional search in the new direction. The procedure continues until some stopping criterion is satisfied.

It is possible to obtain computer calculations of the maximum, minimum, and mean midplane doses, and the given dose to each beam necessary to deliver a desired midplane dose.

One interesting feature of the work by Leavitt et al. is that they compare their computer calculations with experimental measurements. By means of an ionization chamber in a water phantom they measured beam profiles. A Masonite phantom was constructed to simulate a patient and used to measure optimized and unoptimized midplane dose distribution by thermoluminescent dosimetry. Their measured midplane doses agreed with computer-calculated doses within experimental error. The overall conclusion from their work is that the optimization procedure improved dose uniformity and reduced the midplane dose variation from ±12-13% to ±3-4%.

This concludes the examples of the present section which has shown some of the attempts at improving radiation treatment planning using elementary nonlinear programming.

9.6 Quantitative Study of Relative Radiation Effects and Isoeffect Patterns

In this section the work of Mistry and DeGinder (1978) is examined in some detail. Their objective is to introduce a mathematical procedure for estimating and diagramming cumulative biological effects resulting from various fractionation schemes used in external beam radiotherapy. First, the concept of the radiation effect ratio is introduced. Then follows a discussion of manual and computer methods for producing isoeffect patterns. These features are combined in split course radiotherapy and in fractional radiation effect ratios with weighted isoeffect lines. No specific nominal standard dose (NSD) tolerance dose figures are needed in the calculations. The presentation continues with an investigation of how visual comparison of the distribution of radiation effect ratios makes it a straightforward matter to select a treatment plan the least harmful to critical organs.

The linear and nonlinear programming methods of the previous sections aided in the analysis of a number of treatment plans, but they did not deal with fractionation schemes. For this, and other reasons, there is a need for examining various factors in time-dose fractionation at specific anatomical sites.

Relative radiation effect ratio (RE)

Current radiotherapy practice involves the treatment to tolerance of connective tissues. Therefore it is useful to compare tissue tolerance, partial or otherwise, at any tissue site prescribed for full tolerance. Evidently partial tolerance equals

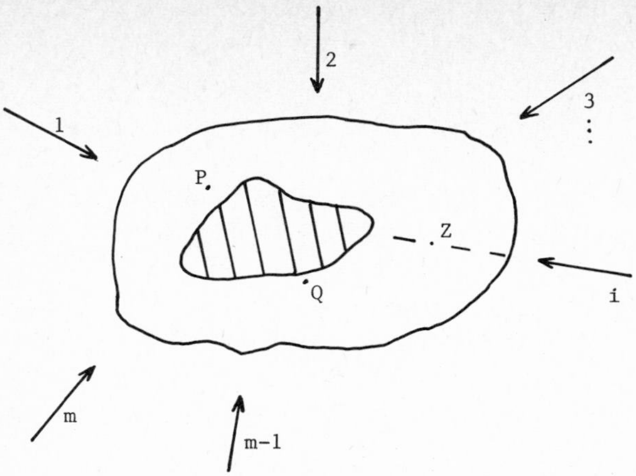

Figure 9.10 Shaded region denotes tumor. The points P, Q and Z are points of interest in healthy tissue. The fields are labelled 1,2,...,m.

full tolerance when n = K; see (9.27).

Consider Figure 9.10 which illustrates an m field treatment plan. Tissue at an arbitrary point P is assumed to have the same tolerance NSD as the tissue at the point Q. If all the fields are treated per session and tissue at the point Q in the vicinity of the tumor receives a tolerance dose in K fractions, then point P, which receives a different dose per fraction requires a different number of fractions K′ to reach tolerance. On using (9.27) the biological dose that point P receives in K fractions is given by

$$\text{RET dose} = (K/K')(\text{NSD}) .$$

The relative radiation effect ratio at P is obtained from (9.26) and written as

$$(\text{RE})_P = K/K'.$$

The Ellis (empirical) formula is given at the beginning of Section 6.2. Introduce the symbols

$$d = \text{dose per fraction, } k = \text{days per fraction,}$$

to an estimated full tissue tolerance. This leads to the "relative radiation effect ratio" or, in short, the RE ratio. It is defined by

$$RE = \frac{\text{partial tolerance dose at tissue site}}{\text{full tolerance dose of tissue}}$$

$$= (\text{RET dose})/(\text{NSD dose}) \tag{9.26}$$

where RET is the rad equivalent therapy. If RE = 1 then the tissue site will have received radiation equal to the tolerance limit on completion of the series of radiation treatments. If RE < 1 then the tissue site has received less radiation than the tolerance limit. However RE > 1 means that atrophy, fibrosis and complications of normal tissue can occur. Note that the relative radiation effect ratio gives a theoretical expected fraction of the full tolerance as the biological effect resulting from radiation.

Isoeffect contour and isoeffect plot

Partial tissue tolerance (PT) is defined by

$$PT = (n/K)(NSD), \tag{9.27}$$

where n is the number of fractions actually given, and, as in earlier chapters, K is the total number of fractions. Then the Ellis formula can be written as

$$NSD = dK^{0.65}\ k^{-0.11}.$$

Let d denote the dose per fraction that the point Q receives and d′ be the dose per fraction that P receives. It follows that

$$(RE)_P = (d'/d)^{1.538}. \tag{9.28}$$

The point P is arbitrarily chosen and receives either the scattered radiation or both the primary and the scattered radiation. Consequently P and Q both get the same number of dose fractions. The RE ratio is independent of k (days per fraction) so long as the number of fractions per week do not alter. If a comparison is made between similar tissue types then the RE ratio is independent of the NSD value. Mistry and DeGinder make the following definitions:

The line connecting points of equal RE ratio is the isoeffect contour.

A plot of isoeffect contours is referred to as an isoeffect plot.

Split course radiotherapy and RE ratio

Assume that the treatment is split into K_1 and $K - K_1$ fractions with a rest period of R days in between them. For the point Q the RE ratio achieved at the end of the split course is given by

$$(RE)_Q^{split} = \frac{1}{K}\left(K_1\left[\frac{T_1}{T_1 + R}\right]^{0.11} + K - K_1\right),$$

where T_1 is the number of days for the first course of treatment and $[T_1/(T_1 + R)]^{0.11}$ is a decay factor. The arbitrary point P in Figure 9.10, which receives the dose per fraction d´, requires K´ fractions to achieve tissue tolerance at P. Hence, at P, the RE ratio achieved after K_1 fractions and a subsequent rest period of R days is the expression

$$\frac{K_1}{K'}\left[\frac{T_1}{T_1 + R}\right]^{0.11} .$$

For the rest of the treatment involving $K - K_1$ fractions an additional RE ratio at the point P is given by

$$(K - K_1)/K'.$$

It follows that the total RE ratio achieved at the end of the split course of radiation treatment for the point P is given by

$$(RE)_P^{split} = \frac{K_1}{K'}\left[\frac{T_1}{T_1 + R}\right]^{0.11} + \frac{K - K_1}{K'}$$

$$= (RE)_P \; (RE)_Q^{split} .$$

The last equation means that the RE ratio at an arbitrary point P changes by the same multiplicative factor $(RE)_Q^{split}$ as that found for the treatment zone where the tissue tolerance was originally specified. At the point P, on completion of the first course of treatment, the RE ratio is

$$(K_1/K)(RE)_P. \tag{9.29}$$

The application of the decay factor $[T_1/(T_1 + R)]^{0.11}$ to the last expression is meaningful so long as (9.29) is less than or equal to unity. If this is the case then the tissue has achieved less than or equal to the tolerance dose during the first course of treatment.

Fractional RE ratios and weighted isoeffect lines

Equation (9.28) can be used in the determination of isoeffect contours from the multifield isodose plot for a multifield treatment plan in which all fields are treated per therapy session. The arbitrary point P receives a varying amount of dose per fraction for those treatment plans in which all fields are not treated at each therapy session. No matter how a multifield treatment plan is carried out the isodose plot of the physical doses in rads as prescribed by total tumor dose, or total given dose from each field, is the same. However, the isoeffect plot is different for each treatment mode.

Consider Figure 9.10 for a multifield treatment plan in which the region containing the tumor receives m fields with only one field treated per treatment session. For the ith field define the following quantities:

M_i ≡ planned number of fractions to be delivered;

d_i ≡ dose per fraction at a reference point Z in the tissue along the central axis of the ith beam;

K_i ≡ number of fractions necessary to reach tissue tolerance at Z;

d_i' ≡ dose per fraction at an arbitrary tissue site, P;

K_i' ≡ number of fractions necessary to reach tissue tolerance at P.

Let $(FRE)_{P,i}$ denote the partial or fractional contribution to the RE ratio at the point P from the ith field on completion of M_i fractions. Then, in symbols,

$$(FRE)_{P,i} = M_i/K_i' \ .$$

This equation can be expressed in the form

$$(FRE)_{P,i} = \frac{M_i}{K_i} \ (RE)_P = \frac{M_i}{K_i} \left(\frac{d_i'}{d_i}\right)^{1.538} , \tag{9.30}$$

by use of (9.28). To obtain the total RE ratio at the point P on completion of the series of treatments perform the summation of the fractional RE ratios from all the fields to obtain

$$(RE)_P = \sum_{i=1}^{m} (FRE)_{P,i} = \sum_{i=1}^{m} \frac{M_i}{K_i} \left(\frac{d_i'}{d_i}\right)^{1.538} .$$

Since d_i' and d_i are the doses received per fraction from the ith field at two different points in tissue, they are proportional to the percentage isodose lines P_i' and P_i respectively passing through these points. It follows that (9.30) can be expressed in the alternative manner

$$(FRE)_{P,i} = (M_i/K_i)(P_i'/P_i)^{1.538} .$$

When a single field is used for the whole treatment then tissue at the depth of maximum dose is the first to reach tolerance. The point on the central axis at that depth can be considered as the reference point where P_i is at the 100% level and K_i equals M_i. An arbitrary point P then has its isoeffect curve evaluated from the quantity $(P_i')^{1.538}$, where P_i' is the percentage isodose line passing through the point P.

Mistry and DeGinder consider four examples to illustrate the significance of their theoretical approach.

The first involves a Cobalt 60 10 x 10 cm field at 80 cm source-skin-distance to treat a tumor at a depth of 5 cm. The tumor region dose is 6000 rads delivered in 6 weeks with five fractions per week.

On the assumption that tissue tolerance is reached at the depth of 5 cm with 200 rads per fraction and 30 fractions then (9.28) can be rewritten in the form

$$RE = [P'/(P \text{ at } 5 \text{ cm})]^{1.538} = (P'/78.5\%)^{1.538},$$

where 78.5% is obtained from an isodose curve (see Mistry and DeGinder (1979) p. 1087 Figure 2). For various values of P′ it is easy to compute the corresponding values of RE. Thus, for a depth of 0.5 cm with P′ = 100% then RE = 1.45. Assume now that tissue tolerance is achieved at 5 cm depth with 200 rad per fraction and 30 fractions. This time,

$$RE = (P'/100\%)^{1.538}.$$

At 0.5 cm depth with P′ = 100% then RE = 1.

Hence the subcutaneous tissue achieves an RE radiation dose which is 45% above the designated tissue tolerance when 6000 rads are delivered at the 5 cm depth. However, when 6000 rads are delivered at 0.5 cm depth the region containing tumor receives 31% less than the designated tissue tolerance (RE = 0.69). On the basis of these numbers a therapist must decide whether to make a compromise or change the treatment to include multifields.

In an example involving parallel opposed alternating fields isoeffect plots indicate why it is best to treat both fields per session and avoid unnecessary high radiation effects. Another example indicates that RE plots provide a way for treating all the fields of a multifield treatment plan per session in order that adverse effects in normal tissue are considerably lessened.

It is evident that the paper by Mistry and DeGinder is a contribution towards the optimization of human cancer radiotherapy.

Chapter 10

RECONSTRUCTIVE TOMOGRAPHY

10.1 Introduction

Many people are familiar with the typical process involved in having an X-ray taken of the chest. Rays from the X-ray source diverge, pass through the chest area, and then impinge onto a photographic film to give a two-dimensional image. This process leads to conventional X-ray pictures in diagnostic radiology. The result can be confusing because all the details of tissue in the path of the rays overlap. Subtle variations in tissue density are usually not reproduced on the X-ray film. As a consequence a number of pictures are often taken from various angles. Yet the exposure of a patient to X-rays must be restricted and it is imperative that all information obtained is fully utilized and interpreted with maximum efficiency.

Roentgen's discovery of X-rays is of profound significance because of their dramatic practical exploitation. Although many technological improvements have been made in such areas as the generation of X-ray photons and better photographic film, his basic principles still apply today.

In the early twenties several radiologists independently devised an alternative X-ray procedure. This procedure is known as tomography and is in widespread usage. For a historical review of tomography see Massiot (1974). The resultant image on the photographic plate is called the tomogram. The principle of tomography is as follows. Assume that it is desired to obtain information on the extent of a lesion at the tip of a patient's rib. An X-ray source moving in an arc sends out photons to the anatomical point of interest, the patient remaining stationary. While this is happening the photographic plate, in synchrony with the source, moves in the opposite direction. (Alternatively, the patient and photographic film are in synchronous motion relative to a stationary X-ray source.) The tomogram gives a display of an anatomical plane which sections the body at a given orientation. Outside of the plane in focus the other layers (or planes) are blurred.

Tomograms are used by radiologists in the diagnosis of disease and by radiation oncologists as an aid to treatment planning for cancer therapy, where it is important to give an accurate location of the tumor relative to nearby anatomical structures. However, tomography does not always produce as great an increase in resolution as the clinician prefers because of the limited dynamic range of radiographic film and partly due to differences between the predicted and the actual imaging properties of the tomographic process. Orphanoudakis and Strohbehn (1976) are interested in improving the quality of tomograms. In particular they develop a mathematical model of conventional tomography which attempts to quantify the imaging properties of the tomographic process. See, also, Orphanoudakis et al. (1978).

Even with conventional tomography the image contrast is very low. It if were possible to exclude interference from the details in other planes and so obtain an image of only the selected plane of interest then this would be an ideal solution.

The interesting thing is that a mathematical basis for the solution to this problem had been published by Radon (1917). He proved that a two-dimensional or three-dimensional object can be uniquely reconstructed from the infinite set of all its projections. His work was in the area of image reconstruction in gravitational theory, and it is not surprising that many were unaware of the potential usefulness of his work in diagnostic radiology. Furthermore similar image reconstruction problems had occurred in such diverse fields as radio astronomy and electron microscopy, Brooks and DiChiro (1975, 1976), and solutions had been independently obtained. Again, workers in these areas did not think of applying their techniques to radiology problems.

The basic problem in diagnostic radiology is concerned with obtaining accurate measurements of the X-ray attenuation coefficient at every point within the object being examined. The attenuation coefficient is defined to be the relative intensity loss per centimeter for a collimated X-ray beam traversing the section of interest. Tissue density in a human head varies between 1.0 and 1.05, in appropriate units, with bone having a density of about 2. Variations of density as small as 0.005 are of medical interest. Bone, therefore, is highly attenuating, while most soft tissues have coefficients slightly greater than that of water. Later, in (10.1), an approximation to the total attenuation along the path of an X-ray is written as a line integral from the X-ray tube to the detector.

In the late fifties Cormack was investigating ways of determining accurate values for the attenuation coefficients and subsequently experimented with a nonsymmetrical phantom of plastic and aluminum. Cormack (1963, 1964) published this work, but it was not noticed; see also Cormack (1973). Present day techniques for determining attenuation coefficients are based on procedures that are superior to the pioneering efforts by Cormack.

The most significant breakthrough since Roentgen's discovery of X-rays occurred in the early seventies. In a brief paper Hounsfield (1973) described a procedure which was the symbiotic interaction between X-ray scanning and digital-computer technology. Hounsfield had calculated the theoretical accuracy of the tomographic approach and had decided that with normal dose levels one should be able to measure the absolute value of the X-ray attenuation coefficient to an accuracy of 0.5 percent. This was about 100 times better than that of conventional methods. His first scanning device was similar to Cormack's. However Hounsfield's method of image reconstruction was much easier to implement than Cormack's method. At EMI Ltd. in the United Kingdom he led the group that developed the EMI Scanner which could generate images of isolated slices of the brain with remarkable discrimination of very small density variations. (See, also, Hounsfield (1976), (1977).) Cormack and Hounsfield shared the 1979 Nobel prize in Physiology or Medicine. See Cormack (1980) and Hounsfield (1980a,b).

The prototype for this Scanner had been in use since 1970 at the Atkinson-Morley Hospital, Wimbledon, England. The first EMI Scanner was installed at the Mayo Clinic in June, 1973 and the second in July at the Massachusetts General Hospital. In a short space of time New et al. (1974) presented a dramatic selection of images of sections of the brain. This was followed by a book, New et al. (1975). The images obtained by the EMI Scanner made a dramatic impact on the medical community as well as the public, and this continues.

Ledley et al. (1974) describe the first computerized axial tomography scanner, which has the capability of scanning every part of the human body.

In the space of a few years improvements have been made in scanners and a number of companies are involved in their development and construction. Numerous articles have been published in the scientific literature. Useful papers include those by Gordon and Herman (1974), Brooks and DiChiro (1975, 1976), Ledley (1976), McCullough and Payne (1977), Smith et al. (1977), Shepp and Kruskal (1978). Books of a specific medical nature include those by New et al. (1975), Gonzalez et al. (1976), Littleton (1976), Norman et al. (1977), Bories (1978), and Gordon (1979).

Scanning time has decreased substantially since the introduction of the "first generation" scanners. For example, third generation (late 1975) scanners have scan times as fast as two seconds. (Second generation scan times were of the order of 20-60 seconds.)

Current scanners can provide an exact contour of some transverse section of the patient and the image provides a distinct reproduction of internal structures and whatever pathologic anatomy may be present. Thus, one can observe hard and soft tumors, cysts, injured or dead tissue, blood clots, etc. Scanners provide an extremely useful diagnostic aid. During the treatment of tumors, and other lesions or abnormalities, regression or change in size can be evaluated with regular scans.

Some have said that the advent of computerized tomography is the beginning of a new era in diagnostic radiological imaging from direct recording on film to quantitative imaging procedures using electronic radiation detectors and computer data processing. Others say that the use of a computer is not (at least in theory) necessary or unique to computerized tomography and suggest that reconstructive tomography is a more technically appropriate name; Brooks and DiChiro (1976).

Our intention here is to describe some of the basic ideas in reconstructive algorithms and to set down some guidelines in connection with selecting the optimal one.

Section 10.2 introduces the basic equation of reconstructive tomography. This is followed by a brief synopsis of the four main approaches utilized in producing algorithms for reconstruction of images from projections.

The basic expression for the projection function in terms of the attenuation coefficient is a Radon transform. Inversion of this type of transform is discussed in a number of places in the mathematics literature. In this Chapter only enough mathematical details, with no rigorous justification of results, are presented to enable the reader to generally follow how some of the results are obtained. This leads naturally to a brief discussion of two approximate methods, in Section 10.3, that can be utilized in numerical work involving digitized data on the projection function.

A particular application of the material in Sections 10.2 and 10.3 to the area of treatment planning occurs in Section 10.4.

It is imperative to restrict the number of scans that a patient receives. This leads to a consideration of the optimization of dose reduction in computerized tomography and is briefly considered in Section 10.5.

Present indications are that reconstructive tomography is going to play an increasingly important role in the development of treatment plans in radiotherapy. A recent survey in this area is by Goitein (1979). It is therefore appropriate that in this Chapter an introduction is given to some of the background of reconstruction algorithms. More detailed discussions can be found in Herman (1979, 1980).

10.2 Reconstruction Algorithms

Figure 10.1 shows a typical situation in the reconstruction of an image from projections. On one end of a frame (or yoke) there is an X-ray tube from which the

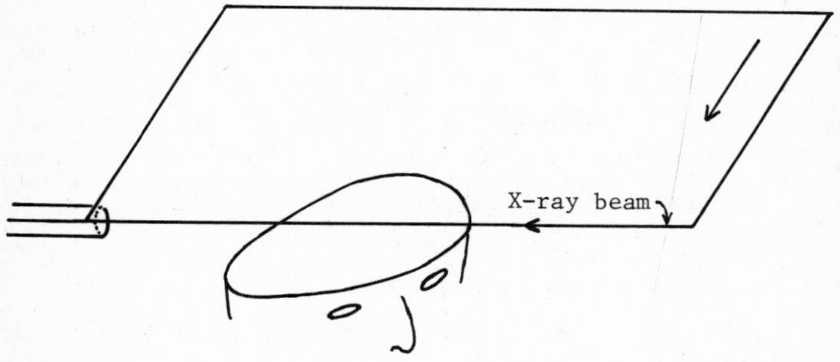

Figure 10.1 Reconstruction from projections using a computer. The X-ray source and X-ray detector are mounted on a yoke which can be moved in the direction of the arrow. The yoke can also be rotated through a series of angles around the head. Initially this procedure was used for brain scans. However it is now possible to use a similar process for scanning the rest of the body.

X-ray photons are collimated and directed through an anatomical slice of the patient towards a scintillation detector. Radiations pass through the anatomical object or plane and do not enter other areas. The numbers of photons emerging at each position are measured and recorded. The yoke is then rotated through a small angle and a further set of measurements recorded. A computer uses the information on the recorded measurements to obtain a distribution of X-ray transmissions in the slice through which the beam passed. This computerized tomographic image can be displayed as a picture on a cathode ray tube.

Consider a beam of photons incident on a uniform slab of matter of constant thickness x. Let I_o denote the incident intensity (that is, the number of photons in the beam prior to interaction with the slab) and let I denote the transmitted intensity. For a beam which is very close to being monoenergetic

$$I = I_o e^{-\mu x}.$$

The quantity μ has units of (1/length) and is referred to as a linear attenuation coefficient. This expression for I is often referred to as Beer's law. When the matter is inhomogeneous the exponent is replaced with a line integral. If, now, x and y represent two rectangular Cartesian coordinates in space then

$$I = I_o \exp\left[- \int_{\text{source}}^{\text{detector}} \mu(x,y)\, d\ell \right],$$

with μ(x,y) denoting the linear attenuation coefficient. Upon rearrangement,

$$-\ell n \frac{I}{I_o} = \int_{\text{source}}^{\text{detector}} \mu(x,y)\, d\ell. \qquad (10.1)$$

The quantity on the left of this equation can be evaluated from experiments and the basic problem of image reconstruction is to determine the "density" μ(x,y). Equation (10.1) is at the foundations of computerized tomography and so it is useful to highlight the main assumptions under which it is derived:

1. The X-ray beam is assumed to be "infinitely thin", and this means that (10.1) is an approximation.

2. The beam is assumed to be monoenergetic, or monochromatic, which means that the physical attenuation coefficient is independent of the energies of the different X-ray photons.

3. The beam consists of a limited number of photons actually transmitted and it is assumed that statistical fluctuations can be ignored.

One of the fascinating features of the papers which have been published concerning (10.1) is the extent to which approximations are used with intuition the only guide to the errors involved.

Figure 10.2 shows the two-dimensional distribution of the linear attenuation coefficient when an X-ray beam is incident edge-on to a slice of matter. During a sequence of exposures the direction of the X-ray beam defines the y´ axis. The integral of μ(x,y) along the straight line path of a photon through the object is referred to as the ray-sum or ray-projection. The projection, or profile, is the complete set of ray sums at a given angle. Projection data are gathered along the x´ axis with θ denoting the angle of rotation. The data on the intensities lead to a known value for $\ell n(I/I_o)$. The projection function f(x´,θ) is defined by the equation

$$f(x',\theta) = -\ \ln(I/I_o).$$

The technique of reconstructing a two-dimensional picture, or cross-section, thus depends on using its one-dimensional projections. By creating a stack of such two-dimensional planes it is possible to produce a full three-dimensional picture, and this is of considerable interest.

By 1979 many improvements had been made so that the resolution in images was as low as 0.375 mm. As time progresses one can anticipate further advances in reduction of the resolution.

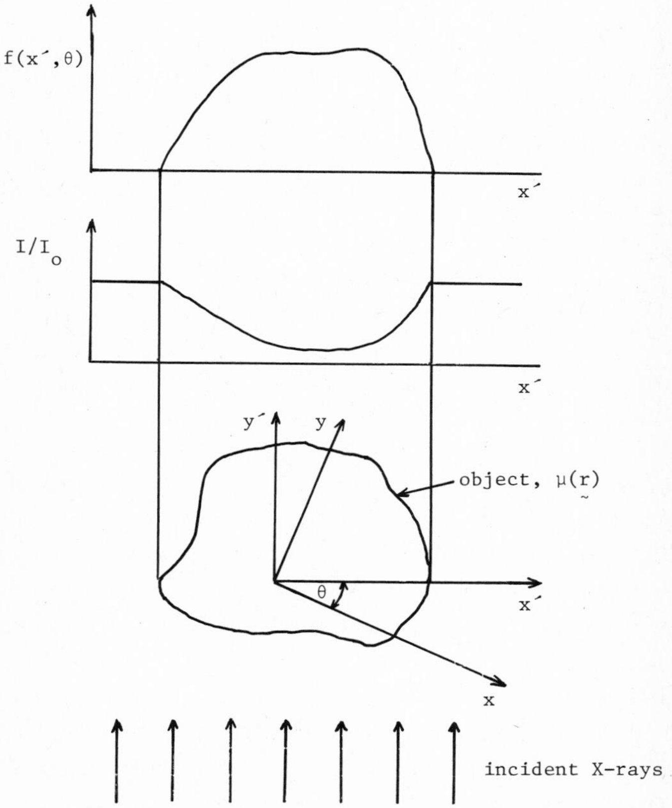

Figure 10.2 Projection function $f(x',\theta)$ for use in computer processing of data.

Since the techniques on imaging are of wide application it is often useful to employ a more general notation. Let $\overline{f}(x,y)$ denote the density function. For transmission imaging $\overline{f} \equiv \mu$, the linear absorption coefficient, whereas, for emission imaging, $\overline{f} \equiv \rho$, the radioisotope concentration. Equation (10.1) can now be expressed in the form

$$f(x',\theta) = \int_L \mu(x,y)\, d\ell, \tag{10.2}$$

where ℓ indicates length along the path L.

Standard formulae for the coordinate transformations indicated in Figure 10.2 are

$$x = x' \cos\theta - y' \sin\theta, \quad y = x' \sin\theta + y' \cos\theta, \tag{10.3}$$

where the x,y axis system is assumed to be fixed.

There are four categories of reconstruction algorithms:

I. Back-projection: The contributions of the rays through each point in the object are added to produce an estimate of the density at the point.

II. Iteration Method: Corrections to an image are made in order to bring it into better agreement with the measured projections.

III. Analytical Reconstruction: A picture and its projections are related by a set of integral equations which can be solved analytically. This category includes Fourier transform analysis.

IV. Series Expansion Approaches: Basis pictures are linearly combined to produce a picture.

It is worthwhile exploring each of these categories in somewhat greater detail.

I. Back-projection (or Summation Method)

The earliest approach at reconstructive tomography utilized an approximation procedure which is commonly referred to as the back-projection method. Simple analog hardware (even a pencil and a straightedge) can be used for the implementation of this procedure. Also, there is no need of a computer or use of sophisticated mathematics, and hence this procedure has a main advantage over other reconstructive techniques. An understanding of back-projection serves as a basis for comprehending more recent (and complex) methods.

Each X-ray transmission path through the object is divided into equally-spaced elements. For simplicity, it is assumed that each of these elements gives an equal contribution to the total attenuation along the X-ray path. The attenuation for each element over all ray paths that intersect the element at differing angular orientations is collected in a sum. Another way of saying this is that, for a given image point, the reconstructed density is the sum of all the ray projections that pass through it.

Reconstructive tomography using back-projection can eliminate unwanted planes. However, the method produces blurred images of sharp features in the object. For more details see Gordon and Herman (1974).

II. Iterative Reconstruction

Iterative processes are commonplace in many types of applications of mathematics and numerical analysis. In tomography, the term iterative refers to the following situation. Select some arbitrary initial image and apply corrections to it to bring it into better agreement with the measured projections. Now apply new corrections (as necessary) until satisfactory agreement is reached. Let the object to be reconstructed be approximated (Figure 10.3) by an array of N cells with f_i, i=1,2,...N denoting the density value in the cell with label i. Note that "cell" in this context

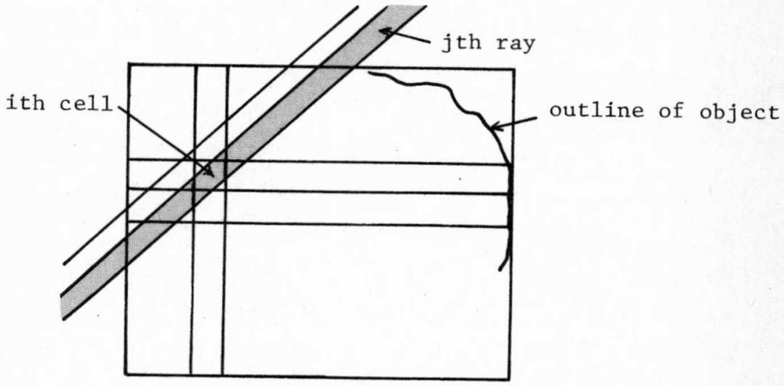

Figure 10.3 Ray geometry for use with iterative construction. Note that a ray is a strip of finite width.

refers to the area of one of the little squares and does not mean biological cell. The projections are divided into strips of finite width called rays. Each cell intersected by a ray contributes to the ray sum so that for the jth ray

$$p_j = w_{1j} f_1 + w_{2j} f_2 + \dots + w_{Nj} f_N, \tag{10.4}$$

where the w's are weighting factors representing the contribution from each cell. This last equation is a discrete version of (10.2) with p_j denoting the measured projection $f(x',\theta)$.

The manner in which (10.4) is used is as follows. An initial set of values is selected for the cell densities. The values $f_i = 0$, $i = 1,\dots,N$ correspond to a blank screen and f_i = constant, $i = 1,\dots,N$, refer to a "gray" screen. Equation (10.4) is used to calculate the projections and the results compared with the actual measured projection values. If a calculated ray-projection is larger than its measured value then each cell that contributed to that ray has its density decreased by some amount until the new calculated ray-sum agrees with the measured value. The first iteration is finished when this process has been applied to each cell and all rays. It is apparent, though, that each new correction destroys any agreement obtained from the earlier corrections. However one can continue the process until any remaining error is acceptable. As each iteration proceeds the measured ray-projections are compared with the calculated ray-projections, and the difference is applied as a correction to those cells that make up the ray.

If the initial values give a blank screen then the first iteration is equivalent to back-projection, since the calculated projections in this case are zero.

There are three variations of iterative reconstruction in current usage (Brooks and DiChiro (1975)):

1. Simultaneous correction (ILST): All projections are calculated at the beginning of an iteration, in one method, and all corrections are made simultaneously. Another method uses an interative least squares technique to dampen out oscillations about the correct solution.
2. Ray-by-ray correction (ART): This technique was utilized in the first version of the EMI Scanner. At the beginning of each iteration one ray-sum is calculated and corrections are applied to all points that contribute to the ray. Now repeat this process for each ray in turn, by incorporating previous corrections in each new calculation, until all rays in every projection have been considered. This completes one iteration. The technique is also known by the title Algebraic Reconstruction Technique (ART).
3. Point-by-point correction (SIRT): This Simultaneous Iterative Reconstruction Technique begins the iteration from a particular point, which is correct for all rays that pass through it. The remaining points are similarly dealt with, excepting that corrections are made during the iteration are embodied in succeeding calculations.

III. Analytical Reconstruction

Cormack (1963, 1964) is credited with the first analytical reconstruction of an X-ray image, even though his method is not in current usage. Analytical methods make use of exact formulas for the reconstructed image density. There are two fundamental categories: Two-dimensional reconstruction using Fourier methods and filtered back-projection.

(a) Direct Fourier Methods

It is appropriate to first investigate the implementation of Fourier integral transform methodology in the reconstruction of images.

Consider (see Figure 10.2) a projection along the y' axis:

$$f(x',\theta) = \int_{-\infty}^{\infty} \mu(x,y)dy',$$

where the source is taken at $-\infty$, the detection unit is at $+\infty$, and coordinates x,y are given by (10.3). The one-dimensional Fourier transform of the projection is

$$F(\xi',\theta) = \int_{-\infty}^{\infty} f(x',\theta)\ \exp(2\pi i\xi'x')dx'.$$

For convenience throughout this and the next section upper case letters denote Fourier transforms and the corresponding lower case letters are quantities in the spatial x,y domain. The symbol ξ' is the spatial frequency variable conjugate to x'. Hence,

$$F(\xi',\theta) = \int_{-\infty}^{\infty}\int_{-\infty}^{\infty} \mu(x,y)dy' \exp(2\pi i\xi' x')dx'.$$

The right-hand side of this equation is like the two-dimensional Fourier transform of $\mu(x,y)$. This suggests, if the interchange in the orders of integration is permissible, that the last equation be written in the form

$$F(\xi',\theta) = \left[\int_{-\infty}^{\infty}\int_{-\infty}^{\infty} \mu(x,y) \exp 2\pi i(\xi' x' + \zeta' y')dx'dy'\right]_{\zeta' = 0}.$$

Let $F\{\mu\}$ denote the two-dimensional Fourier transform of $\mu(x,y)$, then

$$F(\xi',\theta) = [F\{\mu\}]_{\zeta' = 0}. \qquad (10.5)$$

The right-hand side of this equation is the two-dimensional Fourier transform of $\mu(x,y)$ evaluated along the line $\zeta' = 0$ in a two-dimensional frequency plane. The line $\zeta' = 0$ rotates in synchrony with the alteration of the projection angle θ, since ξ' and ζ' are always conjugate to x' and y', respectively. The conclusion from the mathematical result in (10.5) is that $F\{\mu\}$ can be determined at all points from a set of projections over a 180 degree range in θ. This result is worthy of being stated as a theorem which states that the one-dimensional Fourier transform of a one-dimensional projection of a two-dimensional object is mathematically equivalent to one line (or slice) through the two-dimensional Fourier transform of the object itself; see, e.g., Mersereau (1976). Thus, given a knowledge of all one-dimensional projections, it is possible to synthesize the two-dimensional transform of the object. A further inverse two-dimensional transform is then implemented to recover the object itself.

Assume that the projections are known for a number of different orientations then this implies that the Fourier transform of the unknown quantity is available on the "spokes of a wheel" in the Fourier plane. Exact reconstruction requires an infinite number of projections, in general. However, the digital evaluation of the Fourier transform usually requires that a discrete Fourier transform be constructed on samples of the projection functions. Interpolation must be performed to provide the information omitted by taking the limited number of views. When all this is done then the final computation involves an inverse Fourier transform. Discussions on the limitations of the sampled data are provided in Mersereau (1976). Care is also required on the type of interpolation procedure that is used because Fourier components may not be obtained within the desired resolution; Gordon and Herman (1974, p. 124).

It is worthwhile presenting some of the details of the derivation of expressions for the attenuation coefficient μ by means of the Fourier transform approach and generalized functions. This leads to the basic results (10.10) and (10.11).

(b) Approach Using Generalized Functions

From (A 3.1) in Appendix 3 it is possible to replace the line element $d\ell$ in the integral (10.2) to give

$$f(p,\theta) = \int \mu(\underset{\sim}{r})\delta(p - \underset{\sim}{\omega} \cdot \underset{\sim}{r})dx\, dy, \tag{10.6}$$

where, for convenience, the symbol $p \equiv x'$. An integral of this form is referred to as the Radon transform of the quantity $\mu(\underset{\sim}{r})$. Mathematically, the integral is well defined if $\mu(\underset{\sim}{r})$ satisfies the requirement that it be a locally summable function with bounded support. Note that the integration is taken over appropriate ranges of x and y.

Some mathematical details are now presented of the inversion of (10.6) to obtain the attenuation coefficient. Define

$$F(\xi,\theta) = \int_{-\infty}^{\infty} f(p,\theta)\, e^{i\xi p} dp. \tag{10.7}$$

Substitution of $f(p,\theta)$ from (10.6) into the last integral gives

$$F(\xi,\theta) = \int_{-\infty}^{\infty} \int_{-\infty}^{\infty} \mu(\underset{\sim}{r}) \int \delta(p - \underset{\sim}{\omega} \cdot \underset{\sim}{r}) e^{i\xi p}\, dp\, dx\, dy$$

$$= \int_{-\infty}^{\infty} \int_{-\infty}^{\infty} \mu(\underset{\sim}{r}) \exp(i\xi\underset{\sim}{\omega} \cdot \underset{\sim}{r})\, dx\, dy, \tag{10.8}$$

where the ranges of x and y are assumed to be from $-\infty$ to $+\infty$. Write equations for polar coordinates (ξ,θ) in the manner of $x = \xi \cos\theta$ and $y = \xi \sin\theta$ so that $dx\, dy = |\partial(x,y)/\partial(\xi,\theta)|d\xi d\theta$. The Jacobian of the transformation is $|\xi|$ and hence inversion of (10.8) gives

$$\mu(\underset{\sim}{r}) = \frac{1}{(2\pi)^2} \int_{\theta=0}^{\pi} \int_{\xi=-\infty}^{\infty} |\xi|\, F(\xi,\theta) \exp(-i\xi\underset{\sim}{\omega} \cdot \underset{\sim}{r}) d\xi d\theta,$$

or, alternatively,

$$\mu(r,\phi) = \frac{1}{(2\pi)^2} \int_{\theta=0}^{\infty} \int_{\xi=-\infty}^{\infty} |\xi|\, F(\xi,\theta) \exp[-i\xi r \cos(\theta-\phi)] d\xi d\theta. \tag{10.9}$$

The Fourier transform $F(\xi,\theta)$ appears in the integral and it can be replaced by its definition (10.7). Accordingly, assuming that it is permissible to interchange orders of integration, (10.7) and (10.9) become

$$\mu(r,\phi) = \frac{1}{(2\pi)^2}\int_{\theta=0}^{\pi}\int_{p=-\infty}^{\infty} f(p,\theta) \int_{\xi=-\infty}^{\infty} |\xi|\exp\{-i\xi[r\cos(\theta-\phi) - p]\}d\xi dp d\theta$$

$$= \frac{-1}{2\pi^2}\int_{\theta=0}^{\pi}\int_{p=-\infty}^{\infty} \frac{f(p,\theta)}{[p - r\cos(\theta-\phi)]^2}\, dp d\theta, \qquad (10.10)$$

by use of the result 13 in the table of page 359 of Gel'fand and Shilov (1964). A further integration by parts, with respect to the variable p, assuming that $f(p,\theta)$ is well-behaved at $\pm\infty$, gives the result

$$\mu(r,\phi) = \frac{1}{2\pi^2}\int_{\theta=0}^{\pi}\int_{p=-\infty}^{\infty} \frac{\partial f(p,\theta)/\partial p}{r\cos(\theta-\phi) - p}\, dp d\theta, \qquad (10.11)$$

and the principal value of the double integral is understood. The result (10.11) was obtained by use of Fourier transforms in the work by Berry and Gibbs (1970). Instead of $(0,\pi)$ they take $(-\pi/2, \pi/2)$. The results (10.10) and (10.11) are fundamental for the analysis of the behavior of the attenuation coefficient μ.

The inner integral in (10.11) suggests an interpretation in terms of a mathematical filtering of each projection, that is, of all ray sums at a single angle θ. Current scanners have a filter operation that appears to be based on a different, but mathematically equivalent, integral. The contribution of the outer integral is to superimpose all filtered rays. The reconstruction method based on (10.11) is referred to as filtered back-projection, since the superposition process (the outer integral) is equivalent to a back-projection of the filtered ray sums onto the image plane.

IV. Series Expansion Approach

This category of reconstruction algorithm involves the following. Assume that there is available a set of m basis pictures $\{b_i(x,y)\}$ which can be linearly combined to produce an adequate approximation to any picture $k(x,y)$. This implies that real numbers $n_1, n_2, \ldots$ exist such that

$$k(x,y) \approx \sum_{i=1}^{m} n_i\, b_i\,(x,y).$$

For a more complete discussion see Gordon and Herman (1974, pp. 128-134).

10.3 Numerical Approximations for the Attenuation Coefficient

In this section two approximations are derived for the attenuation coefficient which can be utilized in numerical work involving digitized data on the projection function.

Measurements on shadow graphs are most conveniently made by scanning the data at regular intervals along a line on a photograph using a densitometer, or by using some other appropriate device for direct measurement of intensity. Accordingly the data for the projection function can be obtained at a set of equally-spaced points. The discrete nature of this data indicates that it is useful to investigate approximations to the expression for the attenuation coefficient μ suitable for numerical impementation.

The mathematical theory of generalized functions has provided the framework for dealing with a number of different types of improper integrals; e.g. Chapter 9 of the author's book, Swan (1974). A more mathematically complete discussion of the Radon transform and its inverse for use in the determination of the density μ necessitates the use of generalized functions. However, here, it is appropriate to just provide the reader with some references. For example the whole material in Chapter 1 of Gel'fand et al. (1966) deals with the Radon transform. From p. 11 of that reference it is possible to deduce that the finite part of the divergent integral

$$\int_{-\infty}^{\infty} \frac{f(p)}{(p-\ell)^2}\,dp = \int_0^{\infty} \frac{1}{p^2}[f(p+\ell) + f(-p+\ell) - 2f(\ell)]\,dp.$$

The necessary background for this result is provided in the earlier book, Gel'fand and Shilov (1964, pp. 333-335). If this result is applied to (10.10) then, with $\ell = r\cos(\theta - \phi)$,

$$\mu(r,\phi) = -\frac{1}{2\pi^2}\int_{\theta=0}^{\pi}\int_0^{\infty} \frac{1}{p^2}[f(p+\ell,\theta) + f(-p+\ell,\theta) - 2f(\ell,\theta)]\,dp\,d\theta$$

$$= -\frac{1}{2\pi^2}\int_{\theta=0}^{\pi} g(\ell,\theta)\,d\theta, \qquad (10.12)$$

where the quantity $g(\ell,\theta)$ is defined by the equation

$$g(\ell,\theta) = \int_{p=0}^{\infty} \frac{1}{p^2}[f(p+\ell,\theta) + f(-p+\ell,\theta) - 2f(\ell,\theta)]\,dp. \qquad (10.13)$$

Assume that data for the projection function $f(p,\theta)$ are available at a set of equally-spaced points $p = mh$, where h is a small positive number (the step length, as used in numerical quadratures). Consider an approximation to the projection function by means of the equation $f(p,\theta) = f(mh,\theta)$ within the interval $[(m - 1/2)h, (m + 1/2)h]$.

The expression (10.13) can now be represented by a sum of integrals over each sub-interval in the manner

$$g(\ell,\theta) = \sum_{m=1}^{\infty} \int_{(m-1/2)h}^{(m+1/2)h} [f(mh+\ell,\theta) + f(-mh+\ell,\theta)\frac{dp}{p^2}$$

$$- 2f(\ell,\theta)\int_{h/2}^{\infty} \frac{dp}{p^2} + \tau,$$

and τ represents an error term. On writing $\ell = nh$, with n denoting an integer, this last result takes the alternative form, after integration and neglect of the error term,

$$g(nh,\theta) = \frac{4}{h}\sum_{m=1}^{\infty} \frac{1}{(4m^2-1)} [f(mh+nh,\theta) + f(nh-mh,\theta)] - \frac{4}{h} f(nh,\theta).$$

When the appropriate variations in θ are introduced the last expression can be used in (10.12) to give an estimate of the attenuation coefficient.

An alternative approximation expression, suitable for use in numerical work is now derived.

Consider the following integral:

$$q(\nu) = \frac{1}{(2\pi)^2}\int_{-\infty}^{\infty} |\xi| \exp(-i\nu\xi)d\xi. \tag{10.14}$$

When $\nu = \ell - p$ this is the ξ-integral which occurred in the intermediate analysis leading to (10.10). In fact it is possible to write, since $\ell = r\cos(\theta - \phi)$,

$$\mu(r,\phi) = \int_{\theta=0}^{\pi}\int_{p=-\infty}^{\infty} f(p,\theta)q(\ell - p)dpd\theta, \tag{10.15}$$

which is in the form of equation (9) in Ramachandran and Lakshminarayanan (1971). Equation (10.15) indicates that $\mu(r,\phi)$ is the convolution of $f(p,\theta)$ and $q(\nu)$.

The integral (10.14) arose in the investigations of Ramachandran and Lakshminarayanan (1971). They replaced the limits $-\infty$ and ∞ by $-\pi/2h$ and $+\pi/2h$ (where h is the step length introduced earlier in this section) when the integral exists for all values of ν. Define

$$q_h(\nu) = \frac{1}{(2\pi)^2}\int_{-\pi/2h}^{\pi/2h} |\xi| \exp(-i\nu\xi)d\xi,$$

then (10.14) can be rewritten in the manner

$$q(\nu) = q_h(\nu) + \Delta,$$

in which Δ indicates an error term, which tends to zero as h tends to zero. However, it is to be appreciated that in practice one is not at liberty to make h as small as one would prefer. For projection data available at the points $p = mh$ (as before), then

$$\begin{aligned} q_h(mh) &= 1/4h^2, \text{ for } m = 0, \\ &= -1/\pi^2 m^2 h^2, \text{ for } m \text{ odd}, \\ &= 0, \text{ for } m \text{ even}. \end{aligned}$$

Define

$$t(\ell,\theta) = \int_{-\infty}^{\infty} f(p,\theta)\, q(\ell - p)dp,$$

then, for $\ell = nh$, and since $q[(m - n)h] = q[(n - m)h]$,

$$\begin{aligned} t(nh,\theta) &\approx h \sum_{m=-\infty}^{\infty} f(mh,\theta)q[(m - n)h] \\ &= h \sum_{s=-\infty}^{\infty} f[(n + s)h,\theta]\; q(sh) \\ &= h\left[\ldots + \frac{f[(n - 1)h,\theta]}{(-\pi^2 h^2)} + \frac{f(nh,\theta)}{4h^2} + \frac{f[(n + 1)h,\theta]}{(-\pi^2 h^2)} + \ldots\right] \end{aligned}$$

$$= -\frac{1}{\pi^2 h} \sum_{j=-1,-3,\ldots} \frac{f[(n + j)h,\theta]}{j^2} + \frac{f(nh,\theta)}{4h} - \frac{1}{\pi^2 h} \sum_{j=1,3,\ldots} \frac{f[(n + j)h,\theta]}{j^2}.$$

This last result is also obtained in Ramachandran and Lakshminarayanan (1971, equation (14)). Equation (10.15) can now be used to determine $\mu(r,\phi)$. Since

$$\sum_{j=1,3,\ldots} \frac{1}{j^2} = \frac{\pi^2}{8}, \quad \sum_{j=-1,-3,\ldots} \frac{f[(n + j)h,\theta]}{j^2} = \sum_{j=1,3,\ldots} \frac{f[(n - j)h,\theta]}{j^2}$$

the representation for $t(nh,\theta)$ can be rearranged in the form

$$t(nh,\theta) = -\frac{1}{\pi^2 h} \sum_{j=1,3,\ldots} \frac{1}{j^2}\{f[(n + j)h,\theta] + f[(-j + n)h,\theta]-2f(nh,\theta)\}.$$

On comparing this expression with (10.13) it is apparent that (10.13) can be written in terms of the quadrature formula

$$g(\ell,\theta) = h \sum_{j=0,1,2} c_j\, b(j,\ell,\theta) + \sigma$$

in which $b(j,\ell,\theta)$ is the integrand in (10.13) and σ is an error term. The coefficients c_j are defined by

$$c_j = 0 \text{ (j even)}, \quad c_j = 2 \text{ (j odd)}.$$

In the analysis of formulae for use in numerical quadrature, Davis and Rabinowitz (1967), it is known that this special choice of coefficients allows for the error term to be zero, i.e. $\sigma = 0$. What this means is that the approximate result for $t(nh,\theta)$ is a very useful ont to utilize in practice, because of the zero value for the error term.

10.4 Cross-sectional Absorption Density Reconstruction for Treatment Planning

The material in the previous two sections can be used in various areas. In the present Section a particular application of the material to treatment planning in radiology is discussed.

Figure A 3.1 presents a coordinate system in a slice of tissue being scanned by a beam of photons. Information in this figure was used in the derivation of (10.11). At the origin O, Figure A 3.1, r = 0, and hence (10.11) can be written

$$\mu(0) = -\frac{1}{2\pi^2} \int_{\theta=0}^{\pi} \int_{p=-\infty}^{\infty} \frac{1}{p} \frac{\partial f}{\partial p}\, dp\, d\theta. \tag{10.16}$$

Under appropriate assumptions (e.g. if Compton scattering is the dominant attenuation process, and hydrogen concentration is ignored) the attenuation coefficient for a particular radiation is essentially proportional to the local density, ρ. Let σ_o denote the mass attenuation coefficient. The expression (10.16), see Figure A 3.1, can now be expressed in the form

$$\rho(0) = -\frac{1}{2\pi^2 \sigma_o} \int_{p=0}^{C} \frac{1}{p} \frac{\partial}{\partial p} \int_{\theta=0}^{2\pi} f(p,\theta)\, d\theta\, dp. \tag{10.17}$$

For any point O in the slice, the integral with respect to θ is 2π times the angular average of the line integrals on paths which are tangential to a circle of radius p with O as its center. The density at the point O is now the integral of the gradient of these angular averages, normalized by the circumference of the circle at radius p, with the integral evaluated from O out to C, where there is no longer any gradient.

Now introduce the following assumptions:

(i) there are B equally spaced angles θ_j so that $B\Delta\theta = 2\pi$;

(ii) the quantity p^{-1} in (10.17) can be replaced by its linearly interpolated value $2/(p_k + p_{k+1})$;

(iii) the partial derivative with respect to p can be transferred through the integral sign and $\partial f/\partial p$ is approximated by the difference in f-values at the points (p_{k+1},θ_j) and (p_k,θ_j);

(iv) each of the integrations can be represented by the trapezoidal rule of numerical quadrature theory.

Direct implementation of these four assumptions indicates that (10.17) can be cast in the form

$$\rho(0) = -\frac{2}{\pi B\sigma_o}\sum_{k=1}^{n-1}\frac{1}{p_k + p_{k+1}}\sum_j [f(p_{k+1},\theta_j) - f(p_k,\theta_j)], \tag{10.18}$$

which is the representation used by Friedman et al. (1974). The fact that the mathematical analysis of the inverse Radon transform leads to a discussion involving generalized functions indicates that difficulties are encountered with the numerical evaluation of (10.17) as p approaches zero. Friedman et al. suggest that (10.18) be used for $p \geq p_1$, and, for $p < p_1$, they make the approximation

$$\int_0^{p_1}\frac{1}{p}\frac{\partial f}{\partial p}\,dp \approx \frac{1}{2}(\Delta p)[f(p_2,\theta_j) - f(p_{-1},\theta_j)). \tag{10.19}$$

They use the formulae (10.18) and (10.19) in a numerical scheme for reconstructing the effective absorption density distribution. The original image was traversed in equally spaced steps. Onto the number of detectable quanta noise was added by imposing a Gaussian distribution. A comparison was then made of the original and reconstructed density distributions for a vertex view of a phantom patient, having a diameter of 39 cm, in which lungs, ribs, esophageal and bronchial airways, spinal column and tissue homogeneities of both high and low relative densities (representing metastases and emphysema) are present. The reconstruction is quite accurate and is almost identical to the original distribution.

The information on density distributions provides for a satisfactory evaluation of dose distributions. In turn, this influences the design of a radiation therapy plan. The goal is the production of an optimal treatment plan; McCullough (1978).

10.5 Towards the Optimization of Dose Reduction in Computerized Tomography

As mentioned in the introduction to this Chapter, one should try to obtain as much information as possible from the X-ray image, while keeping the dosage to the patient as small as possible. While much attention had been focused on using the fascinating range of new scanners there is a need not to take any more scans than are absolutely necessary, since the patient X-ray doses are comparable to the exposures received prior to the introduction of computerized tomography. Gordon (1976) introduced a number of methods which are effective in reducing the radiation dose to patients and it is worthwhile examining his suggestions in light of the overall objective of this book, which is to try to optimize human cancer radiotherapy. Unfortunately, as Gordon noted, his ten methods are not in general use. Some of the features of these approaches are now presented.

(1) Take fewer views

More work needs to be done in learning, by objective and psychophysical measurements, the smallest number of views that can produce an image whose quality is just adequate for a reliable diagnosis of a given situation.

(2) Reducing motion artifacts

It is often difficult to keep the patient immobilized during a scan, as the present author is well aware from his own experience. One possibility is to require the computer to have a single angle rescanned, or drop, or correct data. Patient motion could be detected by sensors or acoustic probes.

During a body scan motion artifacts are caused by patient breathing. Body scanners could partially compensate for breathing by distorting the internal computer representation of a cross section in synchrony with the breathing cycle.

(3) Tuning the algorithm to the instrument

Computational algorithms may include "models" of the scanner's geometry, which does not correspond to its actual construction, and this can lead to an extensive loss of resolution. The algorithm should be designed for the scanner.

(4) Use of a priori information

For example, if one is not looking for bone pathologies, the bone could be located and its densities constrained to be within the a priori range of densities. A more precise reconstruction of the soft tissues can now be obtained.

One should try to incorporate into algorithms the "constraint" that the X-ray attenuation coefficients are positive.

(5) Radiate only the area of interest

It is possible to use a computational algorithm which allows only the region of interest to be multiply radiated, as in radiation therapy.

(6) Minimize the effects of noise

There is evidence in the literature that nonlinear techniques can produce super-resolution well beyond the classical Rayleigh limit in optics, and the concepts and mathematics involved are of direct application to the reconstruction problem. Improved imagery may be expected to come from analyses in this area.

(7) Energy dependent phenomena

The basic formulae for the absorption coefficient depend on the three assumptions introduced at the beginning of Section 10.2. An X-ray beam has an energy spectrum that alters as it traverses the patient--a "beam hardening" effect. There is also scattering of the beam. If truly monochromatic X-ray sources can be introduced the problems of scattering and beam hardening should be effectively eliminated.

(8) Changes in scanner geometry

A major limitation of fine spatial resolution is the wide sampling aperture of current scanners. When the aperture is narrowed the computational burden significantly increases. Special algorithms can speed up the computations. Optical computing can be much faster.

(9) Other radiation

Gamma rays have the advantage of being nearly monochromatic, and, if sufficient beam intensities could be achieved, they could replace X-rays.

(10) Display of reconstructions

The physician needs to be given appropriate quality images of the computer output. Significant improvement in reconstruction quality could be obtained by using hexagonal masters, instead of square ones, for both the computation and the display. The reason for this is that the resolution of a hexagonally sampled image is more uniform in all directions.

For more details of these methods of dose reduction see Gordon (1976).

The material of this and the previous two sections should aid in providing some guidelines for an "optimal" reconstruction algorithm. However, it is well to keep in mind that the whole area is rapidly expanding, with a typical "exponential increase" in the number of papers in the scientific literature. A recent intensive clinical review is by Ring (1979).

Ultrasound techniques have not been discussed in this book. The future prospects for ultrasound in diagnostic radiology are promising. The integration of ultrasound techniques with computerized tomography has progressed; see, e.g., Moss and Goldberg (1979).

The implementation of heavy particles in reconstructive tomography is under investigation; see, e.g., Holley et al. (1979).

10.6 Other Imaging Technologies

(a) The Dynamic Spatial Reconstructor

In the early spring of 1980 the Mayo Clinic (Rochester, Minnesota) announced that it is involved in building the world's most advanced medical X-ray scanner--the Dynamic Spatial Reconstructor (DSR). This machine costs several million dollars. Not only is the price huge; the machine is about 20 feet long and weighs 17 tons. For the "prototype" there will be 14 X-ray cameras mounted on it, and the design calls for 28. The DSR will take thousands of X-ray pictures in seconds and uncover as much about what is going on inside a patient as a skilled doctor could in hours of surgery. Typically, a patient will be wheeled on a stretcher into the machine where the X-ray cameras will spin around the patient, taking 30,000 pictures in four seconds. The resulting images are processed by a computer and generate moving, clearly focussed, pictures on a television screen. On command, a doctor can ask the computer to "slice" open the heart image on the television screen in order to inspect it from the inside, as it beats. Organs will be able to be seen life-size and in motion and a study of them can be made electronically. Even though a great number of X-rays are involved the radiation exposure to the patient will not exceed that from a conventional scanner. A recent article on the DSR occurs in Computer Medicine, Vol. 10, No. 11, 1980.

(b) The Positron-Emission Tomographic Scanner

Another high-priced machine is the positron-emission tomographic (PET) scanner--it costs about 1.5 million dollars. A chemical compound with a certain biological activity is labeled with a radioactive isotope, which on decay emits a positron (a positive electron). Almost immediately this positron combines with an electron and these two are mutually annihilated, resulting in the emission of two gamma rays. These two gamma rays follow nearly opposing trajectories and interact with the surrounding body tissues, where they are recorded by a circular array of detectors. Thereafter, a mathematical reconstruction algorithm is used to determine the spatial distribution of the radioactivity within the subject at some selected plane. The resulting images can be projected onto a cathode-ray screen. One refinement is that images, recorded at intervals after the administration of the labeled compound, can be color-coded to illustrate differences in the biological activity from point to point. In this way a PET scanner can provide a non-invasive assessment of a number of biochemical processes in the organ that is being visualized. The recent article by Ter-Pogossian et al. (1980) provides a number of color images of the process just described.

(c) Nuclear Magnetic Resonance and Computerized Tomography

Nuclear magnetic resonance measurements can be utilized to approximate the plane integrals of the density $f(x,y,z)$ of hydrogen nuclei in a real object; see, e.g. Lauterbur (1974). In recent years there has been an increase in nuclear magnetic resonance (NMR) diagnostic imaging since NMR is nonionizing and noninvasive in contrast to X-ray computerized tomography; Hinshaw et al. (1978). Various "direct" techniques have been used in NMR to avoid the mathematical inversion process. This has resulted in various technical disadvantages--e.g., only a small volume of the object under investigation is actually radiating spin energy. If it is desired to reconstruct the whole object then mathematical inversion has the advantage of decreasing the data acquisition time.

Radon's inversion of the density $f \equiv f(x,y,z)$ from plane integrals was as follows:

Assume that f is continuous and has compact support. For each unit vector $\underset{\sim}{v}$ and $-\infty < \rho < \infty$ let $p(\rho,\underset{\sim}{v})$ represent the plane whose normal from the origin is $\rho\underset{\sim}{v}$. The plane integral

$$P(\rho,\underset{\sim}{v}) = \int_{p(\rho,\underset{\sim}{v})} f \, dA$$

is the two-dimensional projection of f along $P(\rho,\underset{\sim}{v})$. Here $p(-\rho,-\underset{\sim}{v}) = P(\rho,\underset{\sim}{v})$. For each point q(x,y,z) the point mean value of P over all planes through q is

$$F(q) = \frac{1}{4\pi} \iint_{\underset{\sim}{v} \in S} P[\rho(q),\underset{\sim}{v}]\, dS(\underset{\sim}{v}),$$

where $\underset{\sim}{v} \in S$ indicates that $\underset{\sim}{v}$ runs over the unit sphere S of unit vectors with $dS(\underset{\sim}{v})$ denoting the local element of area on S and ρ(q) being the value of ρ for which $P(\rho,\underset{\sim}{v})$ contains the point q. Although F(q) designates a fourfold integration of f it can be reduced to a threefold integral of f--

$$F(q) = F(x,y,z)$$

$$= \frac{1}{2} \int\int_{-\infty}^{\infty}\int \frac{f(x',y',z')}{[f(x - x')^2 + (y - y')^2 + (z - z')^2]^{1/2}}\, dx'dy'dz',$$

indicating that F(q) is the same as the convolution of f with (1/2r); $F = \frac{1}{2} f * r^{-1}$. This being true, then 2F is the analog of the electrostatic potential due to an electric charge density f. By Gauss' formula, $f = -(1/4\pi)\nabla^2(f * r^{-1})$ and hence

$$f(x,y,z) = -\frac{1}{2}\left[\frac{\partial^2}{\partial x^2} + \frac{\partial^2}{\partial y^2} + \frac{\partial^2}{\partial x^2}\right] F(x,y,z).$$

This last result gives the Radon formula for reconstructing f from a knowledge of P.

Applications of these mathematical results are given by Shepp (1980). He presents a simple algorithm for numerical quadrature of the Radon formula and suggests how one might use it in an application to imaging the nuclear magnetic resonance spin density of an object.

Perhaps the decade of the eighties will see as much advance in nuclear magnetic resonance imaging as the seventies did in reconstructive tomography.

GLOSSARY

Adenocarcinoma: A malignant neoplasm of epithelial cells in glandular or gland like pattern.

Anterior: In front of.

Anoxia: Absence of oxygen in tissues.

Carcinoma: Any of the various types of malignant neoplasm derived from epithelial tissue in several sites, occurring more frequently in the skin and large intestine of both sexes, the bronchii, stomach, and prostate gland in men, and the breast and cervix in women.

Clonogenic surviving fraction: The expected proportion of surviving cells (usually cancerous) after a single radiation dose.

Connective tissue: Any of the tissues of the body that support the specialized elements of parenchyma, e.g. adipose, cartilaginous tissues.

Cybernetic: Relating to the concepts of a communication and control network and its function in maintaining homeostasis.

Damage: Loss or detriment caused by injury.

Event: The passage of a particle through the critical locus of a cell for the effect under consideration.

Field (diagnostic radiology): The projected image of an anatomic organ or region; e.g. a lung field.

Field (therapeutic radiology): The area directly encompassed by an external therapy beam. The word "port" is also used.

Filter: See wedge filter.

Homeostasis: The state of equilibrium in the body with respect to various functions and to the chemical composition of the fluids and tissues (e.g. temperature, heart rate, blood pressure, etc.)

Hot spot: The area circumscribed by the maximum isodose line relative to the line of normalization.

Hyperthermia: Therapeutically induced hyperpyrexia (high fever).

Hypoxia: A state in which a physiologically inadequate amount of oxygen is available to, or utilized by, tissue without respect to cause or degree.

Injury (radiation): Hurt.

Isodose curve: A line connecting multiple points of equal dose within a plane.

Lesion: 1. A wound or injury. 2. A more or less circumscribed pathologic change in the tissues.

Melanoma: A malignant tumor whose parenchyma is composed of anaplastic melanocytes.

Mitotic delay time: The irradiation of cultured cells delays cell division as well as causing extinction of reproductive capacity. One implication is that DNA injury that is less than lethal requires time for repair with the result that cell division is delayed. See Andrews (1978a, pp. 38, 39).

Nominal standard dose: This is a single reference dose for the biological effect of a fractionated course of radiotherapy. This number aids in the comparison of treatment plans having widely different fractionation patterns and overall treatment times. See Ellis (1971).

Osteogen: The substance forming the inner layer of the periosteum from which new bone is formed.

Osteosarcoma: Osteogenic sarcoma.

Oxygenation: Addition of oxygen to any chemical or physical system.

Penumbra: The soft edge of an irradiation field when an isotropic source is used.

Portal: See field.

Posterior: Situated behind, in back of.

Radiosensitizer: Used to sensitize hypoxic cells. A radiosensitizer is generally considered to be a chemical compound that is not a normal metabolite and can diffuse (possibly) to regions of human tumors inaccessible to oxygen. In cancer therapy the term "radiosensitivity" indicates a desire to enhance the effect of radiation.

Regime: A systematic course of radiotherapy treatment involving one or more schedules.

Ret: This is the unit for the nominal standard dose. The rad equivalent therapy (ret) is determined by a formula that converts the rad dose.

Rhabdomyosarcoma: A malignant tumor, usually involving the muscles of the extremities or torso.

Roentgen (Röntgen) rays: Also called X-rays.

Sarcoma: A tumor, usually highly malignant, formed by the proliferation of mesodermal cells; a malignant connective tissue neoplasm.

Schedule: A repetitive application of fractions of equal doses of radiation at equal time intervals over a predetermined treatment time.

Tissue: A collection of similar cells and the intercellular substance surrounding them. There are four basic tissues in the body: (1) epithelium, (2) the connective tissue, including blood, bone and cartilage, (3) muscle tissue and (4) nerve tissue.

Treatment portal: The field of irradiation encompassing the potential tumor-bearing volume. Generally, these are square or rectangular fields defined by the collimators of the treatment.

Uniform fractionation regime: The treatment plan calls for just a single schedule.

Wedge filter: A radiation filter so constructed that its thickness or transmission characteristics vary continuously or in steps from one edge to another.

Weight (beam): Refers to the amount of irradiation energy being deposited at the points of greatest dose in a treatment field.

Chapter 4.

Section 4.3. Model 1: The basic system of kinetic equations from the scheme (4.5) can be expressed in terms of D (under the assumption that $\alpha_i t = k_i D$, i = 1,2,3) in the vector differential equation form (A.1) with

$$\underset{\sim}{X}(D) = \begin{bmatrix} X_1(D) \\ X_2(D) \\ X_3(D) \end{bmatrix}, \quad \underset{\sim}{A} = \begin{bmatrix} -k_1 & 0 & 0 \\ k_1 & -k_2 & 0 \\ 0 & k_2 & 0 \end{bmatrix}, \quad \underset{\sim}{X}(0) = \begin{bmatrix} 1 \\ 0 \\ 0 \end{bmatrix},$$

with $\underset{\sim}{x}(t) \equiv \underset{\sim}{X}(D)$. For the expression given by $\underset{\sim}{A}$ the right-hand side of (A.2) becomes

$$\begin{bmatrix} 1-k_1 D + k_1^2 \frac{D^2}{2!} - \ldots & 0 & 0 \\ P & 1-k_2 D + k_2 \frac{D^2}{2!} \ldots & 0 \\ Q & 1 - (1-k_2 D + k_2 \frac{D^2}{2!} \ldots & 0 \end{bmatrix}$$

where

$$P = \frac{k_1}{k_2-k_1} \left[(k_2 - k_1)D - (k_2^2 - k_1^2) \frac{D^2}{2!} + (k_2^3 - k_1^3) \frac{D^3}{3!} - \ldots\right]$$

$$Q = 1 + \frac{1}{k_2-k_1} \left[-(k_2 - k_1) + k_1 k_2 (k_2 - k_1) \frac{D^2}{2!} - k_1 k_2 (k_2^2 - k_1^2) \frac{D^3}{3!} + \ldots\right]$$

and hence

$$\begin{bmatrix} X_1(D) \\ X_2(D) \\ X_3(D) \end{bmatrix} = \begin{bmatrix} e^{-k_1 D} & 0 & 0 \\ [k_1/(k_2-k_1)](e^{-k_1 D} - e^{-k_2 D}) & e^{-k_2 D} & 0 \\ 1 + [1/(k_2-k_1)](k_1 e^{-k_2 D} - k_2 e^{-k_1 D}) & 1-e^{-k_2 D} & 0 \end{bmatrix} \begin{bmatrix} X_1(0) \\ X_2(0) \\ X_3(0) \end{bmatrix}$$

which gives the solution previously obtained in (4.6), since $X_1(0) = 1$ and $X_2(0) = X_3(0) = 0$.

Now consider the kinetic scheme

$$x_1 \xrightarrow{\alpha} x_2 \xrightarrow{\alpha} x_3 \xrightarrow{\alpha} \ldots x_{n-1} \xrightarrow{\alpha} x_n.$$

For this situation

$$\underset{\sim}{X}(D) = \begin{bmatrix} X_1(D) \\ \cdot \\ \cdot \\ \cdot \\ X_n(D) \end{bmatrix}, \quad \underset{\sim}{A} = \begin{bmatrix} -k & 0 & & & \\ k & -k & & & \\ 0 & k & -k & & \\ & \ddots & \ddots & & \\ & & k & -k & 0 \\ & & 0 & k & 0 \end{bmatrix}$$

with $X_1(0) = 1$, $X_j(0) = 0$, $j = 2,\ldots,n$; also $\underset{\sim}{A}$ is $n \times n$. Direct use of the result (A.3) eventually produces

$$\underset{\sim}{X}(D) = \begin{bmatrix} e^{-kD} \\ k\,De^{-kD} \\ \cdot \\ \cdot \\ \cdot \\ (kD)^{n-1}(e^{-kD})/(n-1)! \\ 1-e^{-kD}[1 + kD + \ldots + (kD)^{n-1}/(n-1)!] \end{bmatrix}$$

The survival function is $1 - X_n(D)$ and agrees with (4.7).

APPENDIX 2

Derivation of the result (5.[illegible]). Define $x(t) = \ln L(t)$ so that (5.6) becomes

$$\frac{dx(t)}{dt} = [illegible] + \ln S \sum_{j=0}^{K-1} [illegible] \qquad (A2.1)$$

Define the Laplace transform of $x(t)$ by the equation

$$X(s) = \int_0^\infty x(t)e^{-st}\,dt. \qquad [illegible]$$

Multiply each side of (A2.1) by e^{-st} and integrate the result with respect to t from 0 to ∞. This gives

$$-x(0) + sX(s) = [illegible]$$

$$X(s) = \frac{x(0)}{s} + [illegible]$$

The inverse transform is

$$x(t) = [illegible]$$

where [illegible]

$$x(0) [illegible] \ln S \sum^{K-1} [illegible]$$

The residue [illegible] $x(0)$ [illegible]

[illegible]

[illegible] $x(0)$

APPENDIX 3

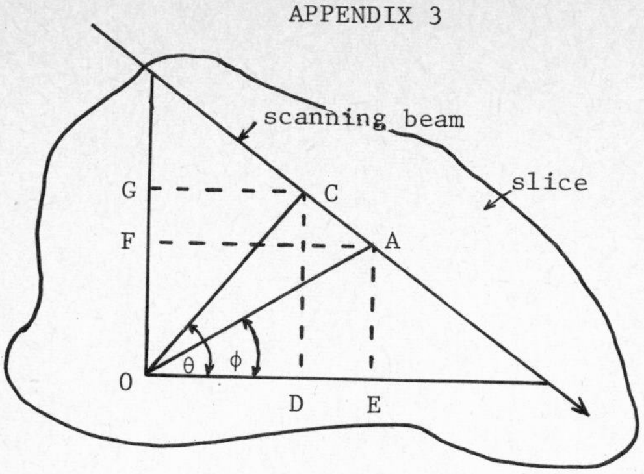

Figure A3

From the diagram:

$$DB = AE = OA \cos EAO = r \sin \phi, \; DC = p \sin \theta,$$

$$DB + BC = DC \Longrightarrow dy = p \sin \theta - r \sin \phi,$$

$$OD = p \cos \theta, \; OD = OE - DE = r \cos \phi - dx$$

$$\therefore dx = r \cos \phi - p \cos \theta.$$

Since $p = r \cos(\theta - \phi)$ the expressions for dx and dy can be expressed in the alternative forms

$$dx = r \sin \theta \sin (\theta - \phi), \; dy = r \cos \theta \sin (\theta - \phi).$$

Now the line element AC = $d\ell$ and

$$\frac{d\ell}{dxdy} = \left[\frac{1}{(dx)^2} + \frac{1}{(dy)^2} \right]^{1/2} = [r \sin \theta \cos \theta \sin (\theta - \phi)]^{-1}.$$

The singular behavior in the denominator of this expression suggests that it is permissible to introduce the generalized function, or Dirac distribution, so that

$$d\ell/dxdy = \delta[p - r \cos (\theta - \phi)],$$

where the argument of the δ-function reflects the fact that $d\ell = 0$, when $p \neq r \cos (\theta - \phi)$.

Let $\underset{\sim}{r}$ denote the vector OA and let $\underset{\sim}{\omega} = (\cos \theta, \sin \theta)$ be the vector at right-angles to the ray. Then $\underset{\sim}{\omega} \cdot \underset{\sim}{r} = r \cos (\theta - \phi)$ and

$$d\ell = \delta(p - \underset{\sim}{\omega} \cdot \underset{\sim}{r})dxdy. \qquad \text{(A3.1)}$$

BIBLIOGRAPHY

1. Abillon, E. 1974. "The Extrapolation Number in the 'm Targets - One Hit' Model." Math. Biosci., 19, 191-200.

2. Abou-Mandour, M., and D. Harder. 1978. "Systematic Optimization of the Double-scatterer System for Electron Beam Field-flattening." Strahlentherapie, 154, 328-332.

3. Ahnström, G., and L. Ehrenberg. 1980. "The Nature of the Target in the Biological Action of Ionizing Radiations." Advances Biol. and Med. Physics, 17, 129-172.

4. Almquist, K.J., and H.T. Banks. 1976. "A Theoretical and Computational Method for Determining Optimal Treatment Schedules in Fractionated Radiation Therapy." Math. Biosci., 29, 159-179.

5. Alper, T., N.E. Gillies and M.M. Elkind. 1960. "The Sigmoid Survival Curve in Radiobiology." Nature, 186, 1062-1063.

6. Alper, T. (editor). 1975. Cell Survival After Low Doses of Radiation: Theoretical and Clinical Implications. New York: J. Wiley.

7. Andrews, J.R. 1968. The Radiobiology of Human Cancer Radiotherapy. Philadelphia: Saunders.

8. Andrews, J.R. 1978a. The Radiobiology of Human Cancer Radiotherapy. Baltimore: University Park Press.

9. Andrews, J.R. 1978b. Position paper for the workshop on Optimization of the Radiobiological Response in Radiation Therapy, sponsored by the International Union Against Cancer and held at the CIBA Foundation in London, Feb. 27 - Mar. 2.

10. Arcangeli, G., F. Mauro, D. Morelli and C. Nervi. 1979. "Multiple Daily Fractionation in Radiotherapy: Biological Rationale and Preliminary Clinical Experiences." Eur. J. Cancer, 15, 1077-1083.

11. Aroesty, J., T. Lincoln, N. Shapiro and G. Boccia. 1973. "Tumor Growth and Chemotherapy: Mathematical Methods, Computer Simulations, and Experimental Foundations." Math. Biosci., 17, 243-300.

12. Athans, M., and P.L. Falb. 1966. Optimal Control. New York: McGraw-Hill.

13. Bacq, Z.M., and P. Alexander. 1961. Fundamentals of Radiobiology, 2nd edn. London: Pergamon Press.

14. Bahr, G.K., J.G. Kereiakes, H. Horwitz, R. Finney, J. Galvin and K. Goode. 1968. "The Method of Linear Programming Applied to Radiation Treatment Planning." Radiology, 91, 686-693.

15. Bahr, G.K., J.G. Kereiakes, H. Horwitz, R. Finney, J. Galvin and K. Goode. 1970. "The Method of Linear Programming Applied to Radiation Treatment Planning." In Year Book of Cancer, pp. 363-367, edited by R.L. Clark and R.W. Cumley. Chicago: Year Book Medical.

16. Bansal, B.N.L., and P.C. Gupta. 1978. "A Stochastic Model for Cell Survival After Irradiation." Biometrics, 34, 653-658.

17. Barendsen, G.W., C.J. Koot, G.R. van Kersen, D.K. Bewley, S.B. Field and C.J. Parnell. 1966. "The Effect of Oxygen on Impairment of the Proliferative Capacity of Human Cells in Culture by Ionizing Radiations of Different LET." Int. J. Rad. Biol., 10, 317-327.

18. Barendsen, G.W. 1979. "Influence of Radiation Quality on the Effectiveness of Small Doses for Induction of Reproductive Death and Chromosome Aberrations in Mammalian Cells." Int. J. Rad. Biol., **36**, 49-63.

19. Baserga, R. 1965. "The Relationship of the Cell Cycle to Tumor Growth and Control of Cell Division: A Review." Cancer Res., **25**, 581-595.

20. Bates, T.D. 1975. "A Prospective Clinical Trial of Post-operative Radiotherapy Delivered in 3 Fractions per Week versus 2 Fractions per Week in Breast Carcinoma." Clin. Radiol., **26**, 297-304.

21. Beckman, F.S. 1960. "The Solution of Linear Equations by the Conjugate Gradient Method." In Mathematical Methods for Digital Computers, pp. 62-72, edited by A. Ralston and H.S. Wilf. New York: J. Wiley.

22. Becquerel, H. 1896. "Emission of the New Radiations by Metalic Uranium." Compt. Rend. Acad. Sci., **122**, 1086-1088.

23. Bellman, R. 1957. Dynamic Programming. Princeton (New Jersey): Princeton University Press.

24. Bellman, R.E., and S.E. Dreyfus. 1962. Applied Dynamic Programming. Princeton (New Jersey): Princeton University Press.

25. Bellman, R., H. Sugiyama and B. Kashef. 1974. "Applications of Dynamic Programming and Scan-rescan Processes to Nuclear Medicine and Tumor Detection." Math. Biosci., **21**, 1-29.

26. Bender, M.A., and S. Wolff. 1961. "X-ray induced Chromosome Aberrations and Reproductive Death in Mammalian Cells." Amer. Nat., **95**, 39-52.

27. Bender, M.A., and P.C. Gooch. 1962. "The Kinetics of X-ray Survival of Mammalian Cells In Vitro." Int. J. Radiat. Biol., **5**, 133-145.

28. Berendsen, G.W., C.J. Koot, G.R. van Kersen, D.K. Bewley, S.B. Field and C.J. Parnell. 1965. "The Effect of Oxygen on Impairment of the Proliferative Capacity of Human Cells in Culture by Ionizing Radiations of Different LET." Int. J. Radiat. Biol., **10**, 317-327.

29. Berry, M.V., and D.F. Gibbs. 1970. "The Interpretation of Optical Projections." Proc. Roy. Soc. (London) Series A. **314**, 143-152.

30. Bestehorn, M., U. Ebert, D. Steinhausen and H. Werner. 1979. "Some Applications of Computational Mathematics to Medical Problems." In Lecture Notes in Mathematics, vol. 704 - Computing Methods in Applied Science and Engineering, pp. 377-391. New York: Springer Verlag.

31. Bett, W.R. 1957. "Historical Aspects of Cancer." In Cancer, Vol. 1, pp. 1-5, edited by R.W. Raven. London: Butterworth.

32. Bjärngard, B.E. 1977. "Optimization in Radiation Therapy." Int. J. Radiation Oncology Biol. Phys., **2**, 381-382.

33. Bjärngard, B.E., and P.K. Kijewski. 1978. "Computer-controlled Radiation Therapy." In Proc. The Second Ann. Symp. on Computer Application in Medical Care, pp. 86-92, edited by F.H. Orthner. New York: Institute of Electrical and Electronics Engineers.

34. Blau, M., and K. Altenburger. 1922. "Über einige Wirkungen von Strahlen, II." Z. Physik, **12**, 315-329.

35. Boone, M.L.M., W.G. Connor, R.S. Heusinkveld and R.E. Morgado. 1976. "New In-

strumentation in Radiation Oncology." CA--A Cancer Jl. for Clinicians, 26, 299-309.

36. Boot, J.C.G. 1964. Quadratic Programming. Amsterdam: North-Holland.

37. Bories, J. (editor). 1978. The Diagnostic Limitations of Computerized Axial Tomography. New York: Springer Verlag.

38. Bourgat, J.F., M. Rivier, A. Dutreix and D. Bernard. 1974. "Optimisation par Ordinateur du Traitement en Télécobalthérapie." J. Radiol. Electrol., 55, 775-779.

39. Bracken, J., and G.P. McCormick. 1968. Selected Applications of Nonlinear Programming. New York: J. Wiley.

40. Brannen, J.P. 1975. "A Temperature- and Dose Rate-Dependent Model for the Kinetics of Cellular Response to Ionizing Radiation." Radiat. Res., 62, 379-387.

41. Braunschweiger, P.G., L.L. Schenken and L.M. Schiffer. 1979. "The Cytokinetic Basis for the Design of Efficacious Radiotherapy Protocols." Int. J. Radiation Oncology Biol. Phys., 5, 37-47.

42. Brogan, W.L. 1974. Modern Control Theory. New York: Quantum.

43. Bronk, B.V. 1976. "Thermal Potentiation of Mammalian Cell Killing: Clues for Understanding and Potential for Tumor Therapy." Advances in Radiat. Biol., 6, 267-324.

44. Bronk, B.V. 1978. Personal communication.

45. Brooks, R.A., and G. DiChiro. 1975. "Theory of Image Reconstruction in Computed Tomography." Radiology, 117, 561-572.

46. Brooks, R.A., and G. DiChiro. 1976. "Principles of Computer Assisted Tomography (CAT) in Radiographic and Radioisotope Imaging." Phys. Med. Biol., 21, 689-732.

47. Brown, B.W., J.R. Thompson, T. Barkley, H. Suit and H.R. Withers. 1974. "Theoretical Considerations of Dose Rate Factors Influencing Radiation Strategy." Radiology, 110, 197-202.

48. Brunton, G.F., and T.E. Wheldon. 1978. "Characteristic Species Dependent Growth Patterns of Mammalian Neoplasms." Cell Tissue Kinet., 11, 161-175.

49. Bryson, A.E., and Y.C. Ho. 1969. Applied Optimal Control. Waltham (Massachusetts): Blaisdell.

50. Buschke, F. 1970. "Radiation Therapy: The Past, the Present, the Future." Amer. J. Roentgenol., 108, 236-246.

51. Buschke, F., and R.G. Parker. 1972. Radiation Therapy in Cancer Management. New York: Grune and Stratton.

52. Caldwell, W.L. 1979. "Principles of Radiation Therapy." In Principles and Management of Urologic Cancer, pp. 205-231, edited by N. Javadpour. Baltimore: The Williams and Wilkins Co.

53. Canon, M.D., C.D. Cullum and E. Polak. 1970. Theory of Optimal Control and Mathematical Programming. New York: McGraw-Hill.

54. Catteral, M., and D.K. Bewley. 1979. Fast Neutrons in the Treatment of Cancer. New York: Grune and Stratton.

55. Cavaliere, R., E.C. Ciocatto, B.C. Giovanella, C. Heidelberger, R.O. Johnson, M. Margottini, B. Mondovi, G. Moricca and A. Rossi-Fanelli. 1967. "Selective Heat Sensitivity of Cancer Cells." Cancer, 20, 1351-1381.

56. Chadwick, K.H., and H.P. Leenhouts. 1973. "A Molecular Theory of Cell Survival." Phys. Med. Biol., 18, 78-87.

57. Chadwick, K.H., and H.P. Leenhouts. 1975. "The Effect of an Asynchronous Population of Cells on the Initial Slope of Dose-effect Curves." In Cell Survival After Low Doses of Radiation, pp. 57-63, edited by T. Alper. New York: J. Wiley.

58. Chadwick, K.H., H.P. Leenhouts, I. Szumiel and A.H.W. Nias. 1976. "Effects of a Platinum Complex and its Combination with Ionizing Radiation on CHO Cells: Interpretation Using the Molecular Theory of Cell Survival." Int. J. Radiat. Biol., 30, 511-524.

59. Chapman, J.D., C.J. Gillespie, A.P. Reuvers and D.L. Dugle. 1975. "The Inactivation of Chinese Hamster Cells by X Rays: The Effects of Chemical Modifiers on Single- and Double-Events." Radiat. Res., 64, 365-375.

60. Cherchas, D.B., and S.S. Ng. 1978. "Optimum Control of Neutron Flux During Nuclear Station Load Following." Automatica, 14, 533-546.

61. Christensen, E.E., T.S. Curry III and J.E. Dowdey. 1978. An Introduction to the Physics of Diagnostic Radiology, 2nd edn. Philadelphia: Lea and Febiger.

62. Clark, C.W. 1976. Mathematical Bioeconomics: The Optimal Management of Renewable Resources. New York: J. Wiley.

63. Clarkson, B.D., T. Ohkita, K. Ota and J. Fried. 1967. "Studies of Cellular Proliferation in Human Leukemia, I. Estimation of Growth Rates of Leukemic and Normal Hematopoietic Cells in Two Adults with Acute Leukemia given Single Injections of Tritiated Thymidine." J. Clin. Invest., 46, 506-529.

64. Clarkson, B.D. 1969. "Review of Recent Studies of Cellular Proliferation in Acute Leukemia." In Human Tumor Cell Kinetics, Monograph 30, pp. 81-120. Washington (D.C.): National Cancer Institute.

65. Clarkson, B.D., J. Fried, A. Strife, Y. Sakai, K. Ota and T. Ohkita. 1970. "Studies of Cellular Proliferation in Human Leukemia, III. Behavior of Leukemic Cells in Three Adults with Acute Leukemia given Continuous Infusions of 3H-thymidine for 8 to 10 Days." Cancer, 25, 1237-1260.

66. Clarkson, B., and S.I. Rubinow. 1977. "Growth Kinetics in Human Leukemia." In Growth Kinetics and Biochemical Regulation of Normal and Malignant Cells, pp. 591-628, edited by B. Drewinko and R.M. Humphrey. Baltimore: Williams and Wilkins Co.

67. Cohen, L. 1960. "The Statistical Prognosis in Radiation Therapy: A Study of Optimal Dosage in Relation to Physical and Biological Parameters for Epidermoid Cancer." Amer. J. Roentgenol., 84, 741-753.

68. Cohen, L. 1968. "Theoretical 'Iso-survival' Formulae for Fractionated Radiation Therapy." Br. J. Radiol., 41, 522-528.

69. Cohen, L., and M.J. Scott. 1968. "Fractionation Procedures in Radiation Therapy: A Computerized Approach to Evaluation." Br. J. Radiol., 41, 529-533.

70. Cohen, L. 1971. "A Cell Population Kinetic Model for Fractionated Radiation Therapy." Radiology, 101, 419-427.

71. Cohen, L. 1973a. "Cell Population Kinetics in Radiation Therapy: Optimization

of Tumor Dosage." Cancer, 32, 236-244.

72. Cohen, L. 1973b. "An Interactive Program for Standardization of Prescriptions in Radiation Therapy." Comp. Prog. Biomed., 3, 27-35.

73. Cohen, L. 1975. "Cell Survival and Iso-effect Contours in Irradiated Tissues." In Biomedical Dosimetry, pp. 355-369. Vienna: International Atomic Energy Agency, IAEA-SM193/69.

74. Cohen, L., and J.L. Redpath. 1977. "Derivation of Survival Kinetic Parameters for Cell Populations by Computer Simulation of Radiobiological Data." Radiat. Res., 69, 387-401.

75. Cohen, L. 1978a. "Dose-time Relationship: Computation of Cell Lethality Following Fractionated Radiation Therapy." Int. J. Radiation Oncology Biol. Phys., 4, 267-271.

76. Cohen, L. 1978b. Personal communication.

77. Cohen, L. 1978c. "Derivation of Cell Population Kinetic Parameters from Clinical Statistical Data (Program Rad 3)." Int. J. Radiation Oncology Biol. Phys., 4, 835-840.

78. Cohen, L., and J.E. Moulder. 1978. "Derivation of Cellular Survival Kinetic Parameters for Experimental Fractionated Irradiation of Rat Skin." Radiat. Res., 76, 250-258.

79. Cohen, L. 1979. Personal communication.

80. Coley, W.B. 1893. "The Treatment of Malignant Tumors by Repeated Innoculations of Erysipelas: With a Report of 10 Original Cases." Am. J. Med. Sci., 105, 487-511.

81. Connor, W.G., E.W. Gerner, R.C. Miller and M.L.M. Boone. 1977. "Prospects for Hyperthermia in Human Cancer Therapy. Part II: Implications of Biological and Physical Data for Applications of Hyperthermia to Man." Radiology, 123, 497-503.

82. Coolidge, W.D. 1913. "A Powerful Roentgen-ray Tube with a Pure Electron Discharge." Physical Rev., 2, 409-413.

83. Cooper, L., and D. Steinberg. 1970. Introduction to Methods of Optimization. Philadelphia: W.B. Saunders Co.

84. Cooper, R.E.M., and B.W. Worthley. 1967. "Computer-based External Beam Radiotherapy Planning II: Practical Applications." Phys. Med. Biol., 12, 241-249.

85. Cooper, R.E.M. 1978. "A Gradient Method of Optimizing External-beam Radiotherapy Treatment Plans." Radiology, 128, 235-243.

86. Cormack, A.M. 1963. "Representation of a Function by its Line Integrals, with Some Radiological Applications." J. Appl. Phys., 34, 2722-2727.

87. Cormack, A.M. 1964. "Representation of a Function by its Line Integrals, with Some Radiological Applications. II." J. Appl. Phys., 35, 2908-2913.

88. Cormack, A.M. 1973. "Reconstruction of Densities from their Projections, with Applications in Radiological Physics." Phys. Med. Biol., 18, 195-207.

89. Cormack, A.M. 1980a. "Early Two-dimensional Reconstruction and Recent Topics Stemming from it." Med. Phys., 7, 277-282.

90. Cormack, A.M. 1980b. "Early Two-dimensional Reconstruction and Recent Topics

Stemming from It." Science, 209, 1482-1486.

91. Cox, E.B., M.A. Woodbury and L.E. Myers. 1980. "A New Model for Tumor Growth Analysis Based on a Postulated Inhibitory Substance." Comp. Biomed. Res., 13, 437-445.

92. Crowther, J.A. 1924. "Some Considerations Relative to the Action of X-rays on Tissue Cells." Proc. Roy. Soc. (London) B, 96, 207-211.

93. Crowther, J.A. 1926. "The Action of X-rays on Colpidium Colpoda." Proc. Roy. Soc. (London) B, 100, 390-404.

94. Crowther, J.A. 1927. "A Theory of the Action of X-rays on Living Cells." Proc. Camb. Phil. Soc., 23, 284-287.

95. Crowther, J.A. 1938. "The Biological Action of X-rays, a Theoretical Review." Br. J. Radiol., 11, 132-145.

96. Curie, P., and M.S. Curie. 1898. "Sur une Substance Nouvelle Radioactive, Contenue dans la Pechblende." Compt. Rend. Acad. Sci., 127, 175-178.

97. Curtis, S.B., G.W. Barendsen and A.F. Hermens. 1973. "Cell Kinetic Model of Tumor Growth and Regression for a Rhabdomyo-sarcoma in the Rat: Undisturbed Growth and Radiation Response to Large Single Doses." Europ. J. Cancer, 9, 81-87.

98. Daellenbach, H.G., and J.A. George. 1978. Introduction to Operations Research Techniques. Boston: Allyn and Bacon.

99. Daniels, R.W. 1978. Introduction to Numerical Methods and Optimization Techniques. New York: Elsevier.

100. Dantzig, G.B. 1970. "Linear Programming and its Progeny." In Applications of Mathematical Programming Techniques, pp. 3-16, edited by E.M.L. Beale. New York: American Elsevier.

101. Davidson, H.O. 1957. Biological Effects of Whole-body Gamma Radiation on Human Beings. Baltimore: Johns Hopkins University Press.

102. Davis, P.J., and P. Rabinowitz. 1967. Numerical Integration. Waltham (Massachusetts): Blaisdell.

103. Delattre, P. 1974. "Systems Approach to Theoretical Models in Radiobiology and Radiotherapy." Int. J. General Systems, 1, 105-117.

104. Delclos, L., E.J. Braun, J.R. Herrera, V.A. Sampiere and E.V. Roosenbeek. 1963. "Whole Abdominal Irradiation by Cobalt 60 Moving-strip Technic." Radiology, 81, 632-641.

105. Delsarte, Ph. 1980. "A Refined Version of Khachian's Algorithm." Philips J. Res., 35, 307-319.

106. Dembo, A.J., J. van Dyk, B. Japp, H.A. Bean, F.A. Beale, J.F. Pringle and R.S. Bush. 1979. "Whole Abdominal Irradiation by a Moving-strip Technique for Patients with Ovarian Cancer." Int. J. Radiation Oncology Biol. Phys., 5, 1933-1942. (A correction to this paper is given in vol. 6, no. 5, 1980 on the page just after the table of contents.)

107. Demicheli, R. 1980. "Growth of Testicular Neoplasm Lung Metastases: Tumor-specific Relation Between Two Gompertzian Parameters." Europ. J. Cancer, 16, 1603-1608.

108. DeMott, R.K., R.T. Mulcahy, and K.H. Clifton. 1979. "The Survival of Thyroid

Cells Following Irradiation: A Directly Generated Single-dose Survival Curve." Radiat. Res., 77, 395-403.

109. Denekamp, J., and J.F. Fowler. 1977. "Cell Proliferation Kinetics and Radiation Therapy." In Cancer, A Comprehensive Treatise, Vol. 6 - Radiotherapy, Surgery and Immunotherapy, pp. 101-137, edited by F.F. Becker. New York: Plenum Press.

110. Denekamp, J., J.F. Fowler and S. Dische. 1977. "The Proportion of Hypoxic Cells in a Human Tumor." Int. J. Radiation Oncology Biol. Phys., 2, 1227-1228.

111. Dessauer, F. 1922. "Über einige Wirkungen von Strahlen, I." Z. Physik, 12, 38-47.

112. Dienes, G.J. 1966. "A Kinetic Model of Biological Radiation Response." Radiat. Res., 28, 183-202.

113. Dienes, G.J. 1971. "Survival Curves and Dose Fractionation: Some General Characteristics." Radiat. Res., 48, 551-564.

114. Dische, S., M.I. Saunders and I.R. Flockhart. 1978. "The Optimum Regime for the Administration of Misonidazole and the Establishment of Multicentre Clinical Trials." Br. J. Cancer, 37, 318-321.

115. Dische, S., M.I. Saunders, I.R. Flockhart, M.E. Lee and P. Anderson. 1979. "Misonidazole--A Drug for Trial in Radiotherapy and Oncology." Int. J. Radiation Oncol. Biol. Phys., 5, 851-860.

116. Dittrich, W. 1957. "Reversible Treffer." Z. Naturforschung, 12b, 536-541.

117. Dorny, C.N. 1975. A Vector Space Approach to Models and Optimization. New York: J. Wiley.

118. Douglas, B.G., and J.F. Fowler. 1975. "Fractionation Schedules and a Quadratic Dose-effect Relationship." Br. J. Radiol., 48, 502-504.

119. Douglas, B.G., J.F. Fowler, J. Denekamp, S.R. Harris, S.E. Ayres, S. Fairman, S.A. Hill, P.W. Sheldon and F.A. Stewart. 1975. "The Effect of Multiple Small Fractions of X-rays on Skin Reactions in the Mouse." In Cell Survival after Low Doses of Radiation, pp. 351-361, edited by T. Alper. London: J. Wiley.

120. Douglas, B.G., and J.F. Fowler. 1976. "The Effect of Multiple Small Doses of X Rays on Skin Reactions in the Mouse and a Basic Interpretation." Radiat. Res., 66, 401-426.

121. Dritschilo, A., J.T. Chaffey, W.D. Bloomer and A. Marck. 1978. "The Complication Probability Factor: A Method for Selection of Radiation Treatment Plans." Br. J. Radiol., 51, 370-374.

122. Dugle, D.L., C.J. Gillespie and J.D. Chapman. 1976. "DNA Strand Breaks, Repair, and Survival in X-irradiated Mammalian Cells." Proc. Nat. Acad. Sci. USA, 73, 809-812.

123. Durand, R.E. 1978. "Effects of Hyperthermia on the Cycling, Noncycling, and Hypoxic Cells of Irradiated and Unirradiated Multicell Spheroids." Radiat. Res., 75, 373-384.

124. Dutreix, J., A. Wambersie and C. Bounik. 1973. "Cellular Recovery in Human Skin Reactions: Application to Dose Fraction Number Overall Time Relationship in Radiotherapy." Europ. J. Cancer, 9, 159-167.

125. Dutreix, J., and A. Wambersie. 1975. "Cell Survival Curves Deduced from Non-quantitative Reactions of Skin, Intestinal Mucosa and Lung." In Cell Survival

after Low Doses of Radiation: Theoretical and Clinical Implications, pp. 335-341, edited by T. Alper. New York: J. Wiley.

126. Elkind, M.M., and H. Sutton. 1960. "Radiation Response of Mammalian Cells Grown in Culture. I. Repair of X-ray Damage in Surviving Chinese Hamster Cells." Radiat. Res., 13, 556-593.

127. Elkind, M.M., and G.F. Whitmore. 1967. The Radiobiology of Cultured Mammalian Cells. New York: Gordon and Breach.

128. Elkind, M.M. 1977. "The Initial Part of the Survival Curve. Implications for Low Dose, Low Dose-rate Radiation Responses." Radiat. Res., 71, 9-23.

129. Elkind, M.M. 1979. "DNA Repair and Cell Repair: Are they Related?" Int. J. Radiation Oncology Biol. Phys., 5, 1089-1094.

130. Ellis, F. 1969. "Dose, Time and Fractionation: A Clinical Hypothesis." Clin. Radiol., 20, 1-7.

131. Ellis, F. 1971. "Nominal Standard Dose and the Ret." Br. J. Radiol., 44, 101-108.

132. Ellis, F. 1974. "The NSD Concept and Radioresistant Tumours." Br. J. Radiol., 47, 909.

133. Epp, E.R., H. Weiss and C.C. Ling. 1976. "Irradiation of Cells by Single and Double Pulses of High Intensity Radiation: Oxygen Sensitization and Diffusion Kinetics." Current Topics in Radiat. Res. Quarterly, 11, 201-250.

134. Fazekas, J.T., and J.G. Maier. 1974. "Irradiation of Ovarian Carcinomas. A Prospective Comparison of the Open-field and Moving-strip Techniques." Am. J. Roentgenol. Radium Ther. Nucl. Med., 120, 118-123.

135. Fertil, B., P. Deschavanne, B. Lachet and E.P. Malaise. 1978. "Survival Curves of Neoplastic and Non Transformed Human Cell Lines: Statistical Analysis Using Different Models." In Sixth Symposium on Microdosimetry, Vol. 1, pp. 145-156, edited by J. Booz and H.G. Ebert. London: Harwood Academic.

136. Finney, D.J. 1971. Probit Analysis, 3rd edn. Cambridge (England): Cambridge Univ. Press.

137. Fischer, J.J. 1969. "Theoretical Considerations in the Optimisation of Dose Distribution in Radiation Therapy." Br. J. Radiol., 42, 925-930.

138. Fischer, J.J. 1971a. "Mathematical Simulation of Radiation Therapy of Solid Tumors. 1. Calculations." Acta Radiol. Ther. Phys. Biol., 10, 73-85.

139. Fischer, J.J. 1971b. "Mathematical Simulation of Radiation Therapy of Solid Tumors. II. Fractionization." Acta Radiol. Ther. Phys. Biol., 10, 267-278.

140. Fischer, J.J. 1971c. "A Computerized Mathematical Simulation of the Radiation Therapy of Solid Tumors." In Computers in Radiology, British J. of Radiology, Special Report Series No. 5, pp. 59-61. London: British Inst. of Radiology.

141. Fischer, J.J., and D.B. Fischer. 1971. "The Determination of Time-Dose Relationships from Clinical Data." Br. J. Radiol., 44, 785-792.

142. Fischer, D.B., and J.J. Fischer. 1977. "Dose Response Relationships in Radiotherapy: Applications of a Logistic Regression Model." Int. J. Radiation Oncology Biol. Phys., 2, 773-781.

143. Fischer, J.J. 1978. "The Role of Computers in Radiation Therapy: Analysis of

Clinical Radiotherapy Data." Radiology, 129, 783-786.

144. Fletcher, G.H. 1978. "The Evolution of the Basic Concepts Underlying the Practice of Radiotherapy from 1949 to 1977." Radiology, 127, 3-19.

145. Fletcher, R., and C.M. Reeves. 1964. "Functional Minimization by Conjugate Gradients." Comput. J., 7, 149-154.

146. Fowler, J.F., and B.E. Stern, II. 1963. "Dose-Time Relationships in Radiotherapy and the Validity of Cell Survival Curve Models." Br. J. Radiol., 36, 163-173.

147. Fowler, J.F., and J. Denekamp. 1977. "Radiation Effects on Normal Tissues." In Cancer, A Comprehensive Treatise, Vol. 6, Radiotherapy, Surgery, and Immunotherapy, pp. 139-180, edited by F.F. Becker. New York: Plenum Press.

148. Fowler, J.F. 1979. "New Horizons in Radiation Oncology." Br. J. Radiol., 52, 523-535.

149. Friedman, M.I., J.W. Beattie and J.S. Laughlin. 1974. "Cross-sectional Absorption Density Reconstruction for Treatment Planning." Phys. Med. Biol., 19, 819-830.

150. Gabutti, V., A. Pileri, R.P. Tarocco, F. Gavosto and E.H. Cooper. 1969. "Proliferative Potential of Out-of-cycle Leukaemic Cells." Nature, 224, 375-376.

151. Gacs, P., and L. Lovasz. 1979. "Khachian's Algorithm for Linear Programming." Report No. STAN-CS-79-750, Department of Computer Science, Stanford University, Stanford, California 94305.

152. Gallagher, T.L. 1967. "Optimization of External Radiation Beams for Therapy Planning." Ph.D. Thesis, Washington University, St. Louis.

153. Garg, S.C. 1977. "Numerical Minimization Methods for Functionals: Comparison and Extensions." University of Toronto Institute for Aerospace Studies Report No. 209 (CN ISSN 0082-5255).

154. Garrett, W.R., and M.G. Payne. 1978. "Applications of Models for Cell Survival: The Fixation Time Picture." Radiat. Res., 73, 201-211.

155. Gass, S.I. 1975. Linear Programming Methods and Applications, 4th edn. New York: McGraw-Hill.

156. Gel'fand, I.M., and G.E. Shilov. 1964. Generalized Functions, Vol. 1. New York: Academic Press.

157. Gel'fand, I.M., M.I. Graev and N. Ya. Vilenkin. 1966. Generalized Functions, Vol. 5. New York: Academic Press.

158. Gerner, E.W., W.G. Connor, M.L.M. Boone, J.D. Doss, E.G. Mayer and R.C. Miller. 1975. "The Potential of Localized Heating as an Adjunct to Radiation Therapy." Radiology, 116, 433-439.

159. Gilbert, C.W. 1975. "Target-type Models for Survival Curves." Br. J. Radiol., 48, 1045-1046.

160. Gilbert, C.W., J.H. Hendry and D. Major. 1980. "The Approximation in the Formulation for Survival $S = \exp -(\alpha D + \beta D^2)$." Int. J. Radiat. Biol., 37, 469-471.

161. Gilbert, H.A., and A.R. Kagan. 1978. Modern Radiation Oncology. Hagerstown (Maryland): Harper and Row.

162. Gillespie, C.J., J.D. Chapman, A.P. Reuvers and D.L. Dugle. 1975a. "The Inactivation of Chinese Hamster Cells by X-Rays: Synchronized and Exponential Cell Populations." Radiat. Res., 64, 353-364.

163. Gillespie, C.J., J.D. Chapman, A.P. Reuvers and D.L. Dugle. 1975b. "Survival of X-irradiated Hamster Cells: Analysis in Terms of the Chadwick-Leenhouts Model." In Cell Survival after Low Doses of Radiation: Theoretical and Clinical Implications, pp. 25-33, edited by T. Alper. New York: J. Wiley.

164. Ginsberg, D.M., and J. Jagger. 1965. "Evidence That Initial Ultraviolet Lethal Damage in Escherichia coli, Strain 15 T A U is Independent of Growth Phase." J. Gen. Microbiol., 40, 171-184.

165. Glicksman, A.S., and J. Hahn. 1974. "Interactive Computer Support for Optimization in the Decision Making Process in the Management of Patients with Cancer." In Radiology, Vol. 2, pp. 662-666, edited by J.G. López, J. Bonmati, R.J. Berry and J.W. Hopewell. Amsterdam: Excerpta Medica.

166. Goitein, M. 1979. "The Utility of Computed Tomography in Radiation Therapy: An Estimate of Outcome." Int. J. Radiation Oncology Biol. Phys., 5, 1799-1807.

167. Gonzalez, C.F., C.B. Grossman and E. Palacios. 1976. Computed Brain and Orbital Tomography. New York: J. Wiley.

168. Gordon, R., and G.T. Herman. 1974. "Three-dimensional Reconstruction from Projections: A Review of Algorithms." Int. Rev. Cytol., 38, 111-151.

169. Gordon, R. 1976. "Dose Reduction in Computerized Tomography." Invest. Radiol., 11, 508-517.

170. Gordon, R. 1979. Treatise on Reconstruction from Projections and Computed Tomography. New York: Plenum Press. (This book is in the preparation stage.)

171. Gor'kov, V.A. 1977. "An Estimation of the Parameters of Asymptotic Curves of Tumor Growth." Vopr. Onkol., 23(3), 51-54; in Russian.

172. Gottfried, B.S., and J. Weisman. 1973. Introduction to Optimization Theory. Englewood Cliffs (New Jersey): Prentice-Hall.

173. Graffman, S., T. Groth, B. Jung, G. Sköllermo and J.-E. Snell. 1975. "Cell Kinetic Approach to Optimising Dose Distribution in Radiation Therapy." Acta. Radiol. Ther. Phys. Biol., 14, 54-62.

174. Graffman, S., T. Groth, B. Jung and G. Sköllermo. 1979. "Equivalence of Quantitative Models for Tumour Response to Ionizing Radiation in Treatment Field Optimisation Procedures." Acta. Radiol. Oncol. Radiat. Phys. Biol., 18, 1-10.

175. Gray, L.H. 1957. "Oxygenation in Radiotherapy. I. Radiobiological Considerations." Br. J. Radiol., 30, 403-406.

176. Green, A.E.S., and J. Burki. 1974. "A Note on Survival Curves with Shoulders." Radiat. Res., 60, 536-540.

177. Hadley, G. 1964. Nonlinear and Dynamic Programming. Reading (Massachusetts): Addison-Wesley.

178. Hagen, U., Th. Coquerelle, L. Mitzel-Landbeck and A. Schön-Bopp. 1980. "Molecular Mechanism of DNA Repair after Ionizing Radiation." Advances in Biol. and Med. Physics, 17, 83-88.

179. Hahn, G.M., J.R. Boen, R.G. Miller, S.F. Boyle and R.F. Kallman. 1965. "Mathematical Models of the Recovery of Mammalian Cells from Radiation Injury with

Respect to Changes in Radiosensitivity." In Cellular Radiation Biology, pp. 411-417. Baltimore: Williams and Wilkins.

180. Hahn, G.M. 1975. "Radiation and Chemically Induced Potentially Lethal Lesions in Noncycling Mammalian Cells: Recovery Analysis in Terms of X-ray- and Ultraviolet-Like Systems." Radiat. Res., 64, 533-545.

181. Hahn, G.M., J. Braun and K. Har-Kedar. 1975. "Thermochemotherapy: Synergism Between Hyperthermia (42°-43°) and Adriamycin (or Bleomycin) in Mammalian Cell Inactivation." Proc. Natl. Acad. Sci. U.S.A., 72, 937-940.

182. Hall, E.J. 1973. Radiobiology for the Radiologist, New York: Harper and Row.

183. Hall, E.J. 1975. "Biological Problems in the Measurement of Survival at Low Doses." In Cell Survival After Low Doses of Radiation: Theoretical and Clinical Implications, pp. 13-24, edited by T. Alper. New York: J. Wiley.

184. Hall, E.J. 1976. Radiation and Life. New York: Pergamon Press.

185. Hall, E.J. 1978. Radiobiology for the Radiologist, 2nd edn. New York: Harper and Row.

186. Hall, E.J., H.R. Withers, J.P. Gerachi, R.E. Meyn, J. Rasey, P. Todd and G.E. Sheline. 1979. "Radiobiological Intercomparisons of Fast Neutron Beams used for Therapy in Japan and United States." Int. J. Radiation Oncology Biol. Phys., 5, 227-233.

187. Hanawalt, P.C., E.C. Friedberg and C.F. Cox (editors). 1978. DNA Repair Mechanisms. New York: Academic Press.

188. Harris, R.J.C. 1976. Cancer, 3rd edn. Baltimore: Penguin Books.

189. Hasdorff, L. 1976. Gradient Optimization and Nonlinear Control. New York: J. Wiley.

190. Hendee, W.R. 1979. Medical Radiation Physics, 2nd edn. Chicago: Year Book Medical.

191. Hendry, J.H. 1979. "A New Derivation, from Split-dose Data, of the Complete Survival Curve for Clonogenic Normal Cells in Vivo." Radiat. Res., 78, 404-414.

192. Henle, K.J., and L.A. Dethlefsen. 1978. "Heat Fractionation and Thermotolerance: A Review." Cancer Res., 38, 1843-1851.

193. Herbert, D., 1977. "The Assessment of the Clinical Significance of Non-compliance with Prescribed Schedules of Irradiation." Int. J. Radiation Oncology Biol. Phys., 2, 763-772.

194. Herman, G.T. (editor). 1979. Image Reconstruction from Projections: Implementation and Applications. New York: Springer Verlag.

195. Herman, G.T. 1980. Image Reconstruction from Projections. The Fundamentals of Computerized Tomography. New York: Academic Press.

196. Hestenes, M.R., and E. Stiefel. 1952. "Method of Conjugate Gradients for Solving Linear Systems." J. Res. Nat. Bur. Standards, 49, 409-436.

197. Hethcote, H.W., and P. Waltman. 1973. "Theoretical Determination of Optimal Treatment Schedules for Radiation Therapy." Radiat. Res., 56, 150-161.

198. Hethcote, H.W., J.W. McLarty and H.D. Thames, Jr. 1976. "Comparison of Mathematical Models for Radiation Fractionation." Radiat. Res., 67, 387-407.

199. Hethcote, H.W. 1978. "A Reconnaissance of Radiotherapy Optimization." Position paper for the workshop on Optimization of the Radiobiological Response in Radiation Therapy, sponsored by the International Union Against Cancer and held at the CIBA Foundation in London, Feb. 27 - Mar. 2.

200. Hidvégi, E.J., J. Holland, C. Streffer and D. van Beuningen. 1978. "Biochemical Phenomena in Ionizing Irradiation of Cells." In Methods in Cancer Research, Vol. XV, pp. 187-278, edited by H. Busch. New York: Academic Press.

201. Hill, B.T. 1978. "Cancer Chemotherapy. The Relevance of Certain Concepts of Cell Cycle Kinetics." Biochim. Biophys. Acta, 516, 389-417.

202. Himmelblau, D.M. 1972. Applied Nonlinear Programming. New York: McGraw-Hill.

203. Hinshaw, W.S., E.R. Andrew, P.A. Bottomley, G.N. Holland, W.S. Moore and B.S. Worthington. 1978. "Display of Cross Sectional Anatomy by Nuclear Magnetic Resonance Imaging." Br. J. Radiol., 51, 273-280.

204. Hodes, L. 1974. "Semiautomatic Optimization of External Beam Radiation Treatment Planning." Radiology, 110, 191-196.

205. Hodes, L. 1976. "Method of Radiation Therapy Treatment Planning." United States Patent No. 3,987,281 (October 19).

206. Holley, W.R., R.P. Henke, G.E. Gauger, B. Jones, E.V. Benton, J.I. Fabrikant and C.A. Tobias. 1979. "Heavy Particle Computed Tomography." In Proc. Sixth Conf. Computer Applications in Radiology and Computer/Aided Analysis of Radiological Images, pp. 64-70. New York: The Inst. of Elect. and Electronics Engineers.

207. Holmes, W.F. 1970. "External Beam Treatment-planning using the Programmed Console." Radiology, 94, 391-400.

208. Hope, C.S., and J.S. Orr. 1965. "Computer Optimization of 4 Mev Treatment Planning." Phys. Med. Biol., 10, 365-373.

209. Hope, C.S., M.J. Laurie, J.S. Orr and K.E. Halnan. 1967. "Optimization of X-ray Treatment Planning by Computer Judgment." Phys. Med. Biol., 12, 531-542.

210. Hope, C.S. 1970. "Computer Optimization of Treatment Planning." In Medical Computing: Progress and Problems, pp. 133-145, edited by M.E. Abrams. New York: American Elsevier.

211. Hope, C.S., and O. Cain. 1972. "A Computer Program for Optimised Stationary Beam Treatment Planning using Score Functions." Computer Prog. Biomed., 2, 221-231.

212. Horn, F., and R. Jackson. 1965. "Discrete Maximum Principle." I and E. C. Fundamentals, 4, 110-112.

213. Hounsfield, G.N. 1973. "Computerized Transverse Axial Scanning (Tomography) Part 1, Description of System." Br. J. Radiol., 46, 1016-1022.

214. Hounsfield, G.N. 1976. "Historical Notes on Computerized Axial Tomography." J. Canad. Assoc. Radiol., 27, 135-142.

215. Hounsfield, G.N. 1977. "The EMI Scanner." Proc. Roy. Soc. (London) Series B, 195, 281-289.

216. Hounsfield, G.N. 1980a. "Computed Medical Imaging." Med. Phys., 7, 283-290.

217. Hounsfield, G.N. 1980b. "Computed Medical Imaging." Science, 210, 22-28.

218. Howard, A., and S.R. Pelc. 1953. "Synthesis of Deoxyribonucleic Acid in Normal and Irradiated Cells and its Relation to Chromosome Breakage." Heredity (Suppl.), 6, 261-273.

219. Hug, O., and A. Kellerer. 1966. "The Stochastics of Radiation Effects." In Biophysical Aspects of Radiation Quality, Technical Report Series No. 58. Vienna: Int. Atomic Energy Agency.

220. Intriligator, M.D. 1971. Mathematical Optimization and Economic Theory, Englewood Cliffs (New Jersey): Prentice-Hall.

221. Ivanov, V.K., A.G. Konoplyannikov, A.M. Petrovsky and E.V. Khenkin. 1977. "Mathematical Modelling in Optimization of Radiation Therapy." Meditsinskaia Radiol., 22, part 5, 27-33; in Russian.

222. Ivanov, V.K. 1978. "Optimization of Radiation Therapy of Malignant Growths." Avtomatika i Telemekhanika, 39, 136-142. (Eng. trans. - Automation and Remote Control, 39, 269-274.)

223. Jameson, D.G., and A. Trevelyan. 1969. "A Computer Approach to Dose Calculation for Supplementary Beam Therapy." Br. J. Radiol., 42, 57-60.

224. Kaplan, H. 1968. "Macromolecular Basis of Radiation-induced Loss of Viability in Cells and Viruses." In Actions Chimiques et Biologiques des Radiations, Vol. 12, 69-94, edited by M. Haissinsky. Paris: Masson.

225. Kaplan, H.S. 1979. "Experimental Frontiers in Radiation Therapy of Cancer." In Radiation Research, pp. 2-14, edited by S. Okada, M. Imamura, T. Terashima and H. Yamaguchi. Tokyo: Japanese Assoc. for Radiation Research.

226. Kappos, A., and W. Pohlit. 1972. "A Cybernetic Model for Radiation Reactions in Living Cells. 1. Sparsely-ionizing Radiations." Int. J. Radiat. Biology, 22, 51-65.

227. Karzmark, C.J., and N.C. Pering. 1973. "Electron Linear Accelerators for Radiation Therapy: History, Principles and Contemporary Developments." Phys. Med. Biol., 18, 321-354.

228. Keller, B.E. 1977. "Mathematical Modeling." Int. J. Radiation Oncology Biol. Phys., 2, p. 823.

229. Kellerer, A., and O. Hug. 1963. "Zur Kinetik der Strahlenwirking." Biophysik, 1, 33-50.

230. Kellerer, A.M., and H.H. Rossi. 1971. "RBE and the Primary Mechanism of Radiation Action." Radiat. Res., 47, 15-34.

231. Kellerer, A.M., and H.H. Rossi. 1978. "A Generalized Formulation of Dual Radiation Action." Radiat. Res., 75, 471-488.

232. Khan, F.M., and J.M.F. Lee. 1979. "Computer Algorithm for Electron Beam Treatment Planning." Med. Phys., 6, 142-144.

233. Kiefer, J. 1970. "Target Theory and Survival Curves." J. theor. Biol., 30, 307-317.

234. Kirk, J., W.M. Gray and E.R. Watson. 1971. "Cumulative Radiation Effect. Part 1: Fractionated Treatment Regimes." Clin. Radiol., 22, 145-155.

235. Kirk, J., and T.E. Wheldon. 1974. "A Mathematical Model for Time-optimisation of Treatment Regimes in Clinical Radiotherapy." In Proc. of the 5th Internat. Confer. on the Use of Computers in Radiotherapy, Hanover, New Hampshire.

236. Kirk, J. 1978. The Cumulative Radiation Effect. Edinburgh: Churchill Livingstone.

237. Klepper, L. Ia. 1966. "Primenenie EVM I Metodov Lineinogo Programmirovaniia Dlia Vybora Optimal'hykh Uslov ñ Distantsionnoi Luchevoi Terapii." Med. Radiol., 11, 8-15.

238. Klepper, L. Ia. 1967. "Primenenie EVM Dlia Rascheta Raspredeleniia Doz Gamma-Izlucheniia Co 60 s uchetom Geterogennosti Sredy." Med. Radiol., 12, 13-20.

239. Klepper, L. Ia. 1969. "Linear Programming in Selecting Optimal Conditions for Radiation Treatment." Med. Radiol., 14, 69-76; in Russian.

240. Kolata, G.B. 1979. "Mathematicians Amazed by Russian's Discovery." Science, 206, 545-546.

241. Kuester, J.L., and J.H. Mize. 1973. Optimization Techniques with FORTRAN. New York: McGraw-Hill.

242. Kuzin, R.A., G.F. Nevskaya, V.I. Popov, V.A. Sakovich, A.V. Shafirkin and V.V. Yurgov. 1971. "Mathematical Description of Radiation Damage and Recovery Processes in the Hemopoietic System." Space Biology and Medicine, 5, 42-47. (Eng. trans of Kosmicheskaya Biologiya i Meditsina, 5, 1971, 29-33.)

243. Lajtha, L.G. 1963. "On the Concept of the Cell Cycle." J. Cell Comp. Physiol. Suppl., 1, 62, 143-145.

244. Landry, J., and N. Marceau. 1978. "Rate-limiting Events in Hyperthermic Cell Killing." Radiat. Res., 75, 573-585.

245. Larson, R.E. 1967. "A Survey of Dynamic Programming Computational Procedures." IEEE Trans. Auto. Contr., Dec., 767-774.

246. Lasdon, L.S., S.K. Mitter and A.D. Waren. 1967. "The Conjugate Gradient Method for Optimal Control Problems." IEEE Trans. Auto. Contr., Vol. AC-12, 132-138.

247. Laurie, J., J.S. Orr and C.J. Foster. 1972. "Repair Processes and Cell Survival." Br. J. Radiol., 45, 362-368.

248. Lauterbur, P.C. 1974. "Magnetic Resonance Zeugmatography." Pure Appl. Chem., 40, 149-157.

249. Lawden, D.F. 1963. Optimal Trajectories for Space Navigation. Washington (D.C.): Butterworth.

250. Lea, D.E. 1955. Actions of Radiations on Living Cells, 2nd edn. London: Cambridge University Press.

251. Leavitt, D.D., D.W. Campbell, J.A. Stryker and G. Sherwood. 1975. "Optimization of Dose Distributions in Moving-strip Therapy using a Minicomputer." Radiology, 116, 159-163.

252. Ledley, R.S., J.B. Wilson, T. Golab and L.S. Rotolo. 1974. "The ACTA-scanner: The Whole Body Computerized Transaxial Tomograph." Comput. Biol. Med., 4, 145-155.

253. Ledley, R.S. 1976. "Introduction to Computerized Tomography." Comput. Biol. Med., 6, 239-246.

254. Lee, E.B., and L. Markus. 1966. Foundations of Optimal Control. New York: J. Wiley.

255. Leenhouts, H.P., and K.H. Chadwick. 1975. "Stopping Power and the Radiobiological Effect of Electrons, Gamma Rays and Ions." In Proc. 5th Symposium on Microdosimetry, 289-310. Vienna: Intl. Atomic Energy Agency (EUR 5452d-e-f).

256. Leenhouts, H.P., and K.H. Chadwick. 1978a. "An Analysis of Radiation-induced Malignancy Based on Somatic Mutation." Int. J. Radiat. Biol., 33, 357-370.

257. Leenhouts, H.P., and K.H. Chadwick. 1978b. "The Crucial Role of DNA Double-strand Breaks in Cellular Radiobiological Effects." Advances in Radiat. Biol., 7, 55-101.

258. Leenhouts, H.P., and K.H. Chadwick. 1978c. "An Analysis of Synergistic Sensitization." Br. J. Cancer, Suppl. III, 37, 198-201.

259. Leitmann, G. 1966. An Introduction to Optimal Control. New York: McGraw-Hill.

260. Leone, C.A. (editor). 1962. Effects of Ionizing Radiations on Immune Processes. New York: Gordon and Breach.

261. Lerch, I.A. 1979. "The Early History of Radiological Physics: 'A Fourth State of Matter'." Med. Phys., 6, 255-266.

262. Levene, M.B., P.K. Kijewski, L.M. Chin, B.E. Bjärngard and S. Hellman. 1978. "Computer-controlled Radiation Therapy." Radiology, 129, 769-775.

263. Littleton, J.T. 1976. Tomography: Physical Principles and Clinical Applications. Baltimore: Williams and Wilkins Co.

264. Lloyd, H.H. 1975. "Estimation of Tumor Cell Kill from Gompertz Growth Curves." Cancer Chemother. Repts., part 1, 59, 267-277.

265. Lokajicek, M., S. Kozubek and K. Prokeš. 1979. "NSD and Cell Survival." Br. J. Radiol., 52, 571-572.

266. Looney, W.B., J.S. Trefil, J.C. Schaffner, C.J. Kovacs and H.A. Hopkins. 1975. "Solid Tumor Models for the Assessment of Different Treatment Modalities: I. Radiation-induced Changes in Growth Rate Characteristics of a Solid Tumor Model." Proc. Nat. Acad. Sci., U.S.A., 72, 2662-2666.

267. Looney, W.B., J.S. Trefil, H.A. Hopkins, C.J. Kovacs, R. Ritenour and J.G. Schaffner. 1977. "Solid Tumor Models for Assessment of Different Treatment Modalities: Therapeutic Strategy for Sequential Chemotherapy with Radiotherapy." Proc. Natl. Acad. Sci., U.S.A., 74, 1983-1987.

268. Madhvanath, V. 1971. "Effects of Densely Ionizing Radiation on Human Lymphocytes Cultured in vitro." Ph.D. thesis. Lawrence Radiation Lab. Report UCRL-20680.

269. Mantel, J., H. Perry and J.J. Weinkam. 1977. "Automatic Variation of Field Size and Dose Rate in Rotation Therapy." Int. J. Radiation Oncology Biol. Phys., 2, 697-704.

270. Maruyama, Y. 1968. "Indirect Effects of Radiation upon Tumor Response In Vivo. A Complex Role." Radiology, 91, 657-668.

271. Maruyama, Y., J.R. van Nagell, Jr., D.E. Wrede, C. Coffey III, J.F. Utley and J. Avila. 1976. "Approaches to Optimization of Dose in Radiation Therapy of Cervix Carcinoma." Radiology, 120, 389-398.

272. Massiot, J. 1974. "History of Tomography." Medica Mundi, 19, 106-115.

273. Mauro, F., and H. Madoc-Jones. 1969. "Age Response to X-radiation of Murine Lymphoma Cells Synchronized in vivo." Proc. Nat. Acad. Sci., U.S.A., 63, 686-691.

274. Mayneord, W.V., and R.H. Clarke. 1975. Carcinogenesis and Radiation Risk: A Biomathematical Reconnaissance. Br. J. Radiol. Supplement No. 12. London: The British Inst. Radiol.

275. McCullough, E.C., and J.T. Payne. 1977. "X-ray-transmission Computed Tomography." Med. Phys., 4, 85-98.

276. McCullough, E.C. 1978. "Potentials of Computed Tomography in Radiation Therapy Treatment Planning." Radiology, 129, 765-768.

277. McDonald, S.C., B.E. Keller and P. Rubin. 1976. "Method for Calculating Dose When Lung Tissue Lies in the Treatment Field." Med. Phys., 3, 210-216.

278. McDonald, S.C., and P. Rubin. 1977. "Optimization of External Beam Radiation Therapy." Int. J. Radiation Oncology Biol. Phys., 2, 307-317.

279. McKenzie, A.L. 1979. "Cell Survival Description of the Cumulative Radiation Effect." Acta Radiol. Oncol. Rad. Phys. Biol., 18, 45-56.

280. McNally, N.J., and P.W. Sheldon. 1977. "The Effect of Radiation on Tumour Growth Delay, Cell Survival and Cure of the Animal Using a Single Tumour System." Br. J. Radiol., 50, 321-328.

281. Mehra, R.K., R.B. Washburn, S. Sajan and J.V. Carroll. 1979. A Study of the Application of Singular Perturbation. NASA Contractor Report 3167. Springfield (Virginia): Scientific and Technical Information Branch.

282. Mendelsohn, M.L. 1965. "The Kinetics of Tumour Cell Proliferation." In Cellular Radiation Biology, pp. 498-513. Baltimore: Williams and Wilkins.

283. Mendelsohn, M.L. 1975. "Cell Cycle Kinetics and Radiation Therapy." In Radiation Research (Biomedical, Chemical and Physical Perspectives), pp. 1009-1024, edited by O.F. Nygaard, H.I. Adler and W.K. Sinclair. New York: Academic Press.

284. Mersereau, R.M. 1976. "Direct Fourier Transform Techniques in 3-D Image Reconstruction." Comput. Biol. Med., 6, 247-258.

285. Meyn, R.E., and H.R. Withers (editors). 1980. Radiation Biology in Cancer Research. New York: Raven Press.

286. Miller, R.C., W.G. Connor, R.S. Heusinkveld and M.L.M. Boone. 1977. "Prospects for Hyperthermia in Human Cancer Therapy. Part 1: Hyperthermic Effects in Man and Spontaneous Animal Tumors." Radiology, 123, 489-495.

287. Mistry, V.D., and W.L. DeGinder. 1978. "Optimization of External Beam Radiotherapy: Quantitative Study of Relative Radiation Effects and Isoeffect Patterns using PC-12 Computer." Int. J. Radiation Oncology Biol. Phys., 4, 1081-1094.

288. Moore II, D.H., and M.L. Mendelsohn. 1972. "Optimal Treatment Levels in Cancer Therapy." Cancer, 30, 97-106.

289. Moss, A., and H. Goldberg (editors). Computed Tomography, Ultrasound and X-ray: An Integrated Approach. New York: Masson.

290. Moss, W.T., W.N. Brand and H. Battifora. 1979. Radiation Oncology: Rationale, Technique, Results. St. Louis: The C.V. Mosby Co.

291. Muntz, E.P., M. Welkowsky, E. Kaegi, L. Morsell, E. Wilkinson and G. Jacobson.

1978. "Optimization of Electrostatic Imaging Systems for Minimum Patient Dose or Minimum Exposure in Mammography." Radiology, 127, 517-523.

292. Muntz, E.P. 1979. "Relative Carcinogenic Effects of Different Mammography Techniques." Med. Phys., 6, 205-210.

293. Nauts, H.C., G.A. Fowler and F.H. Bogatko. 1953. "A Review of the Influence of Bacterial Infection and of Bacterial Products (Coley's Toxins) on Malignant Tumors in Man." Acta Med. Scand. (Suppl. 276): 1-103.

294. Neary, G.J. 1965. "Chromosome Aberrations and the Theory of RBE. 1. General Considerations." Int. J. Radiat. Biol., 9, 477-502.

295. Neufeld, J., H.A. Wright and R.N. Hamm. 1974. "A Comparison of Two-component Models of Cellular Survival." In Symp. Microdosimetry, Vol. 4, pp. 415-436. Vienna: International Atomic Energy Agency.

296. New, P.F.J., W.R. Scott, J.A. Schnur, K.R. Davis and J.M. Taveras. 1974. "Computerized Axial Tomography with the EMI-scanner." Radiology, 110, 109-123.

297. New, P.F., and W.R. Scott. 1975. Computed Tomography of the Brain and Orbit (EMI Scanning). Baltimore: Williams and Wilkins.

298. Newton, C.M. 1971. "What Next in Radiation Treatment Optimization?" In Computers in Radiotherapy - British J. of Radiology, Special Report Series No. 5, pp. 83-89. London: British Inst. of Radiology.

299. Newton, C.M. 1972. "Planning Radiotherapeutic Strategy." Proc. San Diego Biomed. Symp., 11, 189-199.

300. Noble, B.M. 1969. Applied Linear Algebra. Englewood Cliffs: Prentice-Hall.

301. Norman, D., M. Korobkin and T.H. Newton (editors). 1977. Computed Tomography. St. Louis: The C.V. Mosby Co.

302. Norton, L., R. Simon, H.D. Brereton and A.E. Bogden. 1976. "Predicting the Course of Gompertzian Growth." Nature, 264, 542-545.

303. Norton, L., and R. Simon. 1977a. "Growth Curve of an Experimental Solid Tumor Following Radiotherapy." J. Natl. Cancer Inst., 58, 1735-1741.

304. Norton, L., and R. Simon. 1977b. "Tumor Size, Sensitivity to Therapy, and Design of Treatment Schedules." Cancer Treatment Repts., 61, 1307-1317.

305. Norton, L., and R. Simon. 1978. Letter to the editor on Tumor Growth Kinetics, Therapeutic Differentials, and Design of Treatment Schedules. Cancer Treatment Repts., 62, 847-848.

306. Norton, L., and R. Simon. "New Thoughts on the Relationship of Tumor Growth Characteristics to Sensitivity to Treatment." Methods in Cancer Res., 17, 53-90.

307. Nygaard, O.F., H.I.Adler and W.K. Sinclair (editors). 1975. Radiation Research. Biomedical, Chemical, and Physical Perspectives. New York: Academic Press.

308. Order, S.E., J. Kopicky and S.A. Leibel. 1979. Principles of Successful Radiation Therapy. Boston: G.K. Hall and Co.

309. Ormerod, M.G. 1976. "Radiation-induced Strand Breaks in the DNA of Mammalian Cells," In Biology of Radiation Carcinogenesis, pp. 67-92, edited by J.M. Yuhas, R.W. Tennant and J.D. Regan. New York: Raven Press.

310. Orphanoudakis, S.C., and J.W. Strohbehn. 1976. "Mathematical Model of Conventional Tomography." Med. Phys., 3, 224-232.

311. Orphanoudakis, S.C., J.W. Strohbehn and C.E. Metz. 1978. "Linearizing Mechanisms in Conventional Tomographic Imaging." Med. Phys., 5, 1-17.

312. Orr, J.S. 1972. "Optimisation of Radiotherapy Treatment Planning." Comput. Prog. Biomed., 2, 216-220.

313. Orr, J.S., J.F. Malone, C.J. Foster and T.E. Wheldon. 1979. "Repair and Prolonged Hypoxia." Br. J. Radiol., 52, 593-594.

314. Paskin, A., B.V. Bronk and G.J. Dienes. 1967. "Stochastic Models of Cell Proliferation and Cell Response to Radiation." In Recovery and Repair Mechanisms in Radiobiology; Brookhaven Symposia in Biology, No. 20, pp. 169-178.

315. Paterson, R. 1963. The Treatment of Malignant Disease by Radiotherapy, 2nd edn. London: E. Arnold.

316. Payne, M.G., and W.R. Garrett. 1975. "Some Relations between Cell Survival Models having Different Inactivation Mechanisms." Radiat. Res., 62, 388-394.

317. Perelson, A.S., M. Mirmirani and G.F. Oster. 1976. "Optimal Strategies in Immunology I. B-cell Differentiation and Proliferation." J. Math. Biol., 3, 325-367.

318. Perelson, A.S., M. Mirmirani and G.F. Oster. 1978. "Optimal Strategies in Immunology II. B Memory Cell Production." J. Math. Biol., 5, 213-256.

319. Perelson, A.S. 1978. "The IgM-IgG Switch Looked at from a Control Theoretic Viewpoint." In Lecture Notes in Control and Information Sciences, Vol. 6, Optimization Techniques, pp. 431-440. New York: Springer Verlag.

320. Phillips, T.L., and K.K. Fu. 1976. "Quantification of Combined Radiation Therapy and Chemotherapy Effects on Critical Normal Tissues." Cancer, 37, 1186-1200.

321. Pinney, E. 1950. "On a Mathematical Theory of the Reaction of Cells to X-ray Irradiation." Bull. Math. Biophys., 12, 199-206.

322. Polak, E. 1973. "An Historical Review of Computational Methods in Optimal Control." SIAM Review, 15, 553-584.

323. Polyakov, A.I. 1978. "Software for Planning of Remotely Controlled Irradiation Therapy." Eng. Cybernetics, 16 (No. 1), 43-48.

324. Pontryagin, L.S., V. Boltyanskii, R. Gamkrelidze and E. Mishchenko. 1962. The Mathematical Theory of Optimal Processes. Moscow: Fizmatgiz. (English translation - New York: J. Wiley, 1962.)

325. Prasad, S.C. 1978. Relation Between Tolerance Dose and Treatment Field Size in Radiotherapy." Med. Phys., 5, 430-433.

326. Prewitt, J.M.S. 1972. "Programming Systems for Optimal Radiotherapy: Progress and Prospects." In Proc. 2nd Symposium on Sharing of Computer Programs and Technology in Nuclear Medicine, pp. 281-302, Oak Ridge (Tennessee): U.S. Atomic Energy Administration (CONF-720430).

327. Prewitt, J.M.S. 1973. "Optimization Criteria and Strategies for Radiotherapy: 1. Feasibility of an Algorithmic Approach." Proc. San Diego Biomed. Symp., 12, 175-186.

328. Quastler, H. 1963. "The Analysis of Cell Population Kinetics." In Cell Pro-

liferation, pp. 18-36, edited by L.G. Lamerton and R.M.J. Fry. Oxford: Blackwell Scientific.

329. Quintana, V.H., and E.J. Davison. 1970. "A Time-weighted Gradient Method for Computing Optimal Controls." *11th Joint Automatic Control Conference*. New York: Amer. Soc. Mech. Eng.

330. Radon, J. 1917. "Über die Bestimmung von Funktionen durch ihre integralwerte längs gewisser Manningfaltigkeiten." (On the Determination of Functions from their Integrals along Certain Manifolds.) *Ber. Saechs. Akad. Wiss. Leipzig, Math-Phys. Kl.*, **69**, 262-277.

331. Rall, L.B. 1980. Applications of Software for Automatic Differentiation in Numerical Computation. *Computing* Suppl. 2, 141-156. (This publication is also entitled *Fundamentals of Numerical Computation* edited by G. Alefeld and R.D. Grigorieff. New York: Springer-Verlag.)

332. Ramachandran, G.N., and A.V. Lakshminarayanan. 1971. "Three-dimensional Reconstruction from Radiographs and Electron Micrographs: Application of Convolutions instead of Fourier Transforms." *Proc. Nat. Acad. Sci., U.S.A.*, **68**, 2236-2240.

333. Rapp, P.E. 1978. "Biological Applications of Control Theory." In *Continuum Models in Molecular and Cellular Biology*, Chapter 2, edited by L.A. Segel. Cambridge (England): Cambridge University Press.

334. Rapp, P.E. 1979. "Bifurcation Theory, Control Theory and Metabolic Regulation." In *Biological Systems, Modelling and Control*, pp. 1-83, edited by D.A. Linkens. London: P. Peregrinus.

335. Rather, L.J. 1978. *The Genesis of Cancer: A Study in the History of Ideas*. Baltimore: The J. Hopkins Univ. Press.

336. Reboul, J. 1939. "Action des Rayons X sur les Éléments Biologiques; le Facteur de Récupération." *Compt. Rend. Acad. Sci.*, **208**, No. 3, 541-542.

337. Redpath, A.T., B.L. Vickery and D.H. Wright. 1975. "A Set of Fortran Subroutines for Optimizing Radiotherapy Plans." *Computer Prog. Biomed.*, **5**, 158-164.

338. Redpath, A.T., B.L. Vickery and D.H. Wright. 1976. "A New Technique for Radiotherapy Planning using Quadratic Programming." *Phys. Med. Biol.*, **21**, 781-791.

339. Redpath. A.T. 1980. Personal communication.

340. Redpath, J.L., R.M. David and L. Cohen. 1978. "Dose-fractionation Studies on Mouse Gut and Marrow: An Intercomparison of 6-MeV Photons and Fast Neutrons ($\bar{E}$=25MeV)." *Radiat. Res.*, **75**, 642-648.

341. Renner, W.D., T.P. O'Connor and N.M. Paulauskas. 1979. "Computer Assistance in Planning Radiotherapy Seed Implants." *Int. J. Radiation Oncology Biol. Phys.*, **5**, 427-432.

342. Resnick, M.A. 1978. "Similar Responses to Ionizing Radiation of Fungal and Vertebrate Cells and the Importance of DNA Double-strand Breaks." *J. theor. Biol.*, **71**, 339-346.

343. Ring, B.A. 1979. "An Overview: Computed Axial Tomography." *Appl. Radiol.*, **8** (Nov.-Dec., p. 110).

344. Röntgen, W.C. 1895. "Über eine neue Art von Strahlen. Erste mitteilung." *Sitzgsber Physikal-Med Gesellschaft* (Würzburg) 132-141 (Dec. 28).

345. Roux, J.C. 1974. "Irradiation de Chlorelles par des Rayonnements Particulaires." Ph.D. Thesis, University of Grenoble, CNRS A.O. 9896.

346. Roux, J.C., and B. Lachet. 1976. "A Generalization of the Clonal Survival Models: Equations for the Families of Curves Obtained with Fractionated Irradiation." Rad. and Environm. Biophys., 13, 177-186.

347. Rubin, P., and S.K. Carter. 1976. "Combination Radiation Therapy and Chemotherapy: A Logical Basis for their Clinical Use." CA--A Cancer Jl. for Clinicians, 26, 274-292.

348. Rubin, P. (editor). 1978. Clinical Oncology for Medical Students and Physicians, 5th edn. New York: American Cancer Society.

349. Sacher, G.A., and E. Trucco. 1966. "Theory of Radiation Injury and Recovery in Self-renewing Cell Populations." Radiat. Res., 29, 236-256.

350. Sage, Andrew P., and C.C. White, III. 1977. Optimum Systems Control, 2nd edn. Englewood Cliffs (New Jersey): Prentice-Hall.

351. Saunders, E.F., and A.M. Mauer. 1969. "Reentry of Nondividing Leukemic Cells into a Proliferative Phase in Acute Childhood Leukemia." J. Clinic Invest., 48, 1299-1305.

352. Schulz, M.D. 1975. "The Supervoltage Story." Amer. J. Roentgenol., 124, 541-549.

353. Schweitzer, D.G., and G.J. Dienes. 1971. "A Kinetic Model of Population Dynamics." Demography, 8, 389-400.

354. Scott, B.R. 1977. "Mechanistic State Vector Model for Cell Killing by Ionizing Radiation." Rad. and Environm. Biophys., 14, 195-211.

355. Scott, D., A.W. Craig and P.T. Iype. 1976. "Effects of Ionizing Radiations on Mammalian Cells." In Scientific Foundations of Oncology, pp. 427-443, edited by T. Symington and R.L. Carter. Chicago: Year Book Medical.

356. Selman,J. 1977. The Fundemantals of X-ray and Radium Physics, 6th edn. Springfield (Illinois): C.C. Thomas.

357. Shepp, L.A., and J.B. Kruskal. 1978. "Computerized Tomography: The New Medical X-ray Technology." Amer. Math. Monthly, 85, 420-439.

358. Shepp, L.A. 1980. "Computerized Tomography and Nuclear Magnetic Resonance." J. Compt. Assist. Tomog., 4, 94-107.

359. Sievert, R.M. 1941. "Zur Theoretisch-mathematischen Behandlung des Problems der Biologischen Strahlenwirkung." Acta Radiologica, 22, 237-251.

360. Simpson-Herren, L., and H.H. Lloyd. 1970. "Kinetic Parameter and Growth Curves for Experimental Tumor Systems." Cancer Chemother. Repts., Part 1, 54, 143-174.

361. Sinclair, W.K. 1966. "The Shape of Radiation Survival Curves of Mammalian Cells Cultured in vitro." In Biophysical Aspects of Radiation Quality, Technical Report Series No. 58, pp. 21-43, Int. Atomic Energy Agency, Vienna.

362. Sinitsyn, R.V. 1968a. "O Trekh Zadachakh Lineĭnogo Programmirovaniia v Dozimetricheskom Planirovanii Luchevogo Lecheniia." Med. Radiol., 13, 29-36.

363. Sinitsyn, R.V. 1968b. "Raschet Kompensiruiushchikh Fil'trov Dlia Formirovaniia Doznogo Polia pri Distansionnom Mnogopol'nom Obluchenii." Med. Radiol., 13, 58-65.

364. Smith, K.T., D.C. Solmon and S.L. Wagner. 1977. "Practical and Mathematical Aspects of the Problem of Reconstructing Objects from Radiographs." Bull. Amer. Math. Soc., 83, 1227-1270.

365. Smoron, G.L. 1972. "Strip-staggering. Elimination of Inhomogeneity in the Moving-strip Technique of Whole Abdominal Irradiation." Radiology, 104, 657-660.

366. Stear, E.B. 1973. "Systems Theory Aspects of Physiological Systems." In Regulation and Control of Physiological Systems, pp. 496-500. Pittsburth: Instrument Society of America.

367. Stear, E.B. 1975. "Application of Control Theory to Endocrine Regulation and Control." Annals Biomed. Eng., 3, 439-455.

368. Steel, G.G. 1977. Growth Kinetics of Tumours. Cell Population Kinetics in Relation to the Growth and Treatment of Cancer. Oxford: Clarendon Press.

369. Steel, G.G. 1979. "The Utility of Cell Kinetic Data in the Design of Therapeutic Schedules." Int. J. Radiation Oncology Biol. Phys., 5, 145-146.

370. Steel, G.G., and M.J. Peckham. 1979. "Exploitable Mechanisms in Combined Radiotherapy-chemotherapy: The Concept of Additivity." Int. J. Radiation Oncology Biol. Phys., 5, 85-91.

371. Sterling, T.D., and H. Perry. 1964. "Planning Radiation Treatment on the Computer." Annals N.Y. Acad. Sci., 115, 976-999.

372. Sternick, E.S. 1978. "Computers in Radiation Oncology: The Third Decade." In The Second Annual Symposium on Computer Application in Medical Care, pp. 76-85, edited by F.H. Orthner. New York: Inst. Elec. Electr. Eng.

373. Steward, P.S., and G.M. Hahn. 1971. "The Application of Age Response Functions to the Optimization of Treatment Schedules." Cell Tissue Kinet., 4, 279-291.

374. Stoker, M.G.P. 1976. "The Growth of Normal and Neoplastic Cells." Clin. Radiol., 27, 1-7.

375. Strandqvist, M. 1944. "Studien über die Kumulative Wirkung der Röntgenstrahlen bei Fraktionierung." Acta Radiol. Suppl., 55, 1-293.

376. Suit, H.D., and M. Shwayder. 1974. "Hyperthermia: Potential as an Anti-tumor Agent." Cancer, 34, 122-129.

377. Sullivan, P.W., and S.E. Salmon. 1972. "Kinetics of Tumor Growth and Regression in IgG Multiple Myeloma." J. Clinic. Invest., 51, 1697-1708.

378. Swan, G.W. 1974. Applied Separation of Variables, unpublished book manuscript.

379. Swan, G.W. 1975. "Some Strategies for Harvesting a Single Species." Bull. Math. Biol., 37, 659-673.

380. Swan, G.W. 1977. Some Current Mathematical Topics in Cancer Research. Published for the Society of Mathematical Biology by Monograph Publishing on Demand, 300 N. Zeeb Road, Ann Arbor, Michigan 48106.

381. Swan, G.W., and T.L. Vincent. 1977. "Optimal Control Analysis in the Chemotherapy of IgG Multiple Myeloma." Bull. Math. Biol., 39, 317-337.

382. Swan, G.W. 1980. "Optimal Control in Some Cancer Chemotherapy Problems." Int. J. Systems Sci., 11, 223-237.

383. Swan G.W. 1981a. "Optimal Control Applications in Biomedical Engineering--A Survey." *Optimal Control Applications and Methods*, in press.

384. Swan, G.W. 1981b. *Applications of Optimal Control in Biomedical Engineering*, unpublished book manuscript.

385. Swan, G.W. 1981c. "Optimization Concepts in Human Cancer Radiotherapy." Submitted for publication.

386. Swann, W.F.G., and C. del Rosario. 1931. "The Effect of Radioactive Radiations upon Euglena." *J. Franklin Inst*., **211**, 303-317.

387. Tabak, D., and B.C. Kuo. 1971. *Optimal Control by Mathematical Programming*. Englewood Cliffs (New Jersey): Prentice-Hall.

388. Tai, D.T., and Y. Maruyama. 1979. "Application of Linear Programming to Dose Optimization in Intracavitary Implant Therapy." *Acta Radiologica Oncology*, **18**, 357-366.

389. Tannock, I. 1979. "Cell Kinetics and Chemotherapy: A Critical Review." *Cancer Treatment Repts*., **62**, 1117-1133.

390. Tapley, N. duV. (editor). 1976. *Clinical Applications of the Electron Beam*. New York: J. Wiley.

391. Ter-Pogossian, M.M., M.E. Raichle and B.E. Sobel. 1980. "Positron-emission Tomography." *Scient. Amer*., **236** (Oct.), 170-181.

392. Tewfik, F.A., T.C. Evans and E.F. Riley. 1977. "Cell Cycle Kinetics and Control of Solid Tumors in Mice by Fractionated X-irradiation." In *Prevention and Detection of Cancer*, Part I: Prevention - Vol. 1, Etiology, pp. 69-78, edited by H.E. Nieburgs. New York: M. Dekker.

393. Todd, P. 1967. "Heavy-ion Irradiation of Cultured Human Cells." *Rad. Res. Suppl*., **7**, 196-207.

394. Todd, P., J.P. Geraci, P.S. Furcinitti, R.M. Rossi, F. Mikage, R.B. Theus and C.B. Schroy. 1978. "Comparison of the Effects of Various Cyclotron-produced Fast Neutrons on the Reproductive Capacity of Cultured Human Kidney (T-1) Cells." *Int. J. Radiation Oncology Biol. Phys*., **4**, 1015-1022.

395. Tsien, K.C. 1955. "The Application of Automatic Computing Machines to Radiation Treatment Planning." *Br. J. Radiol*., **28**, 432-439.

396. Tsokos, J.O., and C.P. Tsokos. 1977. "A Model for the Statistical Analysis of Cell Radiosensitivity During the Cell Cycle." In *Nonlinear Systems and Applications*, pp. 327-348, edited by V. Lakshmikantham. New York: Academic Press.

397. Turner Jr., M.E. 1975. "Some Classes of Hit-theory Models." *Math. Biosci*., **23**, 219-235.

398. Usher, J.R. 1980. "Mathematical Derivation of Optimal Uniform Treatment Schedules for the Fractionated Irradiation of Human Tumors." *Math. Biosci*., **49**, 157-184.

399. Van Bekkum, D.W. 1975. "Mechanisms of Radiation Carcinogenesis." In *Radiation Research. Biomedical, Chemical and Physical Perspectives*, pp. 886-894, edited by O.F. Nygaard, H.I. Adler and W.K. Sinclair. New York: Academic Press.

400. Van de Geijn, J. 1972a. "Computational Methods in Beam Therapy Planning." *Computer Progr. Biomed*., **2**, 153-168.

401. Van de Geijn, J. 1972b. "EXTDØS 71. Revised and Expanded Version of EXTDØS, A Program for Treatment Planning in External Beam Therapy." Computer Prog. Biomed., 2, 169-177.

402. Van de Geijn, J. 1975. "Backgrounds of Computer-assisted Treatment Planning in Radiation Therapy." Radiologe, 15 , 224-230.

403. Van der Laarse, R., and J. Strackee. 1976. "Pseudo Optimization of Radio-Therapy Treatment Planning." Br. J. Radiol., 49, 450-457.

404. Van Putten, L.M., and P. Lelieveld. 1976. "The Effects of Cytostatic Drugs and Radiotherapy on the Cell Cycle." In Scientific Foundations of Oncology, pp. 136-145, edited by T. Symington and R.L. Carter. Chicago: Year Book Medical.

405. Walter, J., and H. Miller. 1959. A Short Textbook of Radiotherapy for Technicians and Students. Edinburgh: Churchill Livingstone.

406. Walter, J. 1977. Cancer and Radiotherapy, 2nd edn. Edinburgh: Churchill Livingstone.

407. Wambersie, A., J. Dutreix, J. Gueulette and J. Lellouch. 1974. "Early Recovery for Intestinal Stem Cells, as a Function of Dose per Fraction, Evaluated by Survival Rate After Fractionated Irradiation of the Abdomen of Mice." Radiat. Res., 58, 498-515.

408. Warren, S.L. 1935. "Preliminary Study of the Effect of Artificial Fever upon Hopeless Tumor Cases." Amer. J. Roentgenol., 33, 75-87.

409. Wasserman, T.H., T.L. Phillips, R.J. Johnson, C.J. Gomer, G.A. Lawrence, W. Sadee, R.A. Marques, V.A. Levin and G. Van Raalte. 1979. "Initial United States Clinical and Pharmacologic Evaluation of Misonidazole (Ro-07-0582), a Hypoxic Cell Radiosensitizer." Int. J. Radiation Oncol. Biol. Phys., 5, 775-786.

410. Watson, J.D. 1972. "Molecular Biological Approach to the Cancer Problem" In The Biological Revolution. Social Good or Social Evil, pp. 169-184, edited by W. Fuller. New York: Doubleday.

411. Weinkam, J., and T. Sterling. 1972. "A Versatile System for Three-dimensional Radiation Dose Computation and Display, RTP." Comp. Prog. Biomed., 2, 178-192.

412. Wheldon, T.E., and J. Kirk. 1975. "Optimal Radiotherapy of Radioresistant Tumours." Br. J. Radiol., 48, 870-871.

413. Wheldon, T.E., and J. Kirk. 1976. "Mathematical Derivation of Optimal Treatment Schedules for the Radiotherapy of Human Tumours. Fractionated Irradiation of Exponentially Growing Tumours." Br. J. Radiol., 49, 441-449.

414. Wheldon, T.E., J. Kirk and J.S. Orr. 1977. "Optimal Radiotherapy of Tumour Cells Following Exponential-quadratic Survival Curves and Exponential Repopulation Kinetics." Br. J. Radiol., 50, 681-682.

415. Wheldon, T.E. 1978. "Optimal Control Strategies in the Radiotherapy of Human Cancer." In Cell Kinetics and Biomathematics, edited by A.-J. Valleron and P.D. MacDonald. New York: Elsevier.

416. Wheldon, T.E., and G.F. Brunton. 1978. Letter to the editor on Tumor Growth Kinetics, Therapeutic Differentials, and Design of Treatment Schedules. Cancer Treatment Repts., 62, 845-846.

417. Wheldon, T.E. 1979. "Optimal Fractionation for the Radiotherapy of Tumour

Cells Posessing Wide-shouldered Survival Curves." Br. J. Radiol., **52**, 417-418.

418. Whitmore, G.F., S. Gulyas and J. Botond. 1965. "Radiation Sensitivity Through the Cell Cycle and its Relation to Recovery." In Cellular Radiation Biology, pp. 423-441. Baltimore: Williams and Wilkins.

419. Wickwire, K. 1977. "Mathematical Models for the Control of Pests and Infectious Diseases: A Survey." Theor. Pop. Biol., **11**, 182-238.

420. Wideröe, R. 1966. "High-energy Electron Therapy and the Two-Component Theory of Radiation." Acta. Radiol. Ther. Phys. Biol., **4**, 257-278.

421. Wideröe, R. 1971. "Quantitative and Qualitative Aspects of Radiobiology and their Significance in Radiation Therapy." Acta. Radiol. Ther. Phys. Biol., **10**, 605-624.

422. Wideröe, R. 1977. "Theories about Radiobiological Effects." Kerntechnik, Isotopentechnik und -chemie, **19**, 237.

423. Wideröe, R. 1978. "A Comparison of Radiation Effects on Mammalian Cells in vitro Caused by X-rays, High Energy Neutrons and Negative Pions. Theoretical Considerations Based upon the Two Component Theory of Radiation." Rad. and Environm. Biophys., **15**, 57-75.

424. Withers, H.R. 1975. "The Four R's of Radiotherapy." Advances in Radiation Biology, Vol. 5, pp. 241-271.

425. Withers, H.R. 1977. "Response of Tissues to Multiple Small Dose Fractions." Radiat. Res., **71**, 24-33.

426. Withers, H.R., H.D. Thames, Jr., B.L. Flow, K.A. Mason and D.H. Hussey. 1978. "The Relationship of Acute to Late Skin Injury in 2 and 5 Fraction/Week X-ray Therapy." Int. J. Radiation Oncology Biol. Phys., **4**, 595-601.

427. Wolbarst, A.B., E.S. Sternick, B.H. Curran and A. Dritschilo. 1980a. "Optimized Radiotherapy Treatment Planning using the Complication Probability Factor (CPF)." Int. J. Radiation Oncology Biol. Phys., **6**, 723-728.

428. Wolbarst, A.B., E.S. Sternick, B.H. Curran, R.J. Kosinski and A. Dritschilo. 1980b. "A Fortran Program for the Optimization of Radiotherapy using the Complication Probability Factor (CPF)." Computer Prog. Biomed., **11**, 94-104.

429. Wolfe, C.S. 1973. Linear Programming with Fortran. Glenview (Illinois): Scott, Foresman.

430. Worthley, B.W., and R.E.M. Cooper. 1967. "Computer-based External Beam Radiotherapy Planning I: Empirical Formulae for Calculation of Depth-doses." Phys. Med. Biol., **12**, 229-240.

431. Zeitz, L., and J.M. McDonald. 1978. "Pitfalls in the Use of in vitro Survival Curves for the Determination of Tumour Cell Survival with Fractionated Doses." Br. J. Radiol., **51**, 637-639.

432. Zimmer, K.G. 1961. Studies on Quantitative Radiation Biology. London: Oliver and Boyd.

433. Zirkle, R.E. 1952. "Speculations on Cellular Actions of Radiations." In Symposium on Radiobiology. The Basic Aspects of Radiation Effects on Living Systems, pp. 333-356, edited by J.J. Nickson. New York: J. Wiley.

INDEX